Functional Strategies for the Management of Gastrointestinal Disorders:

Principles and Protocols for Healthcare Professionals

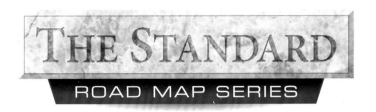

THE STANDARD
ROAD MAP SERIES

Functional Strategies for the Management of Gastrointestinal Disorders:

Principles and Protocols for Healthcare Professionals

By Thomas G. Guilliams Ph.D.

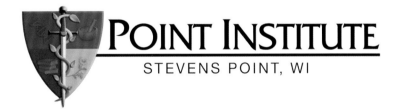

POINT INSTITUTE
STEVENS POINT, WI

The Point Institute was founded by Thomas Guilliams, Ph.D. as an independent research organization focused on examining and disseminating information about the use of natural therapeutic options for treating and preventing chronic disease. Along with therapies generally defined as lifestyle interventions, the Point Institute specializes in the evidence and application of nutraceuticals (dietary supplements, herbs, vitamins, minerals, etc.) as therapeutic and preventative agents in clinical practice.

ISBN: 978-0-9856158-3-3

ATTENTION CORPORATIONS, UNIVERSITIES, COLLEGES, AND PROFESSIONAL ORGANIZATIONS: Quantity discounts are available on bulk purchases of this book for educational or gift purposes, or as premiums for increasing magazine subscriptions or renewals. Special books or book excerpts can also be created to fit specific needs. For information, please contact the Point Institute at info@pointinstitute.org.

Acknowledgements

To the integrative and functional medicine community, those that have taught me, and those that I have been privileged to teach: Your dedication to your patients, your commitment to learn more, to ask probing questions, and to thoughtfully consider new ways to heal has inspired me to do this work. May it add confidence to continue moving us toward a healthier future.

I am greatly indebted to a number of people for inspiring the ideas behind this work, and for the practical efforts that helped me to get this project finished and ready for publication. I could not have accomplished this without their help.

First, I would like to acknowledge the research assistance of Lindsey Drake (soon to have her masters in nutrition). She spent countless hours searching for, reading, and summarizing hundreds of publications that were used as the scientific basis for this work. In particular, her help was invaluable for the sections on the microbiome, probiotics, H. pylori and GERD, though she helped throughout several other sections as well.

Very special thanks go to Rachel H., the designer of the figures and layout of this Road map. The wonderful figures she has created are extremely helpful in explaining the complexity of this topic, as most readers will already have noticed by thumbing through the book (perhaps before reading this acknowledgement). I also want to thank Olivia M. for her help in copyediting each page; the work is much better after you smoothed over the rough patches. Also, to those who helped proof the final copies, Liz, Dave, Olivia, and Lindsey: You found hundreds of little changes and mistakes our readers won't have to encounter. Any remaining mistakes or errors are my own.

Finally, I am grateful to my wonderful family. You are a constant source of joy and wonder. This project was the longest so far, and the most difficult to finish; you helped me to persevere to the end. You have taught me much about life and made me a better person in the process. May God richly bless you in health and in life, and may He grant you the generosity to bring these blessings to others.

Table of Contents

Table of Contents

Table of Contents

Table of Contents

Preface

The fundamental role of the gastrointestinal tract in health and disease has been appreciated since ancient times, as it has played a vital role in the diagnostic and therapeutic schemes of most traditional forms of medicine. But what those ancients could only have speculated, that the GI tract is in some way involved in nearly every facet of human physiology, is now being uncovered in the very latest scientific discoveries. The information on the role of the gut microbiome alone has radically altered our understanding of the pathophysiology of metabolic, immune and psychiatric disorders in ways that could not have been predicted even a few decades ago. For us, these discoveries are even more exciting, as they reinforce the notion that the vast majority of gastrointestinal dysfunctions, whether organic or functional in origin, can often be managed through lifestyle and nutrient support of the core functions of the GI tract.

However, the exhilaration of hearing one new revelation after another is soon replaced by the daunting task of making sense of this avalanche of new information, not to mention forming a balanced and evidence-based approach for clinical application. After all, when does this new information merely confirm what we have already known (with better mechanisms to explain what is seen clinically), and when does it change diagnostic and therapeutic paradigms? This publication seeks to help answer those questions.

Like our previous Road maps, this project is limited in scope. Our goal is not to replace modern textbooks on gastroenterology, but to introduce a framework that allows the clinician to form coherent functional strategies to manage chronic gastrointestinal dysfunctions through the support of core gastrointestinal functions. We summarize these core functions in a manner accessible to the functional and integrative medical practitioner, while also evaluating the evidence for the commonly used diagnostic and therapeutic strategies within these communities. In addition, we hope to introduce these ideas to practitioners and students outside the functional and integrative communities.

In today's world, scientific research and the interpretation and application of that research is constantly changing. For instance, the Rome IV publications were just being published as we finalized our manuscripts, and we were only able to incorporate some of this new information for the reader, especially as it pertains to irritable bowel syndrome. Plans for a second edition to expand on this work are already being discussed to fill in the inevitable gaps a project such as this creates.

We welcome your input. If you know of reputable scientific information that would challenge or modify our recommendations, we ask that you communicate with us via email at info@pointinstitute.org so that we can evaluate the information and consider revising our recommendations. Before sharing your insights, please be sure you have the most recent edition of this guidebook, or have read any updates or addendums posted on our website (www.pointinstitute.org) or through the retailer of this guidebook.

Lifestyle-Based Therapy: Our Core Philosophy

Our core philosophy is simple: the human body has an amazing ability to maintain its own health when provided with the right amounts and types of healthy signals. When harmful signals are removed and appropriate signals are enhanced, cells and organ systems are capable of creating a healthy outcome. Lifestyle-based therapy (i.e., Lifestyle Medicine) provides the tools and incentives to help individuals assess and prioritize the signals in their own lives that require changing, and offers a bridge of support through the journey to a healthier outcome.

For many of today's clinicians, implementing lifestyle medicine means understanding chronic disease prevention and intervention from a different perspective, one that fully integrates the relationship between lifestyle inputs ("signals") and the patient's ability to convert these signals into healthy outcomes. As Hippocrates understood it nearly 2,400 years ago, *"Everyone has a physician inside him or her, we just have to help it in its work. The natural healing force within each one of us is the greatest force in getting well."* Voltaire put this more bluntly in the 18th century when he said, *"The art of medicine consists of amusing the patient while nature cures the disease."*

Lifestyle-based therapy mandates a patient-centered philosophy; it requires assessing all the signals that influence the health of each individual (unlike clinical trials that view patients in cohorts) and recognizes that each individual has a different capacity to translate signals and change behaviors. In this model, clinical success is dependent on a trusting relationship between an engaged clinician and an empowered patient.

Physiological Resilience and Metabolic Reserve

When we enter into a different model or paradigm of thinking, we often need to change the way we describe common phenomena using different nomenclature. While the name we give to chronic diseases might depend on the organ system or tissues involved, such as atherosclerosis, osteoarthritis, inflammatory bowel disease, Alzheimer's disease, type 2 diabetes or cancer, the chronic dysfunction involved in each of these conditions is ultimately caused by the presence of harmful signals that overwhelm tissues' ability to self-heal, or the absence of healthy signals that promote tissue recovery. The Lifestyle Synergy Model we promote is designed to help protect all tissues and organs from the effects of chronic disease and is described by two layers of resistance against poor lifestyle signals: physiological resilience and metabolic reserve.

Physiological resilience is the capacity of each cell or organ system to withstand the necessary (and immediate) changes that create the rhythm of a healthy organism. The ability of arteries to dilate when blood flow increases, the ability to quickly dispose of excess glucose after a meal, or the ability to increase and decrease cortisol when a stressful situation arises

and resolves are just a few examples of physiological resilience. Each of these systems, and thousands more, are like coiled springs or rubber bands capable of being stretched for a particular physiological purpose, then designed to snap back to their original status, ready for the next physiological challenge. Some systems are stretched and snap back in an instant, such as nerve conductivity, while others take hours, like blood-glucose control. Some follow a circadian cycle, such as the HPA axis, and others a monthly cycle, menstruation for example. The GI tract is no exception. Upon ingestion of a meal, dramatic and immediate functional changes occur to help digest and absorb nutrients that then return to a "resting" status in the fasted state.

When inappropriate or overwhelming signals begin to overpower our physiological resilience, the stretching of that system does not immediately resolve. Perhaps the best example of this is the slow progression of impaired glucose tolerance/insulin resistance, which is sometimes referred to as the "metabolic continuum." Note in Figure 1 the "stretching" of the post-prandial glucose affects the area under the curve (AUC) of glucose much more than the change in the eventual

Blood Glucose Excursions in People with Type 2 Diabetes, Impaired (IGT) and Normal Glucose Tolerance

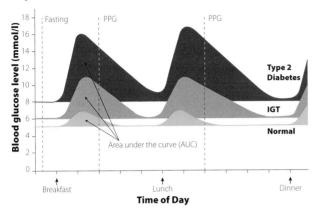

Changes in β-Cell Function Over Time (UKPDS Data)

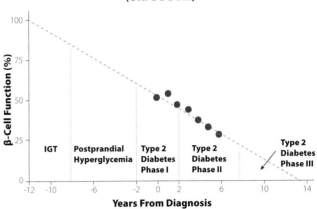

Figure 1 : Blood glucose excursions based on glucose tolerance
These three curves show the relative blood glucose excursions in response to typical meals throughout the day for individuals with normal glucose tolerance, impaired glucose tolerance, and diagnosed type 2 diabetes. Fasting glucose is usually measured after an overnight fast, while post-prandial glucose (PPG) is typically measured 2 hours after consuming a meal. Note the large difference in the area under the curve (AUC) for glucose in these types of individuals, relative to the much smaller differences in fasting glucose levels.

Figure 2 : Pancreatic β cell function through the progression of type 2 diabetes
As metabolic reserve slowly diminishes due to the strain of insulin resistance and oxidative stress, beta cell dysfunction steadily progresses. Dashed line shows extrapolation forward and backward from years 0 to 6 based on HOMA data from UKPDS. From Lebovitz H. *Diabetes Rev.* 1999; 7:139-53.

fasting state. By the time a patient is deemed to be a "type 2 diabetic," the ability to reach normal fasting levels is compromised by changes in peripheral insulin sensitivity and pancreatic insulin capacity—a depletion of their metabolic reserve.

If **physiological resilience** defines the immediate capacity of cells, tissues and organ systems to respond to changes in physiological need, **metabolic reserve** defines the long-term capacity of tissues and organ systems to withstand repeated (chronic) changes to physiological needs. It is, in essence, the stored-up "reserve" available for each metabolic and organ system to maintain and rebuild its physiological resilience. As with any reserve, its capacity is vulnerable to depletion, but also capable of being resupplied and strengthened.

For instance, related to the day-to-day physiological resilience that permits glucose disposal is the long-term metabolic reserve in pancreatic beta cell function. In fact, by the time a person is diagnosed with type 2 diabetes, up to half of pancreatic beta cell function is already depleted (see Figure 2). Peripheral insulin sensitivity and beta cell function are critical long-term metabolic reserve functions that can influence meal-to-meal physiological function. As we shall see throughout this guidebook, glucose metabolism and insulin sensitivity are also influenced by numerous gastrointestinal functions (and dysfunctions), including the metabolic capacity of the gut microbiome.

Another well-known model that shows the principles of physiological resilience and metabolic reserve is bone mineral density. The constant back-and-forth of bone remodeling (osteoclast/osteoblast function) responds to the immediate circumstances of the individual such as nutrient availability, hormone status and weight-bearing activities (physiological resilience). During menopause, these internal and external signals usually favor changes that lead to a loss in bone mineral density. The eventual outcome for

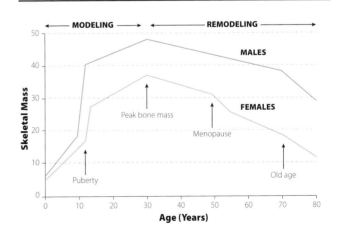

Figure 3 : Bone mass in women and men over time
The general shape of this curve is similar in all women, but the height of peak bone mass and the slope of the bone loss later in life is determined by thousands of lifestyle decisions over her lifetime.

the individual is partly determined by the immediate changes in bone mineral density, but is greatly influenced by peak bone mass, or the level of bone mass built during the previous 50 years (see Figure 3). The level of bone mineral (metabolic) reserve available when menopause starts will greatly impact the likelihood of osteoporosis. While building some bone mineral reserve can be done after menopause, the ability to build the reserve in the years between puberty and age 30 is far greater.

Overall, a lifestyle-based therapeutic approach should be designed to assess an individual's physiological resilience and metabolic reserve using a variety of dynamic/functional tests and knowledge of the patient's history, prioritizing therapies known to specifically support the tissues and organ-systems for which the individual shows weakness.

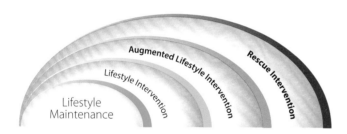

Lifestyle as Intervention

The approach in this guidebook recognizes many patients are well down the road of manifesting outcomes of dysfunction, where the *prevention* of chronic disease seems to be too late. Our premise is that the same processes (building metabolic reserve and supporting physiological resilience) that protect tissues from the onset of chronic damage are even more vital when these tissues are metabolically stressed to the point they manifest dysfunction and result in the diagnosis of a clinically defined "disease." While clinicians and patients may need to augment their lifestyle interventions with targeted therapies or even rescue interventions, the promotion of healthy signals designed to elicit healthy outcomes (lifestyle signals) should always remain the foundation of programs designed to support long-term health outcomes.

Therefore, implementation of lifestyle medicine within a wide range of clinical starting points requires a hierarchy of therapies that span early prevention to late intervention. Our Prevention to Intervention Hierarchy defines four stages along this continuum: Lifestyle Maintenance, Lifestyle Intervention, Augmented

Lifestyle Intervention and Rescue Intervention (see Table 1). Here is a brief description of each:

Lifestyle Maintenance: Eating right, keeping fit, sleeping well, and avoiding signals that sap our vitality are healthy life signals that maintain our metabolic reserve. Done properly, this is the default healthy lifestyle that we hope to impart to the next generation before they experience the diseases coincident with poor lifestyle choices.

Lifestyle Intervention: This is what most clinicians and patients think about when they describe lifestyle medicine or therapy. Using the same signals that maintain our health, we are now more intentional about the therapy, increasing both the specificity and dose of the lifestyle signal. For instance, we are much more specific about dietary choices or changes, becoming fit, modulating stress and kicking bad habits known to be harmful to our health. There is still a strong reliance on the body's capacity to build or rebuild metabolic reserve, but there is a greater focus on risk prevention based on a person's specific vulnerability.

Augmented Lifestyle Intervention: Having discovered many of the specific mechanism(s) that link our lifestyle decisions to our health, we are now capable of designing therapies to target those mechanisms. These therapies are the heart of functional medicine—things like nutritional and nutraceutical therapy, osteopathic or chiropractic manipulation, detoxification protocols and many more. For instance, recognizing the role of beneficial microbes found in our foods and environment, we may consider the therapeutic role of adding foods that contain live bacterial cultures, or augment the diet with probiotic supplements for a more potent therapeutic outcome.

Rescue Intervention: These are interventions now commonplace in our modern medical system: drugs and surgery as reasonable tools to rescue the patient and to prevent organ damage, major debility or death. However, when the same paradigm of rescue interventions is used to ameliorate chronic conditions, a person's metabolic reserve and physiological resilience are rarely enhanced. In fact, they are often depleted. Since the pharmaceutical burden weighs heavily on most patients diagnosed with chronic diseases, wise clinicians who intend to use lifestyle therapies as the core of their intervention strategy must understand how to manage patients who have been treated with, or are currently on, these rescue therapies.

The Prevention to Intervention Hierarchy

	Lifestyle Maintenance	Lifestyle Intervention	Augmented Lifestyle Intervention	Rescue Intervention
Vitamin D & Bones	Sunlight: Work and Play	Sun Therapy/ Diet	Vitamin D Supplement	Osteoporosis Drugs
Antioxidant Defense	Wholesome, Diverse Diet	↑Fruits & Veggies	Supplement Vitamins C and E/ Quercetin etc.	N/A
Back Health	Normal Physical Activity	Exercise and Flex Training	Chiropractic/ Physical Therapy	Surgery/Pain Medications
Joint Health	Physical Activity/Hydration	Weight Loss/ Flexibility	Glucosamine/ Chondroitin Sulfate	Drugs, Knee Replacement
Cancer Prevention	Wholesome, Diverse Diet	↑Fruits & Veggies (Cruciferous)	Supplement Sulforophane or I3C	Antineoplastic Drugs
Detoxification	Wholesome Living	Avoidance/ Organic Focus	Supplement Agents that ↑Detoxification	Drugs to Combat Toxin Symptoms

Table 1: This table shows examples of the relationship between each stage of the Prevention to Intervention Hierarchy. Notice that as we move from left to right along the continuum, the intention is to add signals, not replace them. For instance, the key to cancer prevention from a dietary standpoint is to eat a wholesome and diverse diet with many signals that support immune function and build the metabolic reserve that protects DNA from damage. Some individuals with higher risk or family history may choose to be more specific about increasing their "dose" of certain fruits and vegetables to maximize the dietary signals that help prevent cancer. An example of augmented lifestyle therapy is the use of concentrated phytonutrient supplements derived from these plants (e.g., sulforophane from broccoli) that have been tested for their ability to reduce cancer. In every case, a wholesome and diverse diet sets the foundation for each point along the continuum. Note that rescue interventions rarely trigger the same sorts of mechanisms as those designed to be triggered by lifestyle signals.

The Seven Spheres of Lifestyle Signals

If nearly every aspect of our physiology can be modulated by the lifestyle and environmental signals around us, we could easily define thousands of different signals. In a clinical setting, this vast number of potential variables can overwhelm the therapeutic decision-making process. It is helpful, therefore, to consider signals that can be defined in a limited number of categories. For this purpose, we define seven categories, or spheres, of signals based loosely on origin. Since some lifestyle decisions are complex, they may include signals from multiple categories.

The signals interpreted by and generated by the gastrointestinal system affect nearly every metabolic pathway and chronic disease pathway. Therefore, the lifestyle interventions mentioned throughout this guide will often be categorized by having come from one or more of these seven spheres.

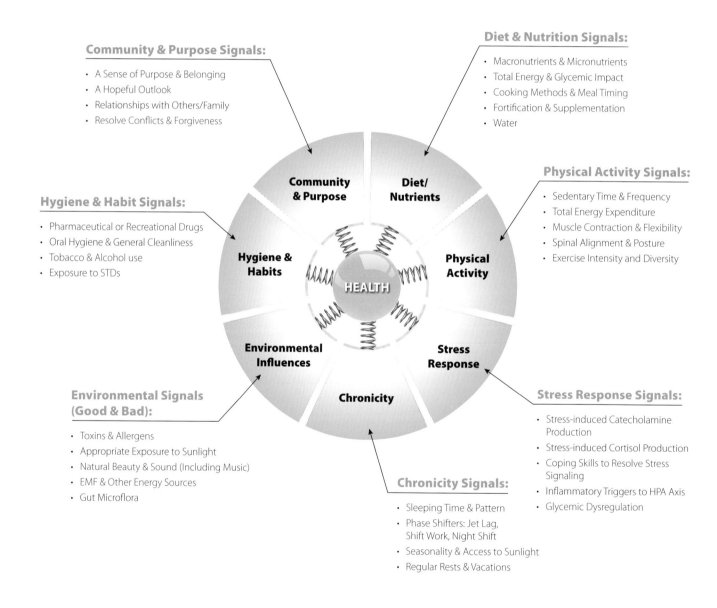

Community & Purpose Signals:

- A Sense of Purpose & Belonging
- A Hopeful Outlook
- Relationships with Others/Family
- Resolve Conflicts & Forgiveness

Diet & Nutrition Signals:

- Macronutrients & Micronutrients
- Total Energy & Glycemic Impact
- Cooking Methods & Meal Timing
- Fortification & Supplementation
- Water

Hygiene & Habit Signals:

- Pharmaceutical or Recreational Drugs
- Oral Hygiene & General Cleanliness
- Tobacco & Alcohol use
- Exposure to STDs

Physical Activity Signals:

- Sedentary Time & Frequency
- Total Energy Expenditure
- Muscle Contraction & Flexibility
- Spinal Alignment & Posture
- Exercise Intensity and Diversity

Environmental Signals (Good & Bad):

- Toxins & Allergens
- Appropriate Exposure to Sunlight
- Natural Beauty & Sound (Including Music)
- EMF & Other Energy Sources
- Gut Microflora

Stress Response Signals:

- Stress-induced Catecholamine Production
- Stress-induced Cortisol Production
- Coping Skills to Resolve Stress Signaling
- Inflammatory Triggers to HPA Axis
- Glycemic Dysregulation

Chronicity Signals:

- Sleeping Time & Pattern
- Phase Shifters: Jet Lag, Shift Work, Night Shift
- Seasonality & Access to Sunlight
- Regular Rests & Vacations

Crossroads in GI Health:
A Functional Approach for Functional Disorders

Gastrointestinal symptoms are some of the most frequently experienced by all subjects and one of the most common reasons individuals seek medical care. Some of these symptoms are acute and self-limiting, while others linger for years or even decades without resolution. Often, individuals describe seeking the help of numerous physicians and treatment modalities over many years, without significant relief. Unfortunately, millions more suffer silently, believing their symptoms are "normal." As they attempt to avoid foods or situations that trigger their symptoms or self-medicate with antacids, over-the-counter laxatives and analgesics, they always keep one eye on the nearest available restroom.

At the same time, clinicians often find GI complaints to be difficult to diagnose and treat, especially in patients who have experienced years of symptoms and unsuccessful remedies. Many other clinicians are frustrated by the overuse of drugs and surgery in the attempt to relieve GI complaints, as these remedies often have no relationship to the root cause(s) of the dysfunctions experienced by the patient. Clinicians are well-aware that a wide range of GI complaints occur in individuals with no discernable organ dysfunction or disease. In recent decades, conditions such as irritable bowel syndrome have fallen into phenomena deemed "functional bowel disorders" to acknowledge that while no discernable organ or tissue defect has been discovered, some overall dysfunction within the GI tract is present.

In fact, over the past few decades, a whole new designation has been given to a wide-range of GI conditions, now referred to as functional gastrointestinal disorders (FGIDs). These disorders have been divided into different categories (for adults and children) using criteria developed by the Rome Foundation (see Table 2 for Rome IV FGIDs).[1] They are generally classified based on "symptom clusters" that remain consistent across clinical and populations with these disorders.

Table 2: Rome IV Functional Gastrointestinal Disorders

Functional Gastrointestinal Disorders

A. Esophageal Disorders
B. Gastroduodenal Disorders
C. Bowel Disorders
D. Centrally Mediated Disorders of Gastrointestinal Pain
E. Gallbladder and Sphincter of Oddi (SO) Disorders
F. Anorectal Disorders
G. Childhood Functional GI Disorders: Neonate/Toddler
H. Childhood Functional GI Disorders: Child/Adolescent

A1. Functional chest pain
A2. Functional heartburn
A3. Reflux hypersensitivity
A4. Globus
A5. Functional dysphagia
B1. Functional dyspepsia
    B1a. Postprandial distress syndrome (PDS)
    B1b. Epigastric pain syndrome (EPS)
B2. Belching disorders
    B2a. Excessive supragastric belching
    B2b. Excessive gastric belching
B3. Nausea and vomiting disorders
    B3a. Chronic nausea vomiting syndrome (CNVS)
    B3b. Cyclic vomiting syndrome (CVS)
    B3c. Cannabinoid hyperemesis syndrome (CHS)

B4. Rumination syndrome
C1. Irritable bowel syndrome (IBS)
    IBS with predominant constipation (IBS-C)
    IBS with predominant diarrhea (IBS-D)
    IBS with mixed bowel habits (IBS-M)
    IBS unclassified (IBS-U)
C2. Functional constipation
C3. Functional diarrhea
C4. Functional abdominal bloating/distension
C5. Unspecified functional bowel disorder
C6. Opioid-induced constipation
D1. Centrally mediated abdominal pain syndrome (CAPS)
D2. Narcotic bowel syndrome (NBS)/
    Opioid-induced GI hyperalgesia
E1. Biliary pain
    E1a. Functional gallbladder disorder
    E1b. Functional biliary SO disorder
E2. Functional pancreatic SO disorder
F1. Fecal incontinence
F2. Functional anorectal pain
    F2a. Levator ani syndrome
    F2b. Unspecified functional anorectal pain
    F2c. Proctalgia fugax
F3. Functional defecation disorders
    F3a. Inadequate defecatory propulsion

    F3b. Dyssynergic defecation
G1. Infant regurgitation
G2. Rumination syndrome
G3. Cyclic vomiting syndrome (CVS)
G4. Infant colic
G5. Functional diarrhea
G6. Infant dyschezia
G7. Functional constipation
H1. Functional nausea and vomiting disorders
    H1a. Cyclic vomiting syndrome (CVS)
    H1b. Functional nausea and functional vomiting
        H1b1. Functional nausea
        H1b2. Functional vomiting
    H1c. Rumination syndrome
    H1d. Aerophagia
H2. Functional abdominal pain disorders
    H2a. Functional dyspepsia
        H2a1. Postprandial distress syndrome
        H2a2. Epigastric pain syndrome
    H2b. Irritable bowel syndrome (IBS)
    H2c. Abdominal migraine
    H2d. Functional abdominal pain - NOS
H3. Functional defecation disorders
    H3a. Functional constipation
    H3b. Nonretentive fecal incontinence

According to the Rome Foundation, the symptoms associated with various FGIDs are related to combinations of physiological phenomena, such as increased motor reactivity, enhanced visceral hypersensitivity, altered mucosal immunity (inflammation), changes in gut microbiota, or altered regulation of the gut by the central nervous system (including psychological and sociocultural factors).[2] FGIDs are the third most common GI diagnosis during an ER visit across the United States, and over 10% of FGID-related emergency visits result in hospitalization.[3] Not surprisingly, it is quite common for a single individual to have symptoms associated with at least two different FGIDs (e.g., IBS-D and functional diarrhea), or an FGID with another gastrointestinal diagnosis (e.g., IBS and IBD or functional dyspepsia and GERD).[4,5,6] This guidebook is not designed to give a detailed review of each FGID, but will discuss the criteria for several as we navigate our way through several topics, including IBS (page 189), functional dyspepsia (page 25), and functional constipation (page 53).

Functional Medicine

Almost parallel in time with the development of the Rome criteria, a paradigm of medicine has been emerging that acknowledges core body functions (and, therefore, dysfunctions) are ultimately at the root of all complex chronic disease and healing potential. This new paradigm of medicine is generally referred to as "functional medicine," though many others within the broader integrative medical community practice a similar paradigm under different banners.[†] While defined differently by various groups, functional medicine essentially combines the importance of patient-centered preventative care with the understanding of the complex interconnections between organ systems. This form of medicine allows clinicians to begin to understand the complex network connecting each body system through a web of physiology and biochemistry. No longer is each body system isolated from the other; instead, the emphasis is on what connects the systems together; and what common relationships (and

deficiencies) help explain a patient's chronic conditions. In essence, this form of medicine asks, "What are the common threads connecting the symptom patterns seen in a patient experiencing chronic illness?" rather than merely "How can we differentiate one disease from one another?" The result is therapies focused on root causes of complex and chronic disease patterns that are tailored to specific patients.

As this paradigm has been emerging, research has greatly advanced the way we understand gastrointestinal functions and related disorders. For instance, many studies have illuminated the complex interaction of the immune system, neuroendocrine system and microbial environment within the gut, detailing how these newly discovered interactions are fundamentally related to core GI functions. Obviously, these advances in understanding have profound implications on the diagnosis and treatment of gastrointestinal disorders. While older models of gastroenterology defined discreet independent disorders, this new approach defines several shared fundamental functions, to be at the root of many, seemingly unrelated, GI disorders. When we combine these scientific advances along with the understanding of the biological individuality of each patient, we are at the heart of functional and lifestyle medicine. In the end, regardless of the name given to the medical tradition or the diagnostic code placed into the chart, this paradigm allows clinicians to treat patients (rather than diseases) and target root causes (rather than merely their manifesting symptoms).

Heal the Gut First

The gastrointestinal (GI) tract represents our most intimate contact with the external environment. In our lifetimes we will consume between 30-50 tons of food and host more microbial cells in our gut than human cells in the rest of our body. The GI tract is tasked with the responsibilities of extracting the appropriate nutrients we need to thrive, maintaining an appropriate balance of helpful and harmful microbes, and acting as a conduit for waste removal. At the same time, the healthy GI tract prevents the entrance of harmful substances into the body. Is it any wonder this delicate balance in the gut is often disturbed, leading to GI symptoms, disorders and syndromes for which many seek medical care?

It is not surprising, then, that one of the most common phrases used within naturopathic, functional and related integrative medical communities is "heal

---

†   The Institute for Functional Medicine (IFM) has championed the functional medicine model and has published the Textbook of Functional Medicine to define their perspective on how to practice within this paradigm. The principles and protocols shared within this book are, in our view, generally complimentary to those of IFM or other organizations teaching similar approaches- though they may differ in nomenclature and specific details.

the gut first." This idea reminds clinicians of the front-line role the GI system plays in nearly every facet of health. It is rare to find an individual with any chronic condition without some related GI system dysfunction. Conversely, patients with major GI disorders will manifest symptoms that are systemic. On top of this, all other recommended therapies involving foods, beverages, supplements or drugs require a predictable interface with the GI system and related detoxification pathways. Therapies that may work in a healthy GI environment may be neutralized or even exacerbate the condition for which they are intended to help when GI function is disrupted. "Heal the gut first" is a reminder that GI dysfunction can lead to many, seemingly unrelated, chronic conditions that may be best addressed after (or along with) known GI dysfunctions.

Core Functions of the GI System

Within this Road map, GI functions will be grouped into five core areas based on function: **Digestion, Elimination, Protective Barrier, Microbial Ecosystem,** and **Neuroendocrine.** These core functions are discrete and different, though most are interrelated and highly dependent upon one another. We will briefly define these core functions here, though each will be expanded greatly throughout this text.

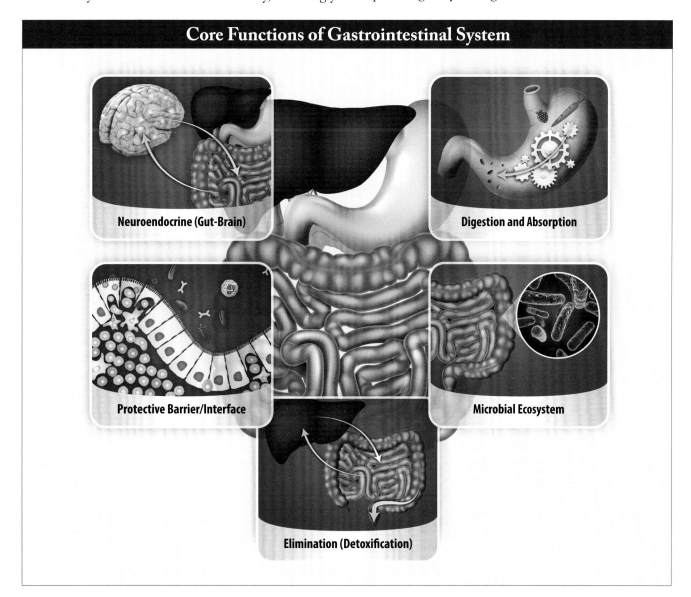

Core Functions of Gastrointestinal System

Neuroendocrine (Gut-Brain)

Digestion and Absorption

Protective Barrier/Interface

Microbial Ecosystem

Elimination (Detoxification)

Figure 4: The five categories of core gastrointestinal functions used within this Road map. See text for more details.

Digestion (and Absorption)

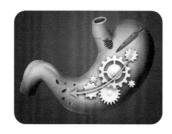

Perhaps the most obvious of all its functions, the GI tract is tasked with digesting and absorbing the nutrients within the food and beverages we consume. Through a complex coordination of enzymes, acids, bile salts, peristaltic action, transporters, and microbial biotransformation, our GI tract must take complex foodstuffs and deconstruct them into macronutrients (protein, carbohydrate, fat) and micronutrients (vitamins, minerals, phytonutrients, etc.) that can be transported into the body. Each step in the processes of digestion is important, as it only requires a deficiency in one or a few micronutrients to lead to a metabolic dysfunction.

Since the GI tract is exposed to 30-50 tons of food in the average lifetime, the types of food we eat are extremely important in maintaining proper GI health. The Standard American Diet, or SAD (sometimes called MUD, the Modern Urban Diet), is associated with nearly every chronic illness discovered, including most chronic GI complaints. Highly processed foods with high amounts of refined carbohydrates, hydrogenated fatty acids, food additives and preservatives, and low in fiber, natural colors and phytonutrients are typical of this dietary pattern. These poor dietary patterns are pro-inflammatory, place a significant burden upon the detoxification reserve capacity, and reduce bowel transit time, all of which can generate a downward spiral of gastrointestinal complaints and dysfunction. On top of this, many individuals have undiagnosed food allergies that continue to mediate ongoing immunological reactivity, further weakening the barrier function of the gut.

We will outline the types of diets and eating patterns known to be beneficial for the prevention and treatment of a range of digestive disorders, including discussions of a variety of ways to specifically improve digestion and absorption of nutrients. In addition, several ways clinicians can test a patient for poor digestive function will be listed.

Elimination

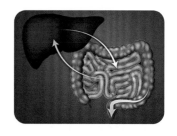

The process of elimination can be nearly as important as digestion. Ridding the body of the unusable portions of foods as well as the toxic metabolites stored and produced in the body is a critical function of the GI system. Healthy liver detoxification (biotransformation), bile production and regular bowel movements are hallmarks of a healthy GI tract. Proper elimination also helps regulate bowel transit time, which has an effect on proper digestion and absorption, water and electrolyte balance, and healthy microbial function. Constipation is one of the most common GI symptoms for which people seek a remedy. Stool frequency and morphology have been used to define overall health for millennia.

Details will be given about healthy detoxification and ways in which clinicians can encourage patients to avoid unhealthy toxins and allergens encountered in their diets, as well as nutritional and supplementary strategies to increase detoxification efficiency. We will also review the efficacy and safety of lifestyle and non-pharmacological approaches for preventing and treating constipation.

Protective Barrier

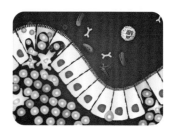

While we think of the GI tract as a digestive and absorptive organ, maintaining proper mucosal barrier function is vital for both GI and system-wide health. The GI tract is specifically equipped to balance the need for massive absorption of nutrients, while preventing the passage of unwanted particles or organisms into the body. The lumen of the gut contains numerous entities that should never reach the blood stream or lymphatic system, such as large antigenic/allergenic food particles, toxins, harmful microorganisms and their metabolites. The integrity of the mucosal barrier is maintained by a single layer of tightly fitted columnar epithelial cells that comprise a surface area the size of a doubles tennis court. As we shall outline later, greater than 70% of the immune system is closely associated with the GI tract in specialized lymphatic compartments within the mucosa and in the intercellular space along the epithelium. The barrier protection can be compromised by a number of factors such as dysbiosis, inflammation, food allergies and immune system dysregulation.

We will outline the consequences of barrier disruption that leads to gastrointestinal permeability (i.e., leaky gut), discussing both the common causes and ways to prevent and treat barrier disruptions. We will also describe the role of the gut-associated lymphoid tissue in maintaining the barrier function, describing ways to improve gut-immune function (and overall immune function), a role closely tied to both the microbiome and the neuroendocrine functions of the GI system.

Ecosystem for Gut Microbiome

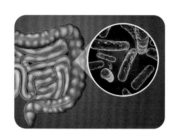

The human GI tract is host to at least 100 trillion individual microorganisms, from at least 1,000 different identified subspecies of bacterial and yeast alone. Over the past decade, research has been uncovering the interrelationship between proper human metabolism and the signals and metabolites that are generated from this internal microbial ecosystem. In fact, by some measures these microorganisms represent one of the most metabolically active systems within the human body— affecting glycemic control, cholesterol and amino acid metabolism, short-chain fatty acid production (e.g., butyrate for colon cell energy), and vitamin synthesis. Proper microbial balance helps regulate immune function and maturation, prevent overgrowth of harmful organisms, and regulate bowel motility.

Dysbiosis, the generic name given to any number of potential imbalances within the gut microbial environment, can lead to a wide range of GI pathologies and create vulnerabilities within the immune and detoxification systems, resulting in system-wide effects. This guidebook will overview the current scientific understanding of the human gut microbiome as it pertains to human metabolism, health and disease, while reviewing the known lifestyle, diet and non-pharmacological approaches (e.g., probiotics and prebiotics) for modulating the gut microbiome in the prevention and treatment of GI-related outcomes.

Neuroendocrine

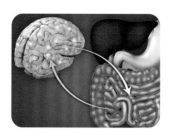

Since the GI system maintains a critical interface with the external environment, there are a number of signaling mechanisms designed to coordinate its function with the rest of the body. The enteric nervous system of the gut interacts in a coordinated fashion with the central nervous system to control a number of gastrointestinal functions. Beyond these basic neuronal connections, a number of endocrine signaling processes occur within the gastrointestinal tract to modulate gastric secretions, mucosal immune functions, microbial signaling, and a collection of functions usually labeled as "gut-brain" interactions. For instance, the strong connection between HPA axis stress and GI function is primarily mediated through the neuroendocrine functions within the GI tract.

As with all the other core functions of the GI system, the neuroendocrine functions of the gut are integrally entwined with the other core functions described above. Throughout the text, we will explain various aspects of the cells and functions which coordinate the neuroendocrine functions of the GI system within the other core functions already mentioned.

Functional Testing and GI Function

Within the functional and integrative medical community, a wide variety of laboratory tests are performed to help the clinician assess basic GI function within patients and to decipher complex gastrointestinal dysfunctions. Some of these tests are commonly used by a wide range of physicians or GI specialists, while others are more commonly used by clinicians trained within functional or integrative clinical models. Throughout various sections of the text, we will include a discussion of the available laboratory tests that may help a clinician confirm (or rule out) a particular GI dysfunction.

4 R (or 5R) Approach to GI Therapy

Over that past decade or so, one of the most commonly taught approaches for healing GI-related dysfunctions within the functional and integrative medical community is the "4R" or "5R" approach (championed by the Institute for Functional Medicine and outlined in their *Textbook of Functional Medicine*[1]). Essentially, the 4R approach is a step-wise therapeutic framework for dealing with a wide range of gastrointestinal conditions. The four main steps include "Remove," "Replace," "Re-inoculate," and "Repair." While these components don't specifically coordinate with the core functions we have outlined in this guidebook, this therapeutic strategy is generally complementary to the principles and protocols discussed throughout this Road map. For that reason, we will briefly describe and comment on this approach here.

REMOVE

The natural inclination in the treatment of patients is to ask, "What can be *given* to the patient?" In the case of the many chronic GI symptoms, however, often the best medicine is what can be removed. By eliminating pathogenic organisms (bacteria, viruses, fungi, parasites), toxic burden and reactive foods, patients can realize profound impacts on numerous GI-related (and non-GI-related) conditions. Unfortunately, it is often difficult to determine what needs to be removed in order

REMOVE *(Important First Step in 4R Model)*
Promote Elimination and Detoxification

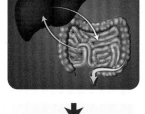

Remove Allergens and Toxins
- Elimination diet
- Detoxification protocol

Remove Harmful Organisms
- Stool testing for pathogens
- Eliminate pathogens

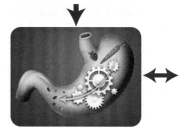 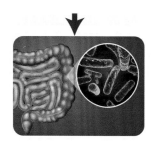 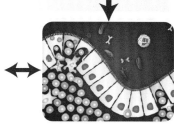

REPLACE
Promote Digestion and Absorption

- Supplement or stimulate
  - Stomach acid
  - Digestive enzymes
  - Bile for fat absorption
  - Easy to absorb nutrients

RE-ESTABLISH
(Re-inoculate)
Ecosystem for Microbiome

- Microbiome-friendly diet
- Avoiding certain drugs/antibiotics
- Probiotics
- Prebiotics

REPAIR
Barrier Function/ Immune Interface

- Reduce gut inflammation
- Provide nutrients for GI cells
- Improve tight junctions
- Increase signals for immune modulation

SUPPORTING NEUROENDOCRINE (GUT/BRAIN) FUNCTION
- Modulate the effects of HPA axis/stress
- Control neurotransmitter synthesis and function
- Manage satiety signals from gut
- Coordinate signals from microbiome, immune system, bowel transit to and from the CNS

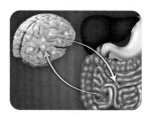

to help restore a patient's health, so this is often accomplished in two steps.

First, and perhaps most importantly, the patient must remove the incoming toxic and immunological burden. This is often accomplished by using an elimination diet focused on limiting common allergenic foods and decreasing or eliminating food toxins (pesticides, herbicides, preservatives, etc.). If possible, combining this with a protocol that allows for the gentle removal of toxins stored by the body (i.e., detoxification), will decrease the GI burden even further. Secondly, clinicians must look for signs and symptoms of pathogenic organisms living within the GI tract (bacterial, viral, parasitic, etc.). By asking specific questions about the patient's health history and the judicious use of pathogenic stool tests, clinicians can identify particular pathogens that must be removed before further healing of the gut can be accomplished. While the next steps within the 4R program can often be accomplished simultaneously, removing harmful inputs and residents of the GI tract is a key first step prior to moving forward.

REPLACE

Within the 4R model, this step involves replacing those factors which might be necessary to help a patient digest and absorb food nutrients (usually through special dietary principles or supplementation). The primary factors around which most therapies are focused are stomach acid, bile and digestive enzymes. Supporting these factors can be accomplished by paying careful attention to food selection and food preparation techniques, avoidance of certain foods, drugs and lifestyle habits that diminish proper digestion, as well as through mealtime supplementation. Detailed discussion of these supporting therapies can be found starting on page 25.

RE-INOCULATE

The third step in the 4R model typically involves the introduction of good bacteria to the GI tract via foods or dietary supplementation. Since it may be a slight misnomer to refer to the introduction of a handful of probiotic strains into the GI milieu (containing hundreds of sub-species of commensal organisms) as "re-inoculate," it may be better to think of this as a means to re-establish an environment that is more friendly to healthy commensal organisms. Along with probiotics (in fermented foods, fortified foods and beverages, supplementation in capsules and tablets), this may also include prebiotic fibers intended to improve the microbiome and the commensals living within it. Extensive information about the use of probiotics and prebiotics in the maintenance of a healthy commensal GI microbial community is included starting on page 114.

REPAIR

Many chronic GI perturbations result in some sort of damage to the gut mucosa, especially those that create ongoing inflammation leading to breaches in the barrier function and immune system overstimulation. The "repair" part of this model describes steps that can be taken to replenish the necessary building blocks for mucosal tissues to repair themselves. This might include the use of natural anti-inflammatory agents (and avoiding inflammatory foods), ingredients that support GI mucus production, nutrients known to be beneficial for either enterocytes or colonocytes, or natural therapies that support immune and liver function.

References

1. This model of GI healing is defined as the "4R Model" in the 2010 edition of the *Textbook of Functional Medicine*, published by IFM. Lectures by IFM staff and others describe a 5th "R," though sometimes this has been listed as "Re-balance" and other times as "Relieve."

References

1. Drossman DA, Hasler WL. Rome IV-Functional GI Disorders: Disorders of Gut-Brain Interaction. *Gastroenterology.* 2016 May;150(6):1257-61.
2. Drossman DA. The functional gastrointestinal disorders and the Rome III process. *Gastroenterology.* 2006 Apr;130(5):1377-90.
3. Myer PA, Mannalithara A, Singh G, et al. Clinical and economic burden of emergency department visits due to gastrointestinal diseases in the United States. *Am J Gastroenterol.* 2013 Sep;108(9):1496-507.
4. Ford AC, Bercik P, Morgan DG, et al. Characteristics of functional bowel disorder patients: a cross-sectional survey using the Rome III criteria. *Aliment Pharmacol Ther.* 2014 Feb;39(3):312-21.
5. Burgell RE, Asthana AK, Gibson PR. Irritable bowel syndrome in quiescent inflammatory bowel disease: a review. *Minerva Gastroenterol Dietol.* 2015 Dec;61(4):201-13.
6. Rasmussen S, Jensen TH, Henriksen SL, et al. Overlap of symptoms of gastroesophageal reflux disease, dyspepsia and irritable bowel syndrome in the general population. *Scand J Gastroenterol.* 2015 Feb;50(2):162-9.

Functional Support for Digestion and Absorption

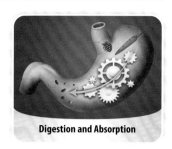

Digestion and Absorption

The old adage "you are what you eat" was meant to be a reminder that our daily food habits will have an effect (directly or indirectly) on our body composition and health.[†] As we shall explore, this is partly true, though it is a bit more complicated when we get into the details. Perhaps we might say that we are what we absorb, since eating foods and absorbing or utilizing their nutrients is not always the same thing; especially in subjects with poor digestion. Reduced nutrient absorption, however, is just one facet of poor digestive health. In fact, various symptoms related to the digestive process (i.e., indigestion/dyspepsia) are some of the most commonly experienced by individuals worldwide; and the use of prescription, OTC and dietary supplements to aid digestion or relieve dyspeptic symptoms is rampant in the United States. This section of the guidebook will discuss both the fundamental principles of digestion and absorption, along with the most common dysfunctions related to digesting and absorbing nutrients from dietary sources. We will also review ways in which digestion can be improved through the use of lifestyle changes or dietary supplementation.

Indigestion and Functional Dyspepsia

Indigestion (i.e., dyspepsia) is one of the most common adverse gastrointestinal conditions experienced by all people—even if only on occasion. The definition of indigestion is somewhat vague, loosely related to an upset stomach or an adverse digestive outcome. Thus, depending on the criteria used to define dyspepsia, chronic indigestion/dyspepsia is experienced by an estimated 10-40% of the general population (estimates are much higher when heartburn is included in the criteria).[1]

On the other hand, functional dyspepsia as a Rome diagnosis is defined a bit differently and, ironically, is mostly *unrelated* to the processes normally associated with digestion. The Rome definition for functional dyspepsia is now divided into two basic syndromes: the epigastric pain syndrome and the postprandial distress syndrome.[2] The epigastric pain syndrome is defined by intermittent pain or burning in the epigastrium at least once per week for six months, while the postprandial distress syndrome is defined by bothersome postprandial fullness occurring after normal-sized meals at least several times per week for six months. Subjects with heartburn/regurgitation

are excluded from a diagnosis of functional dyspepsia, according to Rome criteria.

While these definitions of functional dyspepsia may be helpful for advancing clinical trial inclusion/exclusion criteria, there is still disagreement on their utility in clinical research and practice.[3] As with other functional gastrointestinal disorders (FGIDs), functional dyspepsia often overlaps with other FGIDs such as IBS and/or other GI disorders such as GERD.[4,5,6] Commonly, psychological distress (e.g., anxiety) is associated with functional dyspepsia, although abnormal pain processing or gastric motility and relaxation are also considered to be common as well.[2]

This section will cover the support of "digestive function" within the traditional context of breaking down and absorbing food nutrients. Often, dysfunctional digestion and absorption is called maldigestion/malabsorption to distinguish this from the symptoms that may (or may not) be associated with poor digestion (i.e., dyspepsia/indigestion). We will discuss each phase of digestion first, discussing specific cases of malabsorption along the way.

[†] This phrase appears to have been popularized in the 1920s by the nutritionist Victor Lindlahr, who promoted what he called the Catabolic Diet. In a 1923 edition of the *Bridgeport Telegraph*, he is quoted as saying "Ninety per cent of the diseases known to man are caused by cheap foodstuffs. You are what you eat." He would later publish a book by this name in 1942.

Poor Digestion: What Are The Consequences?

Inadequate digestion and absorption of food nutrients, supplemental nutrients, or therapeutic compounds (e.g., phytonutrients, pharmaceuticals) can lead to a range of clinical consequences. Some of these consequences result in GI-related symptoms, while others result in systemic signs and symptoms that are frequently missed (since many nutrient deficiencies often go undiagnosed). Therefore, it is important to understand the two primary ways in which poor digestion and absorption can affect GI health (see Figure 5).

The first is simply the decreased absorption of necessary nutrients into the body, reducing the availability of these nutrients within GI or other tissues. While we often attribute this to poor food selection, it is also true that poor digestion can render certain food nutrients unavailable to certain individuals, even when they are abundant in their diet (e.g., B12 malabsorption in the elderly). The second major way that poor digestion and absorption can affect GI function is by allowing unprocessed food particles

(usually macronutrients) to be improperly accessed by gut microbes, or to trigger immune reactivity. This can lead to symptoms usually experienced as GI-related discomfort after eating (gas, bloating, nausea, urgent diarrhea, burping, stomach pain, etc.). When severe enough, these effects can lead to changes in the balance of the microbiota (dysbiosis) or in bowel transit time, both of which can further alter nutrient absorption.

While the consequences of poor digestion and absorption are fairly easy to understand, there are many potential contributing factors that reduce the efficiency of the digestive process, some of which are further exacerbated by poor nutrient bioavailability or the fermentation of improperly digested macronutrients. In other words, the consequences of poor digestion can be a cyclical and compounding problem if not addressed in a timely manner. Figure 5 shows some of primary contributing factors that clinicians should keep in mind when determining the potential cause(s) of a person's poor digestion or absorption, most of which will be covered in this section.

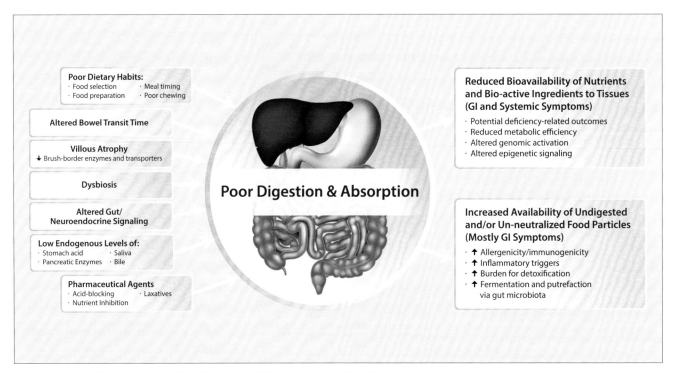

Figure 5: Causes and Consquences of Poor Digestion and Absorption. As the figure illustrates, there are a number of potential causes that may contribute to poor digestion and absorption of important nutrients from food or dietary supplements (macronutrients, micronutrients, phytonutrients etc.). The consequences of poor digestion can be a result of the lack of nutrient availability to the tissues, or a consequence of undigested nutrients as substrates for unwanted outcomes.

The Process and Regulation of Digestion and Absorption

Many textbooks describe the details of food digestion and absorption; we do not intend to duplicate that information here. However, there are numerous steps in the regulation of the digestive process that we outline in the following figures to help the reader understand the numerous mechanisms used to control this important process.

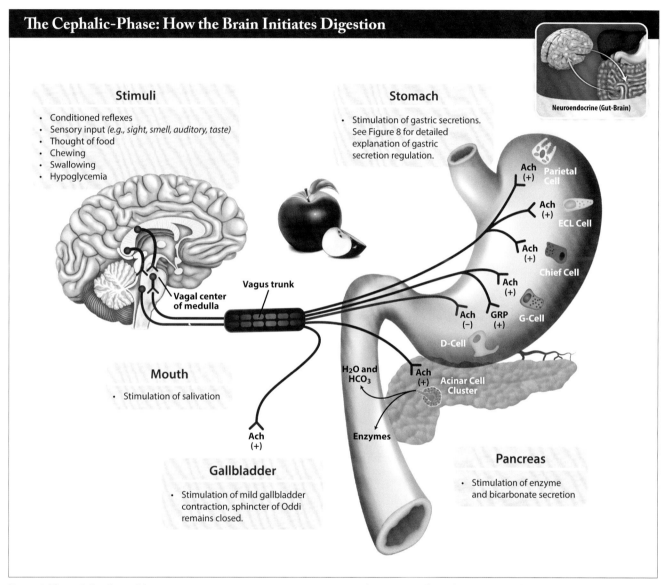

Figure 6: The cephalic phase of digestion is a secretomotor anticipatory response to a diverse range of stimuli that prepares the digestive tract to receive a meal. Stimuli for the cephalic phase include sensory inputs (e.g., sight, smell, auditory, tactile sensations of food), thoughts of food, chewing, swallowing, hypoglycemia, and other conditioned reflexes (e.g., Pavlov's dogs). This stimulatory information is relayed to the dorsal vagal complex of the brain, which propagates parasympathetic action potentials via the vagus nerve to the enteric nervous system. During the cephalic phase, gastric secretion is stimulated through the vagal release of acetylcholine (Ach) which stimulates the parietal, ECL, chief and G-cells; while inhibiting gastric D-cells. Gastrin-releasing peptide (GRP) is also released during vagal stimulation which acts on the G-cells to release gastrin (see Figure 8 for further details related to gastric secretion regulation). Vagal innervation of the pancreas stimulates the release of bicarbonate, water and enzymes from the acinar cells. It should be noted that while pancreatic secretion is initiated in the cephalic phase, pancreatic secretion is mostly stimulated by stomach contents entering the duodenum. Finally, vagal innervation stimulates rhythmic, weak contractions of the gallbladder, though the sphincter of Oddi remains closed during the cephalic phase. The cephalic phase is associated with an increase in salivary secretions as well, but this response does not appear to be under vagal control. Gut motility may also be under cephalic control. Other factors such as an individual's emotional state, personal food preferences and the complexity of stimulatory signals can inhibit or enhance the cephalic response to a given stimulus.

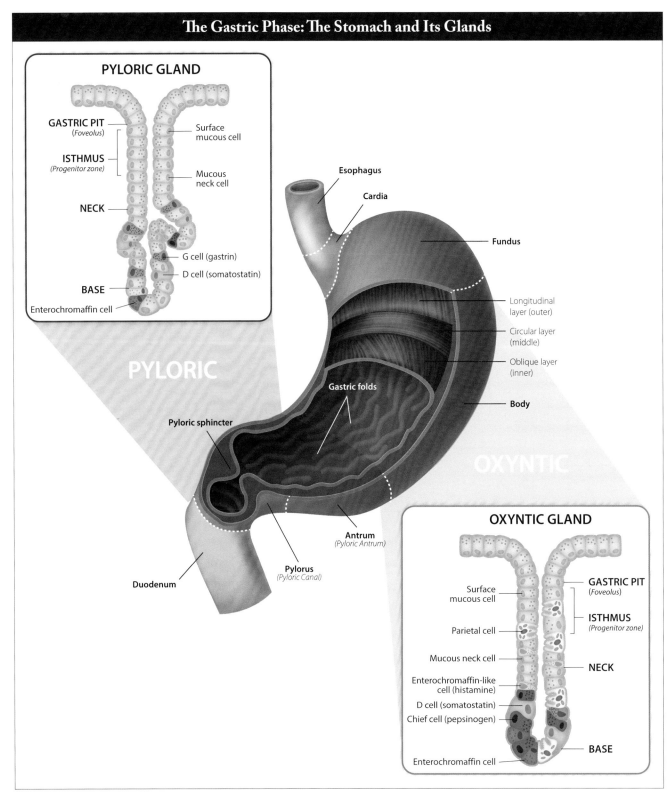

Figure 7: This figure shows the basic design of the stomach, with its basic anatomical sections (cardia, fundus, body, antrum and pylorus), the three muscle layers that allow for mixing in all directions, and the gastric folds that allow for increased surface area within the lumen. The insets show the two main types of glands (i.e., gastric pits) that are generally located in different areas of the stomach (note shaded areas). The cells within these glands control the production of HCl, mucus, pepsinogen etc. Note that acid-producing parietal cells are absent from the pyloric glands and gastrin-producing G-cells are absent from the oxyntic glands. See Figure 8 for interaction between these cells in the regulation of gastric acid production.

Figure 8: Parietal Cell Regulation: How Stomach Acid is Controlled

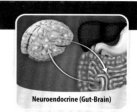

Gastric acid secretion is tightly regulated by four positive modulators for acid release (i.e., acetylcholine (Ach), gastrin releasing peptide (GRP), histamine and gastrin), and one negative modulator of acid release (i.e., somatostatin). Further, there are three pathways through which acid secretion is regulated; direct neuroendocrine, hormonal, and paracrine signaling pathways. As the figure and explanations below outline, this process has a number of checks and balances designed to ensure the proper amount of acid is produced at the appropriate time. The use of proton-pump inhibitors which directly inhibit the ability of the parietal cell to produce and secrete acid, completely inhibits this process and leaves the individual without the ability to properly control stomach pH. For a discussion of the negative consequences of PPI overuse, see page 219.

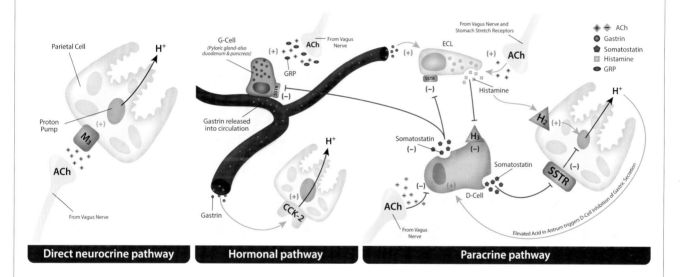

Direct neurocrine pathway | **Hormonal pathway** | **Paracrine pathway**

Direct Neuroendocrine Pathway

The neurotransmitter acetylcholine (Ach) is released from the vagus nerve as part of the cephalic phase of digestion or during the process of eating a meal. Ach acts on muscarinic M3 receptors on the parietal cell which triggers a number of secondary signals (e.g., Ca^{++}, phosphorylation) to activate the proton pump to produce HCl. Proton pump inhibitors (PPIs) function by irreversibly inhibiting the proton pump blocking this, and all other pathways, controlling the function of the proton pump.

Hormonal Pathway (Indirect)

Ach and the gastric neurotransmitter GRP are released from the vagus or enteric nerves. GRP stimulates endocrine G-cells to release the hormone gastrin into the circulation. Gastrin interacts with the parietal cell directly by binding to the CCK-2 receptor on the parietal cell, which triggers a number of secondary signals (e.g., Ca^{++}, phosphorylation) activating the proton pump. Gastrin also indirectly increases acid production by stimulating the enterochromaffin-like (ECL) cells to release the paracrine modulator histamine.

Paracrine Pathway

In addition to gastrin, histamine release by the ECL cell is also stimulated by Ach released by the vagus nerve. Histamine acts in a paracrine fashion to regulate acid secretion by the parietal cell in two ways; first, histamine binds to the H2 receptor on the parietal cell directly stimulating acid secretion (via cAMP signaling pathways). Secondly, histamine acts indirectly by interacting with the H3 receptor on the endocrine D-cells to inhibit somatostatin release; Ach from the vagus nerve also inhibits somatostatin release from the D-cell. When the pH of the antrum falls too low, indicating elevated acid production, there is a mechanism to shut down acid production. The endocrine D-cell becomes stimulated by the elevated acid, and stimulates the release of somatostatin which acts in a direct and indirect fashion to reduce acid secretion. Somatostatin acts directly on the parietal cell via the SSTR receptor, and indirectly by inhibiting both the ECL cell and the G-cell via its receptor, SSTR.

Inadequate Stomach Acid (Hypochlorhydria/Achlorhydria)

An inadequate level of stomach acid (regardless of the root cause) is likely to result in a number of nutritional and digestive issues. For instance, a reduction in gastric acid secretion (elevated stomach pH) prevents adequate denaturing of folded proteins, limiting access to certain proteases, thereby resulting in poor protein digestion and increased food allergenicity.[7] A low-acid environment will result in reduced absorption of key micronutrients such as calcium, iron, folic acid, vitamins B6 and B12.[8,9] Also, since gastric acid helps to eliminate harmful ingested microorganisms and hinders bacterial overgrowth in the stomach and small bowel; low stomach acid can increase the risk for SIBO (see page 231) and specific microbial overgrowth from organisms like *Clostridium difficile* (see also Consequences of PPI Overuse on page 219).[10,11,12] While most of these consequences of low stomach acid are undisputed, there is much less agreement on the prevalence of this condition in the general population, how to test for such a condition and, especially, whether there is an appropriate therapy for low stomach acid.

Low stomach acid (hypochlorhydria) and absence of stomach acid (achlorhydria) are not often clearly defined (and often not distinguished between) within the various publications using these two terms. Also, since a variety of different mechanisms are used to measure stomach acid and pH (gastric intubation, catheter electrodes, radio-telemetric capsules and pH-sensitive tablets), different cut-off points have been used to define hypochlorhydria and achlorhydria in such studies, the majority of which were published decades ago. Generally, a fasting gastric pH of <3.0 is considered "normal," while values above 3.0 are deemed to be gradually more hypochlorhydric. True achlorhydria results in a gastric pH above 7 characterized by very limited acid production when stimulated by gastrin or histamine (e.g., chronic atrophic gastritis).[13]

Debate concerning the prevalence of hypochlorhydria within the general population is noted in the literature. While aging is regularly associated with decreased gastric acid production, fasting hypochlorhydria is reported to be less common (~10% or less) in elderly Americans and very common (>60%) in elderly Japanese subjects.[14,15,16] Neither of these reports actually measured stomach pH directly, as both relied on urinary measures of pH-sensitive substances after ingestion (quinine and riboflavin, respectively). However, while *fasting* gastric pH is likely

an important marker for achlorhydria, especially when this condition is related to chronic atrophic gastritis, the gradual "functional" decline in gastric acid secretion during and after consuming a meal (a biomarker rarely reported in the literature) may be a much more important biomarker.

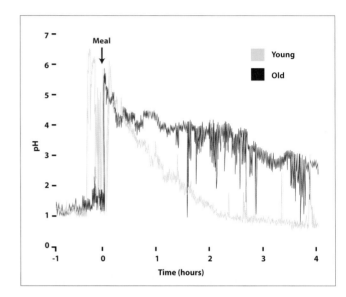

Figure 9: Functional Hypochlorhydria in Older Subjects. Meal-time stomach acid pH, measured by Heidelberg capsule, is shown for a typical older and younger individual. Note that while the pH of the stomach rapidly becomes more acidic in the younger subject, there is a >4 hour delay in reaching pre-meal stomach acid levels in the older individual. See text below for more details. Figure modified from Berardi et al.[17,18]

Interestingly, such studies were performed by researchers at the University of Michigan nearly two decades ago. The researchers reported on the fasting, mealtime and postprandial stomach pH levels in healthy young and elderly subjects (Figure 9).[17,18] Gastric pH levels were measured using a tethered radio-telemetric capsule (Heidelberg) in 15-second intervals. After 12 hours of fasting, gastric pH was measured for one hour before a "standard meal"[†] and continuously for another four hours (post-prandial). In the fasted state, the average gastric pH was similar in both the younger (mean age 25 years) and the older (mean age 71 years) subjects, with a slight statistical trend toward lower pH (more acid) in

---

†   The "standard meal" used in this early 90s report was a 6 oz. hamburger, 2 slices of bread, 2 oz. of hash browns, 1 oz. of tomato, some lettuce, mayo and ketchup and 8 oz. of milk (1,000 calories).

the elderly subjects. However, it should be noted that while none of the younger subjects had a fasting pH >5.0 (their definition of achlorhydria), 11% of the elderly subjects had a fasting gastric pH >5.0, similar to what has been reported in other studies. Using this fasting data alone, one might conclude that ~90% of elderly subjects have similar (or more potent) gastric acid production compared to younger subjects. But, while both groups saw an expected rise in stomach pH upon consumption of the meal, the time required to re-acidify the gastric contents was much slower in the older subjects. For instance, while the average pH after consuming the meal was similar in young and old subjects (5.0 and 4.9, respectively), the time it took to re-acidify the stomach to a pH of 3.0 was 42 minutes in the younger subjects and 89 minutes in the older subjects, averaging nearly an hour longer to reach a pH of 2.0 (16.4% of the elderly subjects did not return to pH of 2.0 within four hours).

These data suggest that a subtle diminution of gastric acid secretion (along with reduced levels of intrinsic factor and pepsin activation) may gradually increase with aging, which cannot be readily detected in the fasted state (i.e., independent of atrophic gastritis/achlorhydria). This extended mealtime/postprandial hypochlorhydria may contribute to poor protein digestion, reduced micronutrient absorption, increased risk of dysbiosis, SIBO, or other symptoms associated with functional dyspepsia. Based upon this notion of progressive "functional" hypochlorhydria in older subjects, it is common for integrative and functional medicine clinicians to recommend oral supplementation of "gastric acid" in the form of betaine HCl (often with pepsin) to help reduce meal-time stomach pH (see page 33 or below).

The Role of Hypochlorhydria in GERD

While the most common treatment for acid reflux-related symptoms are agents that reduce the production of gastric acid (e.g., PPIs and H2 blockers), there is little evidence that the average subject with symptoms of gastric acid reflux produces excess amounts of gastric acid. In fact, researchers at USC studied the gastric and esophageal pH of 1,582 patients with symptoms suggestive of GERD and found they had an average fasting gastric pH that was slightly higher (less acidic, pH 1.7) than normal subject (average pH of 1.5) and that 11%

of these patients actually had fasting hypochlorhydria.[19] Also, while they did find esophageal reflux (measured as % of time with esophageal pH<4) increased when the gastric pH was lower, they also reported that patients with hypochlorhydria had paradoxically more supine reflux and more prolonged reflux episodes than patients with normal gastric pH. The authors speculate that, despite lower gastric acid production, these subjects may have poor esophageal clearance of refluxed acid.

Since the prevalence of both hypochlorhydria and GERD increase with age, and GERD is not typically associated with acid hypersecretion, clinicians should therefore not assume acid-suppressing drugs are addressing the root cause of GERD, even if they appear to be managing its symptoms. (see GERD section on page 223). Likewise, while it may seem paradoxical that low stomach acid can result in symptoms associated with acid reflux, hypochlorhydria should not be ruled out in older subjects suffering symptoms of GERD, especially with increased supine-associated acid reflux. Where the prevalence of hypochlorhydria is higher (e.g., Japan), low stomach acid production has been shown to be related to delayed gastric emptying and dyspepsia (especially in female subjects).[20]

Supplementing "Acid" to Improve Digestion: What is the Evidence?

The debate about the utility of supplementing acid is related to the debate about the relationship between endogenous stomach acid production and gastrointestinal outcomes. While conventional medical literature routinely suggests that the amount of stomach acid production is more than adequate for the purposes of digestion in healthy subjects, "functional" hypochlorhydria may be much more common in older subjects (see page 30) and the rampant use of drugs to suppress acid production increases the frequency of mealtime hypochlorhydria in many subjects. Therefore, it is common within the functional and integrative medicine community to recommend supplementing agents that directly or indirectly increase stomach acid during a meal.

Bitters

The use of bitter-tasting plants or plant extracts to promote digestion and/or relieve digestive complaints is common in many herbal medicinal traditions. Some of the best known and commonly used bitters in the Western herbal traditions are gentian, artichoke leaf, endive and bitter greens (dandelion leaf, wild lettuce, milk thistle, chicory), though there are many others used in other traditions. Some of these herbal extracts are delivered in alcohol as concentrated "bitters," although the bitter constituents found in beer are also known to stimulate gastric acid secretion, as does small quantities of ethanol.[21] Bitter herbs such as gentian root (*Gentiana lutea*) and wormwood (*Artemisia absinthium*) have long been noted to improve both gastric and salivary secretions, though recent scrutiny on the mechanisms of these classic bitters suggests other mechanisms may account for their benefit against dyspepsia.[22] While many patients will benefit from the use of bitters before or during a meal, there is little in the way of systematic research to suggest specific preparations and doses.

Coffee/Caffeine

Coffee consumption (regular and decaffeinated) is associated with increased dyspepsia and heartburn related symptoms, though brewed coffee itself is not strongly acidic having a pH 5-6.[23] *In vitro* research has identified several compounds in brewed coffee that can stimulate gastric acid secretion, some of which are altered by the roasting process.[24,25] While some clinicians recommend patients with GERD avoid drinking coffee, the gastric acid stimulating effects of coffee may be beneficial in subjects with functional (or postprandial) hypochlorhydria, though the magnitude of the gastric pH changes associated with coffee during or after a meal have not been carefully studied.

Betaine HCl

Perhaps the most popular and direct way to lower stomach pH is mealtime supplementation with betaine HCl, a hydrochloride compound of betaine base or trimethylglycine (TMG, a form also available as a dietary supplement without HCl, and used primarily as a methyl donor/homocysteine lowering agent). Betaine HCl readily releases H+ in an aqueous environment (approximately 0.65 mmol/ 100 mg), so it is important that supplements are in the form of capsules or tablets when ingested. Betaine HCl is sold as a dietary supplement in the United States and is most often measured in milligrams; however, some recommendations still use "grains" to measure this compound. One grain of betaine HCl is equal to 65 mg.

The most common recommendation for the use of betaine HCl supplements is combined with the empirical test for low stomach acid where betaine HCl capsules or tablets are increasingly given during meals until such time as an uncomfortable sensation is noticed by the patient (see sidebar for typical recommendation).[26] This, along with improvements in symptoms of dyspepsia or laboratory analysis of improved protein digestion (see page 45), acts as an empirical confirmation that low gastric acid production was contributing to poor digestion and/or dyspeptic symptoms. At this time, we are unaware that this popular recommendation has been rigorously tested in a research setting, though thousands of clinicians follow such recommendations with positive anecdotal outcomes.

Only one group has published data that specifically investigated how betaine HCl supplementation alters stomach pH, producing data that may be helpful to the clinician recommending this therapy. These researchers were investigating the ability of betaine HCl to re-acidify the gastric environment in subjects taking proton pump inhibitors, with a specific goal to improve the solubility and efficacy of specific pH-sensitive drugs in such patients.[27,28] Using six healthy volunteers with normal fasting gastric pH (pH <2), hypochlorhydria was induced by giving 20 mg of rabeprazole sodium twice daily with food for four days prior to the study day. On the fifth day, radio-telemetric Heidelberg capsules were positioned in the stomach and each subject was given an additional 20 mg of rabeprazole (PPI). When subject gastric pH remained above 4.0 for a minimum of 15 minutes, they were given 1,500 mg of betaine HCl (two capsules, 750 mg each) with 250 ml of water and monitored for changes in gastric pH for several hours in the fasted state. Gastric pH in all subjects fell rapidly from an average pH 5.2 in the half hour prior to the betaine HCl to an average pH of 0.6 thirty minutes after supplementation. While the gastric acidification was rapid, averaging 6.25 minutes to reach pH<3, the total duration of re-acidification lasted just longer than one hour (average time to rebound to pH>3 was 73 minutes, rebound to pH>4 was 77 minutes, though there was a wide intra-individual range [±30 minutes] for rebound). They later showed that, indeed, betaine HCl co-administered with a pH-sensitive drug (dasatinib) greatly enhanced solubility and absorption in PPI-induced hypochlorhydric subjects.

There are several ways to interpret and apply this information in the clinic. First, these data clearly show the potency of betaine HCl to acidify gastric pH in a short period of time when using 1,500 mg (~23 grains). The rebound time to higher gastric pH reported in these subjects is confounded by the fact that these subjects were on acid-suppressing therapy on the one hand and were fasted on the other. Nonetheless, it may suggest that doses of supplemental betaine HCl may need to be divided and taken throughout the meal since endogenous gastric HCl production is limited in many older subjects with "functional" hypochlorhydria (see Figure 9). These data may also suggest that supplemental mealtime betaine HCl may even be appropriate for subjects on PPI therapy, in order to decrease common PPI side-effects (protein/micronutrient/drug malabsorption, food-borne microbial survival, or slow gastric emptying). Even when given 1,500 mg of betaine HCl, most subjects had returned to their PPI-induced gastric hypochlorhydria in less than 75 minutes on an empty stomach.

Basic Protocol for Using Betaine HCl
(for empiric testing of mealtime hypochlorhydria and for supplementing acid)

This protocol involves giving patients increasing doses of betaine HCl at mealtimes until such time as noticeable discomfort is reported. Patients who have exceeded the necessary dose will experience tingling, heartburn, diarrhea, *or any type of discomfort* including a feeling of unease, digestive discomfort, neck ache, backache, headache, or any new odd symptom. Upon experiencing tingling, burning, or any uncomfortable symptom, patients can neutralize the acid with 1 tsp baking soda in water or milk.

1. Patients with suspected mealtime hypochlorhydria should begin by taking one (1) capsule containing 350–750 mg (~5-12 grains) of betaine HCl with a protein-containing meal[†] (Capsules containing betaine HCl with added pepsin are fine, and may be superior for overall benefit).

2. If no discomfort or burning sensation is noted, patient can begin taking two (2) capsules with each protein-containing meal.

3. If a burning sensation or any discomfort is noted after taking this (or any) dose, patient can neutralize the acid with 1 tsp baking soda in water or milk and discontinue the protocol.

4. If there are no noticeable reactions to the betaine HCl after two days, patients should increase the number of capsules with each meal to three (3).[†]

5. Continue increasing the number of capsules every two days (maximum 3,000 mg of betaine HCl) with each meal if necessary until a dose results in tingling, burning, or any other type of discomfort. At such point, the patient should decrease the dose by one (1) capsule per meal. *If the discomfort continues, they should be instructed to discontinue the betaine HCl supplementation and consult with their healthcare professional.*

6. Once a dose is established, continue this dose at subsequent meals.

7. With smaller meals, less betaine HCl is needed, so a reduced dose may be adequate.

8. Individuals with very moderate HCl deficiency generally show rapid improvement in symptoms and have early signs of intolerance to the acid. This typically indicates a return to normal acid secretion.

Precautions:
Administration of HCl/pepsin is contraindicated in peptic ulcer disease. HCl can irritate sensitive tissue and can be corrosive to teeth; therefore, capsules should not be emptied into food or dissolved in beverages.

[†]   It is important that this be done with a meal of sufficient size (500 calories or more) containing adequate protein. Betaine HCl should not be given on an empty stomach.

The Core of Digestion: Duodenum, Gallbladder, and Pancreas

The intestinal phase of digestion requires a highly coordinated process of gastric emptying, pH adjustment, enzyme and bile secretion and a range of active and passive transport systems. When the acidic and partially digested contents of the stomach begin entering the duodenum, a chain reaction triggers the secretion of digestive enzymes from the pancreas. First, the low pH of gastric emptying causes the release of secretin from duodenal S-cells, which acts to inhibit gastric acid secretion while also stimulating bicarbonate secretion from the pancreas (creating a neutral duodenal pH for maximal pancreatic enzyme activity). Additionally, partially digested macronutrients (fatty acids, amino acids, etc.) then trigger the release of cholecystokinin (CCK) from enteroendocrine cells along the duodenum (sometimes called "I" cells). CCK causes contraction of the gallbladder (propelling bile into the bile duct) and the release of acetylcholine (ACh) from nerve fibers within the pancreas. ACh, along with CCK and other peptide signals, then stimulates the secretion of pancreatic digestive enzymes from the acinar cells of

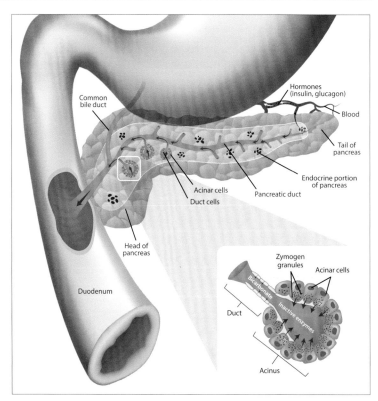

Figure 10: Basic Anatomy of Exocrine Pancreas. This figure shows the basic anatomy of the human pancreas with an inset showing the arrangement of the acini that are designed to produce and secrete the enzymes or pro-enzymes (zymogens) and bicarbonate directly into the lumen of the duodenum. The types of enzymes/proenzymes and their activator is shown in the table below.

Enzymes of the Human Exocrine Pancreas

Enzyme	Proenzyme	Activator	Action
Trypsin	Trypsinogen	Enteropeptidase	Cleaves internal peptide bonds
Chymotrypsin	Chymotrypsinogen	Trypsin	Cleaves internal peptide bonds
Elastase	Proelastase	Trypsin	Cleaves internal peptide bonds
Carboxypeptidase	Procarboxypeptidase	Trypsin	Cleaves last amino acid from carboxyl-terminal end of polypeptide
Phospholipase	Prophospholipase	Trypsin	Cleaves fatty acids from phospholipids such as lecithin
Lipase	None	None	Cleaves fatty acids from glycerol
Amylase	None	None	Digests starch to maltose and short chains of glucose molecules
Cholesterolesterase	None	None	Releases cholesterol from its bonds with other molecules
Ribonuclease	None	None	Cleaves RNA to form short chains
Deoxyribonuclease	None	None	Cleaves DNA to form short chains

Table 3: Pancreatic Enzymes/Proenzymes and their activators and functions.

the pancreas. These enzymes (discussed below) flow into the duodenum along with bile from the bile duct. CCK also slows gastric emptying and acts to promote satiety by binding CCK receptors in the central nervous system.

The majority of the enzymes (by mass) produced in the human pancreas are proteases, primarily trypsin and chymotrypsin (secreted as proenzymes trypsinogen and chymotrypsinogen). Other pancreatic enzymes include pancreatic lipase, pancreatic amylase, pancreatic elastase (secreted as proelastase), and pancreatic nucleases. Though some digestive enzymes are produced in the saliva, stomach and enterocyte brush border, pancreatic enzymes are critical for proper protein, fat and carbohydrate digestion and absorption (see Table 3).

Pancreatic Exocrine Insufficiency

Insufficient production or secretion of pancreatic enzymes leads to various symptoms of maldigestion/malabsorption. Primary pancreatic exocrine insufficiency (PEI, or sometimes EPI) results from chronic pancreatitis, cystic fibrosis, acute necrotizing pancreatitis or pancreatic cancer. Secondary PEI can result from various gastrointestinal surgeries (e.g., gastrectomy, gastric bypass) or GI tract disorders like celiac disease.[29,30] The reduced availability of pancreatic digestive enzymes is most noticeable (and diagnostic) as a reduction in lipase activity resulting in fat malabsorption. Diagnosis of PEI is therefore often tied to fat malabsorption through the cumbersome (and unpleasant) collection of three days of stool samples and strict diet containing 100 gram/day of fat, or a breath test after consuming ^{13}C-labeled mixed triglycerides. These tests are rarely used in the clinical setting.

However, another test that is readily available for most clinicians is fecal elastase 1 (pancreatic elastase measured in fecal samples).[31] In humans, elastase accounts for about 6% of the total pancreatic enzyme output. Because of its stability and low variability within an individual from day to day, fecal levels of elastase have become a helpful biomarker for pancreatic enzyme insufficiency (it is often combined with other digestive-related analytes within commercially available stool tests; see page 45). Generally, fecal elastase 1

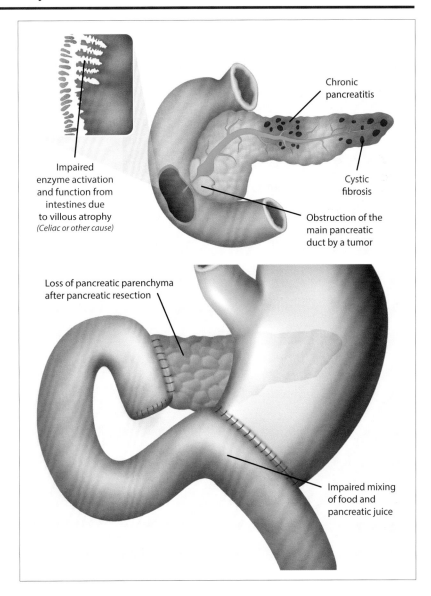

Figure 11: Major Causes of Pancreatic Exocrine Insufficiency. The inability to produce or secrete enough digestive enzymes into the duodenum can be caused by a number of factors inside and outside the pancreas. Regardless, this loss of enzyme activity results in poor digestion which typically manifests first as a reduction in lipid digestion. See text for more details.

levels <100 µg/g are indicative of pancreatic exocrine insufficiency (<15 µg/g high probability of PEI/ chronic pancreatitis). Fecal elastase >200 µg/g usually rules out a diagnosis of PEI. Intermediate levels of fecal elastase (100-200 µg/g) require additional analysis but are consistent with low pancreatic enzyme output (see Figure 12). Clinicians should note that the use of pancreatic enzyme replacement therapy does not interfere with this test since it is specific to human pancreatic elastase (no porcine or bovine cross-reactivity), allowing for follow-up even when giving oral enzyme supplementation (see below). This test should not be confused with the test for neutrophil (or polymorphonuclear) elastase used to measure inflammation, often used to distinguish inflammatory bowel disease from irritable bowel syndrome.

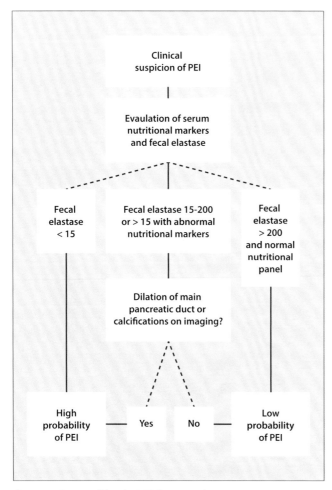

Figure 12: Decision Tree for PEI diagnosis. As this scheme shows, the evaluation of fecal elastase can be an important marker to help a clinician decide whether a subject is likely to have PEI. Additional cut-off points (above 200) may also indicate the need for oral enzyme supplementation- even without a formal diagnosis of PEI. See text for more details.

Along with fecal elastase, some very basic nutrient deficiencies are also a hallmark of pancreatic enzyme insufficiency, such as reduced serum levels of lipid soluble vitamins (A, D, E, and K), retinal-binding protein, calcium, zinc, selenium and apolipoproteins.[29,30] Abnormal serum nutrient profile, along with moderately low fecal elastase 1 levels are indicative of pancreatic exocrine insufficiency, warranting further investigation (see Figure 12).

Aging Changes Pancreatic Function and Output

The relationship between the degenerative processes of aging and reduced pancreatic function has been reported, though it has not been investigated fully. There is a higher incidence of both maldigestive symptoms and functional/postprandial hypochlorhydria in the elderly, although there is limited and contradictory evidence describing the changes of pancreatic exocrine function with age.[32,33,34] In a population-based study of healthy German subjects aged 50-75 years old, 11.5% had fecal elastase levels below 200 µg/g and 5% had levels below 100 µg/g, suggesting a significant level of PEI in subjects with no previously reported pancreatic or digestive complaints.[35]

More recently, fecal elastase 1 levels in healthy elderly subjects (non-diabetics with no known gastrointestinal disease) were compared to levels in healthy young individuals.[36] The average fecal elastase 1 level in the young control subjects (20-28 years old) was 570 µg/g (including one of 53 subjects with levels <200µg/g). Average fecal elastase 1 levels decreased with age; averaging 458 µg/g in subject 60-69 years old, 375 µg/g in subjects 70-79, and 381 µg/g in subjects over 80 years old. The number of subjects with fecal elastase 1 levels <200 µg/g in subjects over 60 years old was 21.7%, more than 10 times the level found in the younger controls, though none had previously been diagnosed with pancreatic deficiencies.

These data, along with postmortem reports, suggest that reduced pancreatic enzyme output and even pancreatic exocrine insufficiency and pancreatitis are more prevalent than clinically reported, especially in older subjects.[37] Other groups with a higher prevalence of low fecal elastase 1 levels (suggestive of reduce pancreatic enzyme output) include subjects with celiac disease,[38] inflammatory bowel disease (IBD),[39] HIV,[40] diabetes (types 1 and 2),[41] and advanced renal disease.[42] Ironically, while pancreatic exocrine insufficiency is often associated with malnourishment and weight loss, some studies show a progressive decline in fecal elastase 1 levels as obesity increases.[43] Therefore, clinicians should be aware that reduced pancreatic enzyme output may be present in subjects with no overt signs of chronic pancreatitis or fat malabsorption, especially in subjects experiencing functional dyspepsia. The role of enzyme supplementation therapy in these subjects will be discussed below.

The Role of Enzyme Replacement Therapy

The primary therapy for pancreatic exocrine insufficiency is oral enzyme replacement. Pancreatic enzyme products (pancreatin, from porcine or bovine sources) have been used for well over 100 years as digestive aids in subjects presumed to have reduced pancreatic enzyme output.[44] Today, numerous FDA-approved pancreatic enzyme products are available for the treatment of pancreatic exocrine insufficiency, as are hundreds of dietary supplement products containing pancreatin-derived enzymes (though no PEI-therapeutic claims are allowed for products labeled as dietary supplements in the United States). In addition, numerous plant, fungal and microbial enzyme products are now available in the United States, mostly as dietary supplements, adding to the available options (and confusion) in selecting an enzyme-replacement product for different patients and purposes. We will discuss each of these in detail below.

Pancreatin

Pancreatin is a concentrate of porcine (most common) or bovine pancreatic juices, standardized to contain minimum activities of lipase, protease, and amylase enzyme activities. The United States Pharmacopeia (USP) has set standards for each of these activities in pancreatin products as follows: each 1 mg of pancreatin 1X contains not less than 25 units each of protease and amylase activity and not less than 2 units of lipase activity. Each unit is defined by a specific enzyme assay using conditions for optimal activity for each enzyme.[45]

Pancreatin 2X contains twice the amount of enzyme activity per mg (50,50,4 units respectively) as that of pancreatin 1X and so on through highly concentrated products, 8X or more, that are commonly used in dietary supplement products sold through healthcare professionals. These products are most often described by their weight in milligrams, the pancreatin concentrate and often, in parentheses, the units of enzyme activity. For instance, 300 mg of pancreatin 8X will provide approximately 60,000 USP protease units, 60,000 USP amylase units, and 4,800 USP lipase units. Some highly concentrated pancreatin products (so called "full strength") may have different ratios of enzyme activities than the standard multiples listed here. For pancreatin activity measurement units, 1 USP unit is equal to 1 NF (National Formulary) unit, while 3 USP units is equal to 1 international unit (IU).[44]

Individual Pancreatic Enzymes

Concentrated powders of trypsin, chymotrypsin, lipase and amylase are also commercially available for use in dietary supplements or pharmaceutical preparations. These ingredients and their activities (USP units) are often listed separately, as they are sometimes used in combination with pancreatin (which already contains these enzymes). Pepsin, an acid-stable protease derived from porcine stomach concentrates, is sometimes added to mixed animal enzyme products designed to help digestion, though it is commonly combined with betaine HCl.

Pancrelipase

Pancrelipase is a special pancreatin concentrate designed to increase the amount of lipase activity, though these products still contain more protease and amylase activity per milligram. The USP monograph defines pancrelipase as containing per milligram: not less than 24 USP units of lipase, and not less than 100 USP units each of protease and amylase.[46] This product can only be derived from porcine sources. This product is specifically created (from pancreatin) to increase the proportional lipase activity, as the primary clinical consideration for most enzyme replacement therapies is fat malabsorption. Pharmaceutical products approved for PEI are almost exclusively those using pancrelipase as the active enzyme ingredient.

Table 4: Fungal Enzymes used in Supplementation

ENZYME	FUNGAL SOURCE	UNIT OF MEASUREMENT	BREAKS DOWN	
Acid Maltase	*Rhizopus oryzae*	MaltU	Starches	The enzyme hydrolyzes the alpha 1,4 and 1,6 glucosidic bonds in starch, glycogen and other polysaccharides, yielding D-glucose.
Alpha-Galactosidase	*Aspergillus niger*	GalU	Sugars	Breaks down disaccharides, trisaccharides and oligosaccharides. Characterized by its ability to hydrolyze the alpha-1-6 linkages in melibiose, raffinose and stachyose.
Amylase	*Aspergillus oryzae*	DU	Starches	This enzyme will randomly hydrolyze the interior alpha-1,4- glucosidic bonds of starch. This enzyme has a dextrinizing action that reduces the viscosity of gelatinous starch, amylose and amylopectin solutions yielding soluble dextrins. Its saccharifying action liberates glucose and maltose.
Bacterial Amylase	*Bacillus subtilis*	BAU	Starches	This enzyme will randomly hydrolyze the interior alpha-d-1,4-glucosidic bonds of starch, yielding soluble dextrins and low levels of glucose.
Amyloglucosidase	*Rhizopus oryzae*	AGU	Starches	The enzyme hydrolyzes the alpha 1,4 and 1,6 glucosidic bonds in starch, glycogen and other polysaccharides, yielding D-glucose.
Beta-Glucanase	*Trichoderma longibrachiatum*	BGU	Fiber	Acts on the interior 1,4-beta-glucosidic bonds of beta glucans containing mixed 1,3- and 1,4-bonds.
Catalase	*Aspergillus niger*	CatU	Hydrogen peroxide	Supplemental catalase works with endogenous catalase to prevent the oxidative effects of hydrogen peroxide, which is a by-product of SOD (Superoxide dismutase) activity, by converting this oxygen radical into water and oxygen.
Cellulase	*Trichoderma longibrachiatum*	CU	Cellulose	It hydrolyzes the beta-D-1,4- glucosidic bonds of cellulose, its oligomers and derivatives.
Cellulase AN	*Aspergillus niger*	CU	Cellulose	It hydrolyzes the beta-D-,4- glucosidic bonds of cellulose, its oligomers and derivatives.
Diastase	*Aspergillus oryzae*	Diastase Activity Units	Starches	This enzyme will randomly hydrolyze the interior alpha-1,4-glucosidic bonds of starch. This enzyme has a dextrinizing action that reduces the viscosity of gelatinous starch, amylose and amylopectin solutions yielding soluble dextrins. Its saccharifying action liberates glucose and maltose.
Glucoamylase	*Aspergillus niger*	AGU	Starches	The enzyme hydrolyzes terminal 1,4-linked alpha-D-glucose residues successively from non-reducing ends of amylose chains to release free glucose. This enzyme also possesses the ability to hydrolyze alpha-1, 6-glucosidic linkages in isomaltose and dextrins.
Hemicellulase	*Aspergillus niger*	HCU	Fiber	Hemicellulase is a mixture of enzymes including polygalacturonate hydrolase, arabinosidase, mannosidase, mannanase and xylanase. It hydrolyzes the interior glucosidic bonds of galactomannoglucans, yielding polysaccharides of lower molecular weight.
Invertase	*Saccharomyces cerevisiae*	SU (not FCC)	Sugars	This enzyme catalyzes the hydrolysis of sucrose into its component parts D-fructose and D-glucose.

DU = Dextrinizing unit, HUT = Hemoglobin Unit Tyrosine base, SAPU = Spectrophotometric acid protease units, PC = Protease Unit, MaltU = Maltase unit, AGU = Amyloglucosidase unit, ALU = Acid lactase units, GalU = Galactosidase units, FIP = Federation Internationale Pharmceutique, Endo-PG = Endo-Polygalacturonase Units, SU = Sumner Units, XU = Xylanase Unit, BAU = Bacterial amylase units, BGU = Beta-gluconase units, CatU = Catalase units, CU = Cellulase units, HCU = Hemicellulase Units, FTU = Phytase units, AP = Aminopeptidase activity units, AJDU = Apple juice depectinizing units

Table 4: Fungal Enzymes used in Supplementation (Continued)

ENZYME	FUNGAL SOURCE	UNIT OF MEASUREMENT	BREAKS DOWN	
Lactase	Aspergillus oryzae	ALU	Lactose	Lactase catalyzes the hydrolysis of the beta-D- galactoside linkage of lactose liberating one mole of D-glucose and one mole of D-galactose.
Lipase	Candida rugosa	FIP Lipase Units	Fats	This lipase catalyzes the hydrolysis of triglycerides of simple fatty acid esters, yielding mono- and diglycerides, glycerol and free fatty acids. This lipase is unique in that it shows no positional specificity and provides effective hydrolysis of fatty acids from all three positions of the triglyceride.
Lipase	Aspergillus niger	FIP Lipase Units	Fats	This lipase catalyzes the hydrolysis of triglycerides of simple fatty acid esters, yielding mono- and diglycerides, glycerol and free fatty acids.
Lipase	Rhizopus oryzae	FIP Lipase Units	Fats	This lipase catalyzes the hydrolysis of triglycerides of simple fatty acid esters, yielding mono- and diglycerides, glycerol and free fatty acids.
Pectinase	Aspergillus niger	endo-PG Units (not FCC)	Pectin	Pectinase is a mixture of pectin methylesterase, which demethylates pectin, and polygalacturonase, which hydrolyzes α-D-1, 4-galacturonide.
Pectinesterase	Aspergillus niger	AJDU (not FCC)	Pectin	Pectinesterase contains both pectin methylesterase, which demethylates pectin, and polygalacturonase, which hydrolyzes β-D-1, 4- galacturonide.
Peptidase	Aspergillus oryzae	HUT	Proteins	This enzyme system contains a very high level of exopeptidase activity. The exo-peptidases liberate amino acids by hydrolysis of the peptide bonds at the terminus of the peptide chain.
Phytase	Aspergillus niger	FTU	Fiber	This enzyme catalyzes the hydrolysis of phytic acid into its component parts, releasing inositol and ortho-phosphate.
Protease 3.0	Aspergillus niger	SAPU	Proteins	This protease is characterized by its ability to hydrolyze proteins under acidic conditions (pH as low as 3). The broad specificity of acid- stable protease enables the enzyme to easily and efficiently hydrolyze most soluble proteins.
Protease 4.5	Aspergillus oryzae	HUT	Proteins	This enzyme preparation is productive throughout a wide range of pH and substrates, and exhibits both exo-peptidase and endo-peptidase activities. The exo-peptidase activities hydrolyze the protein molecule at the terminus of the peptide chain, liberating an amino acid; while the endo-peptidase activities hydrolyze the protein molecule at the interior peptide bonds, liberating peptides of various lengths. In addition, this protease demonstrates significant starch saccharifying alpha-amylase side activity.
Protease 6.0	Aspergillus oryzae var	HUT	Proteins	This enzyme preparation is productive throughout a wide range of pH and substrates, and exhibits both exo-peptidase and endo-peptidase activities. The exo-peptidase activities hydrolyze the protein molecule at the terminus of the peptide chain liberating an amino acid; while the endo-peptidase activities hydrolyze the protein molecule at the interior peptide bonds liberating peptides of various lengths. In addition, this protease demonstrates significant starch saccharifying alpha-amylase side activity.
Protease AM	Aspergillus melleus	AP	Proteins	This enzyme preparation is a complex enzyme preparation of proteases and peptidases, which hydrolyze a wide range of proteins.
Alkaline Protease	Bacillus licheniformis	PC	Proteins	Alkaline protease is a serine endo-protease capable of hydrolyzing a broad range of peptide bonds found in both animal and vegetable source proteins.
Neutral Bacterial Protease	Bacillus subtilis	PC	Proteins	Neutral bacterial protease is an endo-petidase that hydrolyzes the interior bonds of proteins. This protease easily and efficiently hydrolyzes most soluble proteins.
Xylanase	Trichoderma longibrachiatum	XU (not FCC)	Hemicellulose	This enzyme catalyzes the hydrolysis of 1,4 β-D-xylosidic linkages in xylans to produce D-xylose.

Plant-Based Enzymes

The most common plant-based enzymes used in dietary supplements are bromelain (from pineapple stems) and papain (from papaya), both proteases. Papain is also well known as the active protease in meat tenderizers added to break down meat fibers prior to and during cooking.[47] Bromelain, on the other hand, is better known for non-digestive therapeutic effects related to its anti-inflammatory and other properties when consumed away from a meal.[48] Both bromelain and papain are cysteine proteases and have a broader pH activity range (pH of 5.0-8.0) than pancreatic proteases. Unlike pancreatic enzymes, the activity for these enzymes is not yet defined in USP units. Instead, several different units may be used, and currently, the FDA has not specified which unit(s) can or should be used when labeling these ingredients on supplements. Commonly, bromelain and papain will be labeled using gelatin-digesting units (GDUs), milk-clotting units (MCUs), casein-digesting units (CDUs), papain units (PUs) or others. Product labels will usually specify the milligram amount and the activity units in parenthesis as follows: "Bromelain (2,400 GDU/g)......200 mg." It is generally assumed that 1 MCU is equivalent to 0.67 GDU for these enzymes, though the unreliable standardization of the reagents used for these tests makes it difficult to compare products labeled with different enzyme units.

With the exception of individuals allergic to pineapple or papaya, these enzymes are considered safe; however, for use as oral digestive aids, there is little in the way of published data to suggest specific doses. Bromelain and papain are often combined with pancreatin supplements to broaden the pH activity of these products, or added to fungal-derived enzymes preferred by subjects wanting to avoid animal-derived products.

Fungal-Derived Enzymes

In recent years, enzymes isolated from a variety of fungi and yeast have become popular ingredients in products designed to improve digestion; these are sometimes also referred to as microbe-derived enzymes. These enzymes are extracted from a variety of fungal sources including *Aspergillus oryzae, Aspergillus nigra, Kluyveromyces lactis, Trichoderma longibrachiatum, Saccharomyces cerevisiae* and other related subspecies. The enzymes produced by these microorganisms have a much wider range of activities, especially the activities which hydrolyze complex carbohydrates, starches and celluloses (see Table 4 for enzymes and units). In addition, many of these enzymes are active in a more acidic pH range than pancreatic enzymes and are often referred to as "acid-stable."

Fungal-derived enzymes have been used for many years in food preparation (fermentation), and a variety of industrial applications. Several have been studied and marketed for specific purposes, such as alpha-galactosidase for reducing the flatulence related to consuming beans, acid-resistant lipase for improved fat digestion, and lactase (beta-galactosidase) for symptoms related to lactose intolerance.[49,50,51,52,53]

Comprehensive digestive aid products containing fungal-derived enzymes usually list at least a dozen or more specific enzyme activities, and these are often combined with bromelain, papain, and other plant compounds that improve digestion (bitters or bile-stimulating herbs). These combinations are preferred by many vegetarian subjects or those who avoid pork or animal products for religious or cultural reasons. Research into the efficacy of these enzymes for digestive-related outcomes, especially in comparison to pancreatic enzyme supplements, is mostly lacking; though numerous healthcare professionals recommend these enzymes to patients and report positive outcomes.

Approved Products for PEI

There are currently over a dozen different products that are FDA-approved for the treatment of pancreatic exocrine insufficiency (from cystic fibrosis, chronic pancreatitis or other causes). Prior to 2010, the FDA did not regulate the production of pancreatic enzyme products as these types of products (in simpler forms) were available prior to the passage of the first Federal Food, Drug and Cosmetic Act (1938). Even so, the recent change in regulation of these pancreatic enzyme drugs still only pertains to their manufacturing and quality control specifications; and does not yet outline standards of efficacy.[54]

As mentioned previously, these pharmaceutical products are all made using pancrelipase, and most are formulated as enteric-coated beadlets or microspheres, since pancreatic enzymes can be irreversibly inactivated by stomach acid (depending on the stomach pH). They are sold in a variety of dosage units ranging from 3,000-25,000 USP units of lipase activity per capsule.[44,55,56] The costs of these products are notoriously high ($2.50-$4.00 per 10,000 lipase units), where the average recommended dose is 30,000-50,000 USP units of lipase activity per meal.[57] While studies reveal limited benefit in dose escalation, many clinicians still recommend increasing the dose when the initial recommended dose fails to reduce steatorrhea or other signs of fat malabsorption.[58,59] Higher doses are generally recommended with larger meals, while lower doses (10,000-20,000 lipase units) are recommended for snacks.

Head-to-head studies comparing clinically-relevant endpoints using different products have yet to be published, so comparisons of efficacy between similarly dosed products (in terms of lipase units) using different delivery methods (i.e., different microsphere size and enteric-coating formulas) cannot be made. One study, using a total of 40,000 lipase units, showed a slight increase in efficacy when dosed after the meal (four capsules of 10,000 units each), or during the meal (one capsule just before, two during, and one after the meal), compared to taking four capsules at the beginning of the meal.[60] The use of acid-blocking therapy such as PPIs or H2-blockers, has been shown to increase the efficacy of pancrelipase supplements in some patients, though the use of these products may not be recommended for other reasons (see PPI section page 219).[61]

Dietary supplements containing pancreatin, pancrelipase or other enzyme combinations have not been tested and shown to be effective in subjects diagnosed with PEI. Therefore, patients diagnosed with PEI should be treated using an approved pancrelipase-containing product. Research using lipase enzymes derived from other sources (e.g., microbial or fungal) is ongoing, though specific recommendations for these enzymes as substitutes for pancrelipase in subjects with PEI is not yet available.

Digestive Enzymes for Celiac Disease/Gluten Digestion

Patients with diagnosed celiac disease are more likely to experience low pancreatic enzyme output based on reported levels of pancreatic elastase.[62] One study found that 30% of celiac patients with chronic diarrhea had low pancreatic elastase levels.[63] In addition, celiac-related villous atrophy results in decreased activity of brush-border enzymes (e.g., disachharidases), and may also contribute to poor digestion through reduced levels of cholecystokinin and enterokinase activities.[64,65] Celiac patients are therefore candidates for enzyme replacement therapy.

In one recent study, 20 subjects with celiac disease (consuming a gluten-free diet) with both chronic diarrhea and low pancreatic elastase levels (<200 µg/g) were given pancrelipase supplementation and followed for changes in stool frequency and pancreatic elastase for four years.[66] While subjects started with a dose of 10,000 USP units of lipase activity twice per day, this dose was adjusted based on their clinical response. Throughout the four years, the average dose used in these subjects was 45,000 USP units of lipase per day. Of the 20 participants, 18 had significant long-term improvement in their chronic diarrhea demonstrated by reduction in median stool frequency from four per day to one per day. These individuals also reported subjective improvements in consistency and urgency and eight patients discontinued the enzyme supplementation because of resolution of symptoms. Interestingly, the pancreatic elastase levels measured in the stool increased with enzyme supplementation over time; from a median of 90 µg/g stool (15–196), to 212 µg/g stool (15–402) at six months, and 365 µg/g stool (154–>500) at more than 12 months. This suggests an overall improvement of pancreatic exocrine function in these subjects with daily enzyme supplementation.

Researchers have also been investigating the possible therapeutic role of supplementing specific fungal proteases that hydrolyze gluten/gliadin to help reduce gluten-mediated symptoms in celiac or gluten-sensitive subjects. Investigations into these endoproteases, now collectively called glutenases, are on-going as either food processing enzymes (to pre-digest gluten in food products) or oral therapeutic products (dietary supplements or drugs).[67,68] While limited clinical trial data suggest some benefits with these enzymes, there is no current evidence to suggest that subjects with celiac disease or gluten sensitivity will be protected by taking these enzymes while consuming gluten-containing products (intentionally or inadvertently).

Digestive Enzyme Supplementation for Improved Digestion (Non-PEI Indications)

Supplementation with various combinations of digestive enzymes is commonly recommended by functional and integrative medical professionals as it is part of the "replacement" strategy within the "4-R" program taught to thousands of healthcare professionals (see page 22).

The primary products used are: pancreatin (various amounts and strengths), plant derived enzymes, fungal-derived enzymes, and combinations of these ingredients with betaine HCl, bitters, bile or bile-stimulating herbs. Currently, there is almost no published research evaluating various combinations of these enzymes and digestive aids in subjects with undiagnosed pancreatic enzyme deficiency, and therefore it is difficult to recommend specific doses or combinations. Clinicians should work with patients to find a suitable combination that helps to alleviate post-prandial digestive complaints, still the best empirical measure of enzyme supplementation efficacy. Subjects with pancreatic elastase levels between 200-400 µg/g are great candidates for digestive enzyme supplementation.

Bile Stimulants and Bile Supplementation

Digestion and absorption of lipids and fat-soluble vitamins is reduced when bile acid availability is diminished or poorly timed with pancreatic lipase secretion.[69] Bile acids are also important metabolic signaling molecules and play a role in reducing small intestinal bacterial overgrowth.[70,71] It is therefore possible that supplementing the diet with substances that increase bile acid secretion (choleretics/cholegogues), or direct oral supplementation of bile salts, may benefit those with poor fat digestion and absorption. In fact, conjugated bile acids from ox bile extracts or other sources (e.g., synthetic cholylsarcosine) have been tested in subjects with short bowel syndrome, cystic fibrosis and other related liver disease conditions known to affect bile secretion (primary biliary cirrhosis) or resorption.[72] However, most of the published studies using these agents are in few patients, and many are case studies using up to 9 grams/day of conjugated bile acids.[73,74,75,76]

Ox (bovine) bile extract (some standardized to one or more bile acids) is a common ingredient in over-the-counter dietary supplements designed to help digestion (most commonly formulated with enzymes and/or betaine HCl). While there have been no evaluations of these products for therapeutic outcomes (most of these products provide less than 200 mg of ox bile extract per tablet/capsule, though single-ingredient products of 500 mg/capsule are also available), oral intake of ox bile extract in such formulas may provide increased lipid digestion and absorption and is considered to be safe.[77]

Another possible way to increase natural bile production is the use of natural choleretic and chologogues (agents that stimulate bile secretion/synthesis or gall bladder contraction). Besides bile and fat, most of these are herbal/botanical preparations or extracts; commonly from artichoke leaf (*Cynara scolymus*), milk thistle seed (*Silybum marianum*), and dandelion root (*Taraxicum officianale*).[78] Studies on some of these agents in animals and humans have confirmed their historical use in stimulating bile, though not specifically for digestive-related outcomes.[79,80,81,82,83,84] Botanical preparations known as "bitters" are often considered to stimulate bile, though these also lack formal studies (see page 31). The use of these botanicals for digestive complaints, dyspepsia and related conditions is common in Western herbal traditions and many are included in dietary supplements used to improve digestion.

Figure 13: The Biogeography of Nutrient Absorption. This figure illustrates the relative locations for nutrient absorption along the gastrointestinal tract. The fat soluble vitamins (i.e., A, D, E, and K) are shown absorbed in the jejunum but are also absorbed in the duodenum and ileum. Many nutrients (as detailed in the box) are absorbed in a non-location specific manner; these nutrients include: biotin, folate, niacin, riboflavin, thiamin, vitamin B6, vitamin C, calcium, iron, magnesium, molybdenum, and phosphorus. Microbial production of some nutrients occurs and their absorption is mediated by the colonocytes; these nutrients include: biotin, folate, niacin, pantothenic acid, riboflavin, thiamin, vitamin K, and short chain fatty acids (see box). The absorption of most of these nutrients is straightforward; however, the absorption of vitamin B12 is more complex. R-protein (also known as haptocorrin or transcobalamin-1) is a glycoprotein produced in the salivary glands necessary for optimal vitamin B12 absorption. In the stomach R-protein binds to vitamin B12 forming a complex to protect the vitamin from the acidic stomach environment. The R-protein-vitamin B12 complex remains associated until pancreatic proteases cleave the complex in the duodenum. In the duodenum, free vitamin B12 binds to a second glycoprotein produced from the parietal cells of the stomach, called intrinsic factor (IR). The associated IR-vitamin B12 complex is absorbed mostly in the ileum through the intrinsic factor- cobalamin receptor (IFCR) on the enterocyte. Within the enterocyte, IR is degraded and free B12 binds to another protein synthesized by the enterocyte, called transcobalamin II (TC II). The TC II-vitamin B12 complex is released into the bloodstream. Nutrients produced by the colonic microbiota may also be absorbed by colonocytes, though less is known about these pathways.

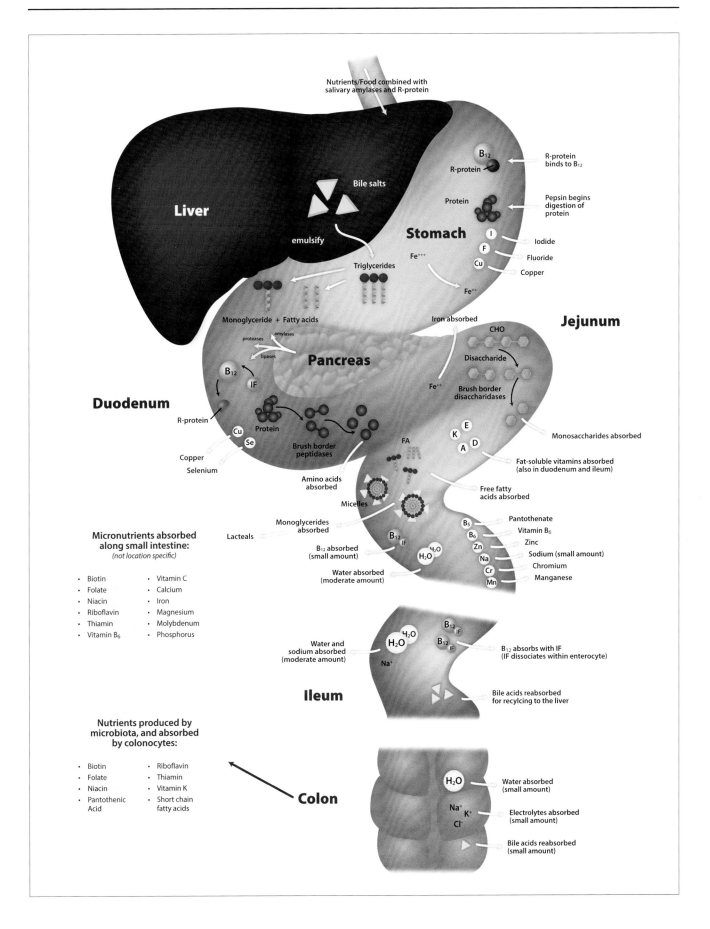

Brush Border Enzymes and Transporters

While pancreatic enzymes are responsible for the majority of carbohydrate and protein macronutrient digestion, the end products of this digestion (i.e., disaccharides and small peptides) are still not readily absorbed. For proper digestion of these molecules, the body relies on enzymes located on the microvilli of enterocytes along the small intestine, called brush border enzymes (e.g., maltase, sucrase, lactase, amino-oligopeptidase, amino peptidases, etc). During times of gastrointestinal inflammation, accompanied by villous atrophy, brush border enzymatic capacity can be greatly diminished and result in inadequate digestion and absorption of carbohydrates and protein.

Brush border enzyme activity for carbohydrate digestion is relatively straightforward (Panel A). In this example, the disaccharide maltose is cleaved into two glucose monosaccharides by the brush border enzyme maltase. These monosaccharides are then transported through the enterocyte by one of several transport mechanisms, and are eventually absorbed into the blood stream. Secondary disaccharide intolerance (e.g., lactose intolerance) that can often result from villous atrophy may resolve once GI inflammation is reduced and normal GI architecture is re-established.

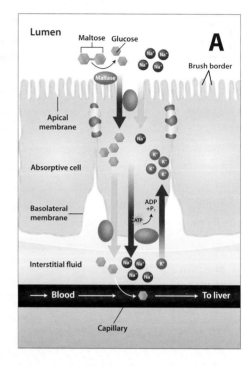

Peptide digestion by brush border enzymes is more complex and involves numerous enzymes and transporters (Panel B). After pancreatic protease activity (e.g., trypsin, chymotrypsin, carboxypeptidases A and B, elastase) dietary proteins are digested into oligopeptides of varying chain length. Since enzymes can only cleave peptide bonds of specific types, the final digestion of small peptides into amino acids requires a diverse set of brush border and endogenous peptidases, often requiring up to 3 or more different peptidases. Amino acids are transported via several different transporters and eventually absorbed from the enterocyte into the bloodstream.

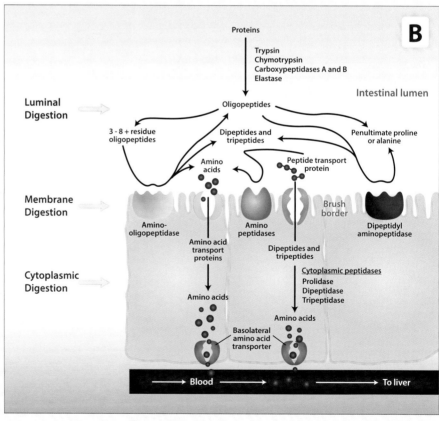

Testing for Poor Digestion

Test for Dietary Habits

- The best analysis of food selection and eating patterns is a food diary. Questionnaires about normal eating patterns (validated food frequency questionnaire) are also helpful.
- **Stool Analysis:** Several analytes within a comprehensive stool test may help reveal diet/digestion/absorption issues. Stool pH and short-chain fatty acid (SCFA) production in particular may reveal slow transit time due to low fiber intake or excessive protein intake.

Test for Nutrient Deficiencies

- While dietary intake is likely to account for much of the nutrient deficiencies seen in patients (assessed through diet diaries, etc.), poor digestion and absorption of nutrient-rich diets can also account for nutrient deficiencies in many subjects.
- Reduced levels of fat-soluble vitamins (vitamins A, D, E, and K) and nutrients (omega-3, CoQ-10) are common in subjects with lipase (pancreatic enzyme) deficiency.
- Reduced levels of calcium, zinc, vitamin B12, folate and protein are common in subjects with low stomach acid.

Test for Food Allergies and Intolerances

- **Elimination Diet:** This is considered the gold standard. By removing the offending food(s), many symptoms will typically disappear within a week or two. Reintroduction of food after three weeks (adding back single food/allergen category at a time) will often trigger symptoms. Once the offending food is determined, avoidance for several months may be required. If re-introduction still elicits negative symptoms the food may need to be avoided long-term.
- **Serum Tests for Cross-Reactivity to Food Allergens:** These tests are available from numerous labs. Blood samples are sent to the lab for IgE and/or IgG cross-reactivity to common food allergens. Test results will indicate a negative or positive reaction.

- **Skin Test:** This classic test will be able to rule out particular allergens (negative result) but a positive skin test does not always indicate that a patient is allergic to that particular food. Eliminating and reintroduction of the suspected food or follow-up serum testing is indicated to confirm.
- **Celiac/Gluten Sensitivity Tests:** Specific lab tests have been developed to test for celiac disease. See page 147 for more details.

Test for Low Stomach Acid

- **Empiric Test:** The easiest (and cheapest) test for low stomach acid is an empiric self-test (though it has not been rigorously studied). By swallowing increasingly more HCl (in the form of a betaine HCl capsule or tablet) with protein containing meals, a person can determine if additional acid is needed and if and when they have enough acid for adequate protein digestion. Typical instructions and precautions for this test are provided on page 33.

Heidelberg and Related Tests

- Tests are available using capsules tethered to a string. These capsules (Heidelberg or "pH Capsules") are swallowed by the patient and suspended into the stomach from where they can transmit a radio signal to a detection device showing the pH of the stomach. Fasting, post-prandial and, most commonly, bicarbonate challenges can be used to determine how quickly the stomach pH returns to acidic conditions and therefore the acid-secreting capacity.
- **Stool Analysis:** Poor protein digestion determined by specific stool analytes may signify poor acid production.
- Positive tests for SIBO (see page 231), H. pylori (see page 205), *Clostridium difficile* (see page 165) or *Candida* overgrowth (see page 239) can also be a sign of low stomach acid production.

Testing for Pancreatic Insufficiency/Malabsorption

Empiric Testing

- Like the addition of HCl for decreased stomach acid, adding digestive enzymes (pancreatin, plant or fungal enzyme products) prior to eating and monitoring changes in symptoms may be an empiric way to discover pancreatic enzyme insufficiency and the need for enzyme supplementation.

- **Stool Testing** (Note: Most of the tests listed below are available together, and are combined with other tests within many available comprehensive stool-testing panels available from several laboratories)

  ° **Pancreatic Elastase I:** Pancreatic elastase 1 (PE1) is a digestive enzyme secreted exclusively by the human pancreas and unlike other pancreatic enzymes, it is highly stable and is not degraded during passage through the gut. Fecal PE1 is a simple, noninvasive method of assessing exocrine pancreatic function, allowing the clinician to establish a prompt and reliable diagnosis with high degrees of sensitivity (63%-100%) and specificity (93%-98%) in suspected cases of pancreatic exocrine insufficiency. PE1 results are not affected by pancreatic enzyme replacement therapy; so patients are not required to stop supplementation prior to providing a sample. Levels below 200 μg/g are low and enzyme supplementation should be considered (levels below 100 μg/g are indicative of pancreatic exocrine insufficiency and indicate the need for approved pancrelipase supplementation). Levels below 400 μg/g are borderline low and are more common in elderly subjects.

  ° **Chymotrypsin:** Chymotrypsin was the first non-invasive exocrine pancreatic test to be discovered and is a reflection of chymotrypsin activity in the pancreas. While it is often still a common analyte in many tests, the use of PE1 is more helpful in analyzing endogenous pancreatic enzyme output. Chymotrypsin is affected by exogenous supplementation which can make it an ideal tool to monitor dosing adequacy. When chymotrypsin values are within the reference range in supplemented individuals, the clinician can be confident that an appropriate dose of digestive enzymes is being administered.

  ° **Vegetable Fibers:** Analysis of vegetable fibers can indicate decreased pancreatic function and malabsorption.

  ° **Putrefactive SCFA:** Valerate, isovalerate and isobutyrate constitute the putrefactive SCFAs. Elevated levels result from anaerobic bacterial fermentation of undigested proteins, polypeptides and amino acids, and suggest hypochlorhydria, exocrine pancreatic insufficiency, and/or protein malabsorption.

  ° **Fecal fat analysis:** Fecal fats include triglycerides, long-chain fatty acids (LCFAs), cholesterol and phospholipids. They are derived predominately from the dietary ingestion of fat, and provide important clues about digestion and absorption. Fat malabsorption can occur from maldigestion and/or impaired uptake of fatty acids, physiological imbalances or disorders that impair lipase activity or bile acid production and release. (see page 35 for why pancreatic elastase is often used in place of fat absorption analysis in subjects with pancreatic exocrine insufficiency).

Optimal Timing for Digestive Enzyme Supplements

Since there are limited ways to test the efficacy of different products designed to improve digestion, there is also limited information to help clinicians define the optimal timing for using such supplements. The limited data available for pancrelipase efficacy in subjects with PEI suggests that consuming pancreatic enzymes after the meal has commenced (perhaps in smaller doses, spaced throughout the meal) or even after finishing the meal may be more effective than consuming the enzymes just prior to the meal.[60] This may allow the enzymes to mix with the meal and exit proportionally into the duodenum, where they are most active. Whether this is true of acid-stable enzymes (fungal-derived or pepsin) is not known. Patients should experiment with different doses and meal-timing to attempt to improve the overall efficacy of their digestive enzyme supplements, recording their post-prandial symptoms as a guide.

Combining Acid and Enzymes:
Should Products Be Enteric Coated?

Since many older individuals experience both reduced gastric acid production and reduced pancreatic enzyme production, supplementation of both acid and enzymes may be a consideration in these subjects. The obvious question then arises: If pancreatic enzymes are harmed by stomach acid, can or should these enzymes be supplemented with acid, and should the enzymes be enteric-coated to protect them from stomach acid?

Addressing the second question first, there is quite a bit of investigation into the enteric coating of pancrelipase products sold as pharmaceuticals. However, these products are not enteric-coated capsules or tablets, but instead, enteric-coated microspheres/beadlets. The reason is simple: an enteric coated capsule or tablet does not mix with and release proportionally with the meal/chyme as it leaves the stomach and enters the duodenum, but enters the duodenum all at once (typically after the stomach is empty, depending on the size of the tablet/capsule). So, while an enteric-coated tablet or capsule will generally protect the enzymes' activities from gastric acid inactivation, this process will also greatly limit the efficacy of the product.

Drug companies have spent large sums of time and money researching ways to optimize enteric-coated microspheres/beadlets to maximize their clinical efficacy. By altering the particle size and enteric-coating material, they have attempted to optimize the protection of the enzymes during gastric mixing, allow for the release of the microspheres with the chyme as it leaves the stomach (over the entire gastric-emptying process) and maximize the release of the enzymatic activity in the duodenum.

Unfortunately, this process has resulted in pharmaceutical products that are extremely expensive with, still, less than optimal efficacy. While we generally suggest that clinicians recommend these types of (FDA-approved) products for subjects with diagnosed pancreatic exocrine insufficiency (see page 40), the use of enteric-coated capsules and tablets (as dietary supplements) are not recommended due to their lack of efficacy (we are not aware of enteric-coated microspheres available as dietary supplements).

Now, we will tackle the question of supplementing betaine HCl with pancreatic enzymes. Research using pancreatin/pancrelipase confirms that, indeed, these enzymes are vulnerable to stomach acid, leading to the enteric-coated microsphere solution for pharmaceutical products mentioned above. Nevertheless, if an individual is using oral betaine HCl to improve digestion and also desires to supplement pancreatic enzymes, they must both be taken with the meal if each is to mix with the food contents. Thus, the efficacy of the pancreatic enzyme supplement will be diminished when consumed with betaine HCl.

Nonetheless, products combining both pancreatic enzymes and betaine HCl have been available for many decades and are preferred by many clinicians and their patients. Ironically, subjects with fasting hypochlorhydria (or meal-time functional hypochlorhydria) may experience the least diminution of pancreatic enzyme supplemental activity, but are also the best candidates for betaine HCl supplementation. Clinicians should first ensure that a subject is likely to need supplementation of both acid and enzymes, and then allow them to experiment with product combinations, doses and timing to improve digestive function. The use of plant enzymes or microbe-derived enzymes, which are more acid-stable, may also be a solution for many when supplementing acid with digestive enzymes.

The Need for Supplementating Dietary Nutrients in Subjects with Poor Digestion

Dietary supplementation of nutrients (macronutrients, micronutrients and phytonutrients) may be important for individuals with poor dietary choices, dietary restrictions, poor digestion or specific metabolic needs. In many cases, nutrients found in dietary supplements (capsules, tablets, powders, fortified foods) are easier to digest and absorb than those found in some foods and are often at higher therapeutic doses. In some cases, higher supplemental doses can compensate for low nutrient absorption of dietary nutrients.

For example, low intrinsic factor levels can hinder the bioavailability of vitamin B12. However, oral intake of 1 mg or more of supplemental cobalamin allows for passive (intrinsic-factor independent) absorption to normalize serum B12 levels. For a complete review of the difference between dietary and supplemental nutrients and the basis and application of dietary supplementation, see our Road map *Supplementing Dietary Nutrients: A Guide for Healthcare Professionals* (Point Institute, 2014).

References

1. Oustamanolakis P, Tack J. Dyspepsia: organic versus functional. *J Clin Gastroenterol*. 2012 Mar;46(3):175-90.
2. Talley NJ, Ford AC. Functional Dyspepsia. *N Engl J Med*. 2015 Nov 5;373(19):1853-63.
3. van Kerkhoven LA, Laheij RJ, Meineche-Schmidt V, et al. Functional dyspepsia: not all roads seem to lead to Rome. *J Clin Gastroenterol*. 2009 Feb;43(2):118-22.
4. Choung RS, Locke GR 3rd, Schleck CD, Zinsmeister AR, Talley NJ. Overlap of dyspepsia and gastroesophageal reflux in the general population: one disease or distinct entities? *Neurogastroenterol Motil*. 2012 Mar;24(3):229-34, e106.
5. Rasmussen S, Jensen TH, Henriksen SL, et al. Overlap of symptoms of gastroesophageal reflux disease, dyspepsia and irritable bowel syndrome in the general population. *Scand J Gastroenterol*. 2015 Feb;50(2):162-9.
6. Fujiwara Y, Arakawa T. Overlap in patients with dyspepsia/functional dyspepsia. *J Neurogastroenterol Motil*. 2014 Oct 30;20(4):447-57.
7. Untersmayr E, Jensen-Jarolim E. The role of protein digestibility and antacids on food allergy outcomes. *J Allergy Clin Immunol*. 2008 Jun;121(6):1301-8.
8. Kassarjian Z, Russell RM. Hypochlorhydria: a factor in nutrition. *Annu Rev Nutr*. 1989;9:271-85.
9. Russell RM, Krasinski SD. Folic acid malabsorption in atrophic gastritis. Possible compensation by bacterial folate synthesis. *Gastroenterology*. 1986 Dec;91(6):1476-82.
10. Schubert ML. Functional anatomy and physiology of gastric secretion. *Curr Opin Gastroenterol*. 2015 Nov;31(6):479-85.
11. McDonald EG, Milligan J, Frenette C, Lee TC. Continuous Proton Pump Inhibitor Therapy and the Associated Risk of Recurrent Clostridium difficile Infection. *JAMA Intern Med*. 2015 May;175(5):784-91.
12. Husebye E, Skar V, Høverstad T, Melby K. Fasting hypochlorhydria with gram positive gastric flora is highly prevalent in healthy old people. *Gut*. 1992 Oct;33(10):1331-7.
13. Feldman M, Barnett C. Fasting gastric pH and its relationship to true hypochlorhydria in humans. *Dig Dis Sci*. 1991 Jul;36(7):866-9.
14. Bhutto A, Morley JE. The clinical significance of gastrointestinal changes with aging. *Curr Opin Clin Nutr Metab Care*. 2008 Sep;11(5):651-60.
15. Morihara M, Aoyagi N, Kaniwa N, Kojima S, Ogata H. Assessment of gastric acidity of Japanese subjects over the last 15 years. *Biol Pharm Bull*. 2001 Mar;24(3):313-5.
16. Hurwitz A, Brady DA, et al. Gastric acidity in older adults. *JAMA*. 1997 Aug 27;278(8):659-62.
17. Dressman JB, Berardi RR, Dermentzoglou LC, et al. Upper gastrointestinal (GI) pH in young, healthy men and women. *Pharm Res*. 1990 Jul;7(7):756-61.
18. Russell TL, Berardi RR, Barnett JL, et al. Upper gastrointestinal pH in seventy-nine healthy, elderly, North American men and women. *Pharm Res*. 1993 Feb;10(2):187-96.
19. Ayazi S, Leers JM, Oezcelik A, et al. Measurement of gastric pH in ambulatory esophageal pH monitoring. *Surg Endosc*. 2009 Sep;23(9):1968-73.
20. Iwai W, Abe Y, Iijima K, et al. Gastric hypochlorhydria is associated with an exacerbation of dyspeptic symptoms in female patients. *J Gastroenterol*. 2013 Feb;48(2):214-21.
21. Walker J, Hell J, Liszt KI, et al. Identification of beer bitter acids regulating mechanisms of gastric acid secretion. *J Agric Food Chem*. 2012 Feb 15;60(6):1405-12.
22. McMullen MK, Whitehouse JM, Towell A. Bitters: Time for a New Paradigm. *Evid Based Complement Alternat Med*. 2015;2015:670504.
23. Boekema PJ, Samsom M, van Berge Henegouwen GP, Smout AJ. Coffee and gastrointestinal function: facts and fiction. A review. *Scand J Gastroenterol Suppl*. 1999;230:35-9.
24. Rubach M, Lang R, Hofmann T, Somoza V. Time-dependent component-specific regulation of gastric acid secretion-related proteins by roasted coffee constituents. *Ann N Y Acad Sci*. 2008 Apr;1126:310-4.
25. Rubach M, Lang R, Bytof G, et al. A dark brown roast coffee blend is less effective at stimulating gastric acid secretion in healthy volunteers compared to a medium roast market blend. *Mol Nutr Food Res*. 2014 Jun;58(6):1370-3.
26. The stepwise increase of betaine HCl as a way to gauge the appropriate supplemental dose (based on empirical sensation of discomfort) has been taught in different ways by many integrative and functional medicine clinicians for decades.
27. Yago MR, Frymoyer AR, Smelick GS, et al. Gastric reacidification with betaine HCl in healthy volunteers with rabeprazole-induced hypochlorhydria. *Mol Pharm*. 2013 Nov 4;10(11):4032-7.
28. Yago MR, Frymoyer A, Benet LZ, et al. The use of betaine HCl to enhance dasatinib absorption in healthy volunteers with rabeprazole-induced hypochlorhydria. *AAPS J*. 2014 Nov;16(6):1358-65.
29. Lindkvist B. Diagnosis and treatment of pancreatic exocrine insufficiency. *World J Gastroenterol*. 2013 Nov 14;19(42):7258-66.
30. Lindkvist B, Phillips ME, Domínguez-Muñoz JE. Clinical, anthropometric and laboratory nutritional markers of pancreatic exocrine insufficiency: Prevalence and diagnostic use. *Pancreatology*. 2015 Nov-Dec;15(6):589-97.
31. Leeds JS, Oppong K, Sanders DS. The role of fecal elastase-1 in detecting exocrine pancreatic disease. *Nat Rev Gastroenterol Hepatol*. 2011 May 31;8(7):405-15.
32. Laugier R, Bernard JP, Berthezene P, Dupuy P. Changes in pancreatic exocrine secretion with age: pancreatic exocrine secretion does decrease in the elderly. *Digestion*. 1991;50(3-4):202-11.
33. Gullo L, Ventrucci M, Naldoni P, Pezzilli R. Aging and exocrine pancreatic function. *J Am Geriatr Soc*. 1986 Nov;34(11):790-2.
34. Vellas B, Balas D, Moreau J, et al. Exocrine pancreatic secretion in the elderly. *Int J Pancreatol*. 1988 Dec;3(6):497-502.
35. Rothenbacher D, Löw M, Hardt PD, et al. Prevalence and determinants of exocrine pancreatic insufficiency among older adults: results of a population-based study. *Scand J Gastroenterol*. 2005 Jun;40(6):697-704.
36. Herzig KH, Purhonen AK, Räsänen KM, et al. Fecal pancreatic elastase-1 levels in older individuals without known gastrointestinal diseases or diabetes mellitus. *BMC Geriatr*. 2011 Jan 25;11:4.
37. Olsen TS. The incidence and clinical relevance of chronic inflammation in the pancreas in autopsy material. *Acta Pathol Microbiol Scand A*. 1978 Sep;86A(5):361-5.

38. Leeds JS, Hopper AD, Hurlstone DP, et al. Is exocrine pancreatic insufficiency in adult coeliac disease a cause of persisting symptoms? *Aliment Pharmacol Ther*. 2007 Feb 1;25(3):265-71.

39. Maconi G, Dominici R, Molteni M, et al. Prevalence of pancreatic insufficiency in inflammatory bowel diseases. Assessment by fecal elastase-1. *Dig Dis Sci*. 2008 Jan;53(1):262-70.

40. Carroccio A, Di Prima L, Di Grigoli C, et al. Exocrine pancreatic function and fat malabsorption in human immunodeficiency virus-infected patients. *Scand J Gastroenterol*. 1999 Jul;34(7):729-34.

41. Hardt PD, Hauenschild A, Nalop J, et al. High prevalence of exocrine pancreatic insufficiency in diabetes mellitus. A multicenter study screening fecal elastase 1 concentrations in 1,021 diabetic patients. *Pancreatology*. 2003;3(5):395-402.

42. Griesche-Philippi J, Otto J, Schwörer H, et al. Exocrine pancreatic function in patients with end-stage renal disease. *Clin Nephrol*. 2010 Dec;74(6):457-64.

43. Teichmann J, Riemann JF, Lange U. Prevalence of exocrine pancreatic insufficiency in women with obesity syndrome: assessment by pancreatic fecal elastase 1. *ISRN Gastroenterol*. 2011;2011:951686.

44. Trang T, Chan J, Graham DY. Pancreatic enzyme replacement therapy for pancreatic exocrine insufficiency in the 21(st) century. *World J Gastroenterol*. 2014 Sep 7;20(33):11467-85.

45. For details on how each assay is performed for the activities of pancreatin, see the USP website: http://www.pharmacopeia.cn/v29240/usp29nf24s0_m60270.html

46. For details on the USP monograph for pancrelipase, see the USP website: http://www.pharmacopeia.cn/v29240/usp29nf24s0_m60320.html

47. Bekhit AA, Hopkins DL, Geesink G, Bekhit AA, Franks P. Exogenous proteases for meat tenderization. *Crit Rev Food Sci Nutr*. 2014;54(8):1012-31.

48. Maurer HR. Bromelain: biochemistry, pharmacology and medical use. *Cell Mol Life Sci*. 2001 Aug;58(9):1234-45.

49. Di Stefano M, Miceli E, Gotti S, et al. The effect of oral alpha-galactosidase on intestinal gas production and gas-related symptoms. *Dig Dis Sci*. 2007 Jan;52(1):78-83.

50. Levine ME, Koch SY, Koch KL. Lipase Supplementation before a High-Fat Meal Reduces Perceptions of Fullness in Healthy Subjects. *Gut Liver*. 2015 Jul;9(4):464-9.

51. Misselwitz B, Pohl D, Frühauf H, et al. Lactose malabsorption and intolerance: pathogenesis, diagnosis and treatment. *United European Gastroenterol J*. 2013 Jun;1(3):151-9.

52. Corazza GR, Benati G, Sorge M, et al. beta-Galactosidase from Aspergillus niger in adult lactose malabsorption: a double-blind crossover study. *Aliment Pharmacol Ther*. 1992 Feb;6(1):61-6.

53. O'Connell S, Walsh G. A novel acid-stable, acid-active beta-galactosidase potentially suited to the alleviation of lactose intolerance. *Appl Microbiol Biotechnol*. 2010 Mar;86(2):517-24.

54. http://www.fda.gov/downloads/drugs/guidancecomplianceregulatoryinformation/guidances/ucm071651.pdf

55. Löhr JM, Hummel FM, Pirilis KT, et al. Properties of different pancreatin preparations used in pancreatic exocrine insufficiency. *Eur J Gastroenterol Hepatol*. 2009 Sep;21(9):1024-31.

56. Berry AJ. Pancreatic enzyme replacement therapy during pancreatic insufficiency. *Nutr Clin Pract*. 2014 Jun;29(3):312-21.

57. Domínguez-Muñoz JE. Chronic pancreatitis and persistent steatorrhea: what is the correct dose of enzymes? *Clin Gastroenterol Hepatol*. 2011 Jul;9(7):541-6.

58. Opekun AR Jr, Sutton FM Jr, Graham DY. Lack of dose-response with Pancrease MT for the treatment of exocrine pancreatic insufficiency in adults. *Aliment Pharmacol Ther*. 1997 Oct;11(5):981-6.

59. Toskes PP, Secci A, Thieroff-Ekerdt R, et al. Efficacy of a novel pancreatic enzyme product, EUR-1008 (Zenpep), in patients with exocrine pancreatic insufficiency due to chronic pancreatitis. *Pancreas*. 2011 Apr;40(3):376-82.

60. Domínguez-Muñoz JE, Iglesias-García J, Iglesias-Rey M, Figueiras A, Vilariño-Insua M. Effect of the administration schedule on the therapeutic efficacy of oral pancreatic enzyme supplements in patients with exocrine pancreatic insufficiency: a randomized, three-way crossover study. *Aliment Pharmacol Ther*. 2005 Apr 15;21(8):993-1000.

61. Bruno MJ, Rauws EA, Hoek FJ, Tytgat GN. Comparative effects of adjuvant cimetidine and omeprazole during pancreatic enzyme replacement therapy. *Dig Dis Sci*. 1994 May;39(5):988-92.

62. Pezzilli R. Exocrine pancreas involvement in celiac disease: a review. *Recent Pat Inflamm Allergy Drug Discov*. 2014;8(3):167-72.

63. Leeds JS, Hopper AD, Hurlstone DP, et al. Is exocrine pancreatic insufficiency in adult coeliac disease a cause of persisting symptoms? *Aliment Pharmacol Ther*. 2007 Feb 1;25(3):265-71.

64. Nieminen U, Kahri A, Savilahti E, Färkkilä MA. Duodenal disaccharidase activities in the follow-up of villous atrophy in coeliac disease. *Scand J Gastroenterol*. 2001 May;36(5):507-10.

65. Nousia-Arvanitakis S, Fotoulaki M, et al. Subclinical exocrine pancreatic dysfunction resulting from decreased cholecystokinin secretion in the presence of intestinal villous atrophy. *J Pediatr Gastroenterol Nutr*. 2006 Sep;43(3):307-12.

66. Evans KE, Leeds JS, Morley S, Sanders DS. Pancreatic insufficiency in adult celiac disease: do patients require long-term enzyme supplementation? *Dig Dis Sci*. 2010 Oct;55(10):2999-3004.

67. Kaukinen K, Lindfors K. Novel treatments for celiac disease: glutenases and beyond. *Dig Dis*. 2015;33(2):277-81.

68. Lähdeaho ML, Kaukinen K, et al. Glutenase ALV003 attenuates gluten-induced mucosal injury in patients with celiac disease. *Gastroenterology*. 2014 Jun;146(7):1649-58.

69. Maldonado-Valderrama J, Wilde P, Macierzanka A, Mackie A. The role of bile salts in digestion. *Adv Colloid Interface Sci*. 2011 Jun 9;165(1):36-46.

70. Boesjes M, Brufau G. Metabolic effects of bile acids in the gut in health and disease. *Curr Med Chem*. 2014;21(24):2822-9.

71. Li T, Chiang JY. Bile acids as metabolic regulators. *Curr Opin Gastroenterol*. 2015 Mar;31(2):159-65.

72. Hofmann AF. Bile acids: trying to understand their chemistry and biology with the hope of helping patients. *Hepatology*. 2009 May;49(5):1403-18.

73. Cheng K, Ashby D, Smyth RL. Ursodeoxycholic acid for cystic fibrosis-related liver disease. *Cochrane Database Syst Rev*. 2014 Dec 15;12:CD000222.

74. Gruy-Kapral C, Little KH, Fordtran JS, et al. Conjugated bile acid replacement therapy for short-bowel syndrome. *Gastroenterology*. 1999 Jan;116(1):15-21.

75. Heydorn S, Jeppesen PB, Mortensen PB. Bile acid replacement therapy with cholylsarcosine for short-bowel syndrome. *Scand J Gastroenterol*. 1999 Aug;34(8):818-23.

76. Rudic JS, Poropat G, Krstic MN, Bjelakovic G, Gluud C. Ursodeoxycholic acid for primary biliary cirrhosis. *Cochrane Database Syst Rev*. 2012 Dec 12;12:CD000551.

77. FDA Website GRAS statement: www.fda.gov/Food/IngredientsPackagingLabeling/GRAS/SCOGS/ucm260943.htm

78. Bone K and Mills S. Principles and Practice of Phytotherapy. Second Edition. Edinburgh, UK: Churchhill Livingstone; 2013.

79. Saénz Rodriguez T, García Giménez D, de la Puerta Vázquez R. Choleretic activity and biliary elimination of lipids and bile acids induced by an artichoke leaf extract in rats. *Phytomedicine*. 2002 Dec;9(8):687-93.

80. Kirchhoff R, Beckers C, Kirchhoff GM, et al. Increase in choleresis by means of artichoke extract. *Phytomedicine*. 1994 Sep;1(2):107-15.

81. Crocenzi FA, Roma MG. Silymarin as a new hepatoprotective agent in experimental cholestasis: new possibilities for an ancient medication. *Curr Med Chem*. 2006;13(9):1055-74.

82. Hagymási K, Kocsis I, Lugasi A, et al. Extrahepatic biliary obstruction: can silymarin protect liver function? *Phytother Res*. 2002 Mar;16 Suppl 1:S78-80.

83. Schütz K, Carle R, Schieber A. Taraxacum--a review on its phytochemical and pharmacological profile. *J Ethnopharmacol*. 2006 Oct 11;107(3):313-23.

84. Vahlensieck U, Hahn R, Winterhoff H, et al. The effect of Chelidonium majus herb extract on choleresis in the isolated perfused rat liver. *Planta Med*. 1995 Jun;61(3):267-71.

Supporting Elimination and Detoxification

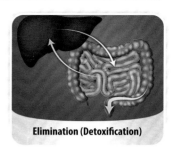

Elimination (Detoxification)

The GI tract is exquisitely designed to quickly and efficiently de-construct complex foods for nutrient absorption, while at the same time acting as the conduit for eliminating a large portion of our dietary and metabolic waste. As mentioned earlier, the process of elimination can be nearly as important as digestion and is prominently featured in the 4R paradigm for healing GI-related dysfunctions ("Remove," see page 22). Ridding the body of the unusable portions of foods as well as the toxic metabolites stored and produced in the body is a critical function of the GI system. These processes can be assessed and improved through basic lifestyle and nutrient therapies. Since the goal of this text is to help the healthcare professional evaluate lifestyle and nutritional strategies to support GI function, this section will essentially focus on three areas: 1) the fundamentals of stool and bowel habit analysis to gauge GI function; 2) ways to prevent and treat constipation, the leading GI complaint in Western society; and 3) the fundamentals of protocols designed to increase metabolic biotransformation (i.e., detoxification). For the "elimination" of specific GI pathogens, see respective chapters on *C. difficile* (page 165), *Candida* (page 239).

Using Stool to Assess Health

One of the most basic non-invasive (and ancient) ways to understand the overall function or dysfunction of the gastrointestinal system is to assess what has been eliminated from it; essentially an assessment and analysis of bowel habits and stool. It is rare to find someone with any sort of significant GI-related dysfunction without some demonstrable alteration in stool frequency, odor or consistency, or a significant finding in one or more stool analyte. However, many clinicians simply do not ask their patients about overall bowel habits and often know little about how to assess stool morphology to discern potential connections to basic GI functions. Whether it is as simple as the Bristol Stool Scale (BSS), or as complex as a metagenomic analysis of the fecal microbiota, what has been eliminated can be very informative to the metabolic functions of, and excretion through, the GI tract.

Bristol Stool Scale: A Marker Of Bowel Transit
The Bristol Stool Scale (BSS) or Bristol Stool Form Scale (BSFS) is a non-invasive and cost effective clinical communication aid designed to estimate colonic transit time based on seven categories of stool shape and form (see chart, page 52). The scale was first published and validated as a surrogate measurement for colonic transit time in 1997 by Dr. Lewis and Dr. Heaton at the

University of Bristol.[1] Use of the scale in conjunction with a patient stool diary has been suggested for the evaluation of constipation and diarrhea in functional bowel disorders.[2] Furthermore, the BSS has been used widely in clinical trials. Variations of the BSS have been proposed for children and infants.[3,4]

Laboratory Stool Testing
The analysis of stool samples for a variety of analytes and/or organisms is readily available from a variety of laboratories serving the integrative and functional medicine community. These tests are designed specifically for, and referenced to, stool samples. They allow for the assessment of a variety of GI functions including: digestion, absorption, metabolism (within the gut or elsewhere), detoxification, immune function, and the presence of commensal, pathobiont or pathogenic organisms (including many parasites). Several labs combine a number of different tests that can be performed using a single stool sample (or set of samples) for clinicians. These are generally referred to as a comprehensive digestive stool analysis (CDSA™)† or comprehensive stool analysis.

---

† CDSA is a trademark of Genova Diagnostics

Bristol Stool Scale

Type 1
Separate hard lumps, like nuts (hard to pass)

Type 2
Sausage shaped, but lumpy

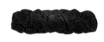

Type 3
Like a sausage or snake, but with cracks on its surface

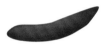

Type 4
Like a sausage or snake, smooth and soft

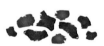

Type 5
Soft blobs with clear cut edges (passed easily)

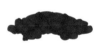

Type 6
Fluffy pieces with ragged edges, a mushy stool

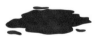

Type 7
Watery, no solid pieces

The scale moves from stool morphology typical of very slow transit time (Types 1 and 2), to those typical of extremely fast transit time or diarrhea (Types 6 and 7, respectively). Types 3 and 4 are generally considered ideal for most individuals, though opinions vary amongst practitioners and patients. While the BSS is only one measure of GI function, it has been shown to be an easy way for clinicians and patients to begin the conversation about bowel habits and elimination frequency. Clinicians can download free BSS charts on a number of websites and they should encourage their patients to print and refer to these charts when completing their dietary habits diary.

Throughout this guidebook, we have discussed numerous stool analytes that may be helpful in diagnosing one or more GI dysfunctions, many of which are part of a comprehensive stool analysis. Clinicians should work with their laboratory to understand their specific guidelines for sampling, shipping, and reference ranges, and also how to interpret the specific tests and patterns indicating specific pathologies or dysfunctions. Comprehensive stool tests are often used as a way to get an overall picture of many different GI functions with a single sample, since many patients find repeated stool sampling for individual tests to be unpleasant. Follow-up tests can then be used months later using a comprehensive test battery, or a few specific analytes.

Stool-based Digestive Test Markers: See page 45
Microbiome Testing of Feces: See page 94

Assessing, Preventing and Treating Constipation

Constipation (defined by patient or clinician) is one of the most frequent GI-related complaints in the Western world, resulting in a growing number of office and emergency room visits each year.[5,6] As we shall see, defining constipation is nearly as difficult as defining "normal" stool frequency; though most would agree that stool frequency less than three times per week would define constipation, some patients would even say that less than once per day defines constipation in need of intervention. In addition to frequency, difficult evacuation of hard, dry stools may constitute the diagnosis of constipation for some.

The regular use of laxatives is another sign that the patient is concerned about constipation, even if they may not meet the requirements for a diagnosis.[7] However, estimates of laxative use (which have been estimated at 10% of the United States population) may not be an adequate way to assess populations, as patients concerned about constipation are prone to underestimate bowel frequency and overuse laxatives.[8] This is why physicians need to take an extensive patient history when assessing the patient's bowel habits. Questions should include what the patient considers "normal" or "regular," duration of constipation, and what remedies have been tried and when. A stool diary which includes time, difficulty in passing, general appearance, and size of stool should be considered along with a food and water diary.

Defining Constipation

As many readers already know, definitions of constipation are not left up to the patient or clinician to decide. There are official criteria for various constipation diagnoses including chronic constipation (CC), chronic idiopathic constipation (CIC), functional constipation (FC), opioid-induced constipation (OIC) and IBS-C. Rome criteria (III and IV) for the diagnosis of functional constipation (which incorporates CC and CIC) requires the following three criteria to be met for the previous three months with symptom onset at least six months prior to diagnosis:[9]

1. Must include two or more of the following:
    a. Straining during more than 25% of defecations
    b. Lumpy or hard stools (BSFS 1-2) in more than 25% of defecations
    c. Sensation of incomplete evacuation in more than 25% of defecations
    d. Sensation of anorectal obstruction/blockage in more than 25% of defecations
    e. Manual maneuvers to facilitate in more than 25% of defecations
    f. Fewer than three spontaneous bowel movements per week

2. Loose stools are rarely present without the use of laxatives

3. Insufficient criteria for IBS

We should note here that there has been some debate as to the diagnostic differences between functional constipation and IBS-C, where the defining symptom distinguishing these symptoms (according to Rome IV) is abdominal pain.[†] However, Rome IV criteria for FC acknowledge that abdominal pain and/or bloating may be present, but are *not predominant* (therefore excluding the necessary criteria for IBS), supporting the concept that FC and IBS-C are disorders that may exist on a continuum with no clear biomarkers to distinguish them (though distinctions in successful treatment between the two suggest some differences in underlying dysfunction).[10,11]

Regardless of how constipation is defined, one should remember that constipation is a symptom of dysfunction, not a disease (though there are four ICD-10 codes for constipation).[‡] The underlying causes of constipation may be quite varied and therefore treatment protocols will vary as well. Causes may include endocrine disorders such as diabetes and hypothyroidism, neurological diseases such as MS, Parkinson's or spinal cord injuries, functional gastrointestinal disorders like IBS, or diseases within the colon/anal area like anal fissures or inflammatory bowel disease. Many drugs (esp. opioids) and surgical interventions will also lead to symptoms of constipation. However, the primary root cause for many suffering with constipation is the dietary habits and lifestyle factors common in the Western culture, even when associated with the other causes listed here. Women, especially petite women within child-bearing age, generally have the highest incidence of constipation, though the elderly frequently report symptoms of constipation.[12]

Bowel Transit Time and the Microbiome

It is known that bowel transit time is one of the factors that greatly influences the diversity of the gut microbiota (at least when analyzing fecal samples).[13,14] When bowel transit time is increased or decreased experimentally in subjects with no dietary changes, dramatic changes in overall stool weight and character have been observed, along with dramatic changes in microbial mass. Along with many other factors, stool frequency and morphology (using BSS) is a strong predictor of GI microbial diversity, perhaps helping to define a person's enterotype (see page 102 for more details). However, a recent study suggests that a long colonic transport time, which is associated with more microbial richness, can alter macronutrient fermentation that is negative for the host.[15] In other words, a longer bowel transit time may allow certain slow-growing bacteria more time to become abundant, though this may alter the metabolic outcome of the microbiome in negative ways. Maintaining a steady turnover of bacteria, and colonic cells, appears to be a healthier milieu achieved by regular bowel movements and transit time.

Conversely, certain species within the GI tract may greatly influence bowel transit time. Besides those organisms causing diarrhea, it is likely certain species

---

†   OIC has been added as a sixth category of Functional Bowel Disorders in the new Rome IV criteria. With the exception of drugs designed to block the effects of opioids, the treatment options should be similar to FC.

‡   There are four different ICD-10 codes used to describe the diagnosis of constipation: constipation-unspecified (K59.00), slow transit constipation (K59.01), outlet dysfunction constipation (K59.02), other constipation (K59.09)

of bacteria can influence bowel transit time. In a small (n=24) pilot study using fecal microbiota transplantation (FMT) in subjects with slow-transit constipation, researchers showed statistically and clinically significant improvements in bowel transit time lasting 12 weeks after the FMT.[16] This suggests a large shift in the gut microbiota can influence bowel transit time. While FMT is not yet approved for treating constipation or slow-transit time, the research in this area is advancing quickly and clinicians should stay abreast of the changing recommendations and regulations regarding FMTs (for more on FMTs, see page 110).

Probiotics for Improved Transit Time or Constipation
Numerous clinical trials have been performed in a variety of patients to assess the effectiveness of probiotics for improving symptoms of constipation or other objective measures of intestinal transit time. A systematic review of 14 eligible clinical trials confirms probiotics reduce whole gut transit time (by about 12 hours), increase stool frequency (by about 1/3 bowel movements/week) and improve stool consistency in subjects with functional constipation.[17] Similar findings have been seen in subjects not suffering from constipation, though the magnitude and statistical significance of these changes are notably smaller.[18]

While several different species and strains of probiotics have been investigated, the number of strains or strain combinations tested in randomized, controlled clinical trials is relatively limited. Nonetheless, the probiotic strains associated with the most positive clinical outcomes related to improved transit time and constipation are various strains of *Bifidobacterium lactis* (technically *B. animalis subsp. lactis*), though a few positive studies have been performed using products containing strains of *L. casei*, *L. rhamnosus* and several other *Lactobacilli* or *Bifidobacterium* strains. Doses ranged from as low as 10 million CFU/day (in yogurt) to as high as 30 billion (usually delivered in dairy preparations, capsules or tablets.) Since almost no strain-to-strain or dose-to dose comparison trials have been done in human subjects with constipation, it is difficult to say which particular species, strains or doses are necessarily more efficacious than other species or doses with fewer (or no) published clinical trials. So, while we generally agree clinicians should recommend probiotics to patients with slow bowel transit time or constipation, our recommendation is generally similar to our overall probiotic recommendation: a multi-strain product containing 20 to 40 billion CFU/day (see page 129 for specifics on probiotics, and see below for prebiotics/fiber supplementation). Trying different strain combinations or doses may help different subjects, or may also be necessary to accommodate different GI-related outcomes in addition to symptomatic relief of constipation.

Improving Constipation through Diet and Lifestyle

"One of the gravest defects of the civilized diet is its lack of raw foods and ballast, or roughage. We eat over-milled cereals, chemicalised sugars, softly cooked vegetables, sloppy seasoned hashes, slushy puddings and soups, pappy porridges, sophisticated and highly-refined concocted dished of all kinds. In such a diet there are no rough irritating substances to stimulate intestinal peristalsis." George Dupain, 1934[19]

Constipation is considered by many to be highly associated with a Western pattern of diet and lifestyle; more specifically, to a diet low in natural fiber and healthful bacteria, and a lifestyle high in stress and sedentary activities. Though many of these factors have been difficult to link specifically with constipation, few have been tested as interventional strategies to improve outcomes in patients.[20]

Fiber: An Essential Component
Dietary fiber is defined as all plant non-starch polysaccharides, with the addition of plant lignans. This includes celluloses, gums, pectins and mucilages. Plant fiber is virtually indigestible using human-derived enzymes alone, and has often been referred to as "roughage." Most dietary fiber is found in fruits, vegetables, legumes and grains. Just like vitamins and minerals, dietary fiber has a daily recommended value (DRV) from the Institutes of Medicine (IOM). The current DRV for dietary fiber is 25 g per day for women and 38 g per day for men.

However, many believe these recommendations are much too low to maintain optimal health, and should be closer to 40 or 50 g per day (respectively). But even using the lower recommended levels, most Americans are not getting adequate levels of dietary fiber. A report from

IOM said that only 3% of Americans are consuming adequate amounts of fiber, and average consumption is only about half the recommended amount of 14 g/ 1,000 calories.[21] In children, recommendations are typically determined by adding five to the child's age to get the recommended grams per day (child age seven = 12 g per day).

Some standard foods are found in Table 5, along with their typical fiber content. As the table shows, dietary fiber can be further divided into soluble and insoluble fiber. This characteristic does not mean true solubility (in the chemical sense), but describes those fibers that are dispersible in water. The soluble fibers, such as pectin and gums, have a very high water-holding capacity and often form a gel when mixed with water. Insoluble fibers hold very little water and will usually fall to the bottom of a glass when mixed in water. Most non-isolated plant fibers (eaten as food) will be a combination of soluble and insoluble fibers. There are some exceptions, especially with some grain seeds and seed husks (e.g., flax and psyllium), which are very high in soluble fibers.

Water-holding capacity, however, is not the only predictor of benefits when adding fiber to the diet. Foods high in fiber are rich in other phytonutrients, some of which are bound within the matrix of the fiber itself. Certain fibers are also important foods for the healthy microbial organisms within the gut, a class of fermentable fibers termed "prebiotics" (see page 108 for more details on prebiotics). In fact, other characteristics, such as viscosity, susceptibility to fermentation, effect on digestive enzymes, bile acid binding capacity and anion exchange capacity, must be added to water-holding capacity to fully gauge the therapeutic benefits of individual fibers. Even the shape of certain fibers is likely to be important, as inert plastic in the "shape" of flakes improved bowel transit time, while plastic as small granules had no effect.[22]

We cannot overestimate the role diet, specifically low dietary fiber intake, is thought to play as a cause of constipation in Western countries.[23] Comparing dietary fiber intake between populations has often correlated positively with stool frequency and weight and, inversely, with colon diseases including some cancers.[24] Likewise, the increase in refinement of sugars and carbohydrates is linked with slowing bowel transit times and altering the ecosystem for the gut microbiota (see page 106 for more details). As we have seen, the decreased intake of fiber as a function of modern food practices is suggested by many to be the leading cause of idiopathic constipation. While this has been empirically shown in adults for more than a century, this has recently been researched specifically in children. In one study in Brazil, children with chronic constipation typically ingested 20 to 30% less fiber than age and gender-matched controls with normal bowel habits.[25]

In a larger sample group of children in Greece, dietary fiber alone was independently and inversely correlated with chronic constipation, despite the child's age or age of onset of constipation.[26] Furthermore, a study done in the United States, showed constipated children were consuming less than one-fourth of the age+5 recommended intake, even though they had been instructed "to eat a high-fiber diet."[27] It appears that in children, as well as in adults, increasing dietary fiber is a difficult lifestyle change many simply decline to make. For example, the use of dietary fiber in patients in elderly care facilities, where less individual control over diet is practiced, has been shown to decrease laxative use and increase bowel frequency.[28] This has also been the case with severe developmentally disabled children.[29]

Fiber Supplementation for Laxative Effects

In general, increasing the intake of fiber-containing foods or specially prepared dietary supplements should is considered the safest laxative for most individuals and should be considered first for the treatment of idiopathic constipation. As was mentioned above, food sources of fiber are preferred (see Table 5), as the additional phytonutrients derived from these foods are beneficial to disease prevention, although many "therapeutic fibers" have additional benefits as well (the non-laxative benefits of fiber are not discussed here). Bulk fibers are also "dietary fibers," although they are usually in concentrated forms and are primarily soluble fibers.

Adequate water intake is necessary when consuming fiber supplements to ensure proper action in the colon. Since many mixed fiber supplements alter bowel transit time, and provide substrates for microbial fermentation, increased gas and bloating is often associated with the first days or weeks of fiber supplementation. Patients should start with a lower dose and increase over several weeks to the long-term recommended or symptom-relieving dose.

Table 5: FIBER CONTENT OF FOODS IN COMMON PORTIONS, IN GRAMS PER SERVING

Food Item	Serving Size	Total Fiber (g)	Soluble Fiber (g)	Insoluble Fiber (g)	Food Item	Serving Size	Total Fiber (g)	Soluble Fiber (g)	Insoluble Fiber (g)
Vegetables (cooked)					**Legumes (cooked)**				
Asparagus	1/2 cup	2.8	1.7	1.1	Black beans	1/2 cup	6.1	2.4	3.7
Beets, flesh only	1/2 cup	1.8	0.8	1.0	Black-eyed peas	1/2 cup	4.7	0.5	4.2
Broccoli	1/2 cup	2.4	1.2	1.2	Kidney beans, light red	1/2 cup	7.9	2.0	5.9
Brussels sprouts	1/2 cup	3.8	2.0	1.8	Lentils	1/2 cup	5.2	0.6	4.6
Corn, whole kernel, canned	1/2 cup	1.6	0.2	1.4	Lima beans	1/2 cup	4.3	1.1	3.2
Carrots, sliced	1/2 cup	2.0	1.1	0.9	Navy beans	1/2 cup	6.5	2.2	4.3
Cauliflower	1/2 cup	1.0	0.4	0.6	Pinto beans	1/2 cup	6.1	1.4	4.7
Green beans, canned	1/2 cup	2.0	0.5	1.5	**Pasta, Rice, Grains**				
Kale	1/2 cup	2.5	0.7	1.8					
Okra, frozen	1/2 cup	4.1	1.0	3.1	Barley, pearled, cooked	1/2 cup	3.0	0.8	2.2
Peas, green, frozen	1/2 cup	4.3	1.3	3.0	Popcorn, popped	3 cups	2.0	0.1	1.9
Potato, sweet, flesh only	1/2 cup	4.0	1.8	2.2	Rice, white, cooked	1/2 cup	0.8	trace	0.8
Spinach	1/2 cup	1.6	0.5	1.1	Spaghetti, white cooked	1/2 cup	0.9	0.4	0.5
Tomato sauce	1/2 cup	1.7	0.8	0.9	Spaghetti, whole wheat, cooked	1/2 cup	2.7	0.6	2.1
Turnip	1/2 cup	4.8	1.7	3.1	Wheat bran	1/2 cup	12.3	1.0	11.3
Raw Vegetables					Wheat germ	3 tbsp	3.9	0.7	3.2
Cabbage, red	1 cup	1.5	0.6	0.9	**Breads and Crackers**				
Carrots, fresh	1, 7 1/2 in. long	2.3	1.1	1.2					
Celery, fresh	1 cup chopped	1.7	0.7	1.0	Pumpernickel	1 slice	2.7	1.2	1.5
Cucumber, fresh	1 cup	0.5	0.2	0.3	Rye	1 slice	1.8	0.8	1.0
Lettuce, iceberg	1 cup	0.5	0.1	0.4	White	1 slice	0.6	0.3	0.3
Mushrooms, fresh	1 cup pieces	0.8	0.1	0.7	Whole wheat	1 slice	1.5	0.3	1.2
Onion, fresh	1/2 cup chopped	1.7	0.9	0.8	**Cereals**				
Pepper, green, fresh	1 cup chopped	1.7	0.7	1.0					
Tomato, fresh	1 medium	1.0	0.1	0.9	All Bran	1/3 cup	8.6	1.4	7.2
Fruits					Benefit	3/4 cup	5.0	2.8	2.2
					Cheerios	1 1/4 cup	2.5	1.2	1.3
Apple, red, fresh w/skin	1 small	2.8	1.0	1.8	Corn flakes	1 cup	0.5	0.1	0.4
Applesauce, canned	1/2 cup	2.0	0.7	1.3	Cream of wheat, regular, dry	2 1/2 tbsp	1.1	0.4	0.7
Apricots, dried	7 halves	2.0	1.1	0.9	Fiber One	1/2 cup	11.9	0.8	11.1
Apricots, fresh w/skin	4	3.5	1.8	1.7	40% Bran Flakes	2/3 cup	4.3	0.4	3.9
Banana, fresh	1/2 small	1.1	0.3	0.8	Grapenuts	1/4 cup	2.8	0.8	2.0
Blueberries, fresh	3/4 cup	1.4	0.3	1.1	Oat bran, cooked	3/4 cup	4.0	2.2	1.8
Cherries, black, fresh	12 large	1.3	0.6	0.7	Oat flakes	1 cup	3.1	1.5	1.6
Figs, dried	1 1/2	3.0	1.4	1.6	Oatmeal, dry	1/3 cup	2.7	1.4	1.3
Grapefruit, fresh	1/2 medium	1.6	1.1	0.5	Puffed Wheat	1 cup	1.0	0.5	0.5
Grapes, fresh w/skin	15 small	0.5	0.2	0.3	Raisin Bran	3/4 cup	5.3	0.9	4.4
Kiwifruit, fresh, flesh only	1 large	1.7	0.7	1.0	Rice Krispies	1 cup	0.3	0.1	0.2
Mango, fresh, flesh only	1/2 small	2.9	1.7	1.2	Shredded Wheat	1 cup	5.2	0.7	4.5
Melon, cantaloupe	1 cup cubed	1.1	0.3	0.8	Special K	1 cup	0.9	0.2	0.7
Orange, fresh, flesh only	1 small	2.9	1.8	1.1	Wheat flakes	3/4 cup	2.3	0.4	1.9
Peach, fresh, w/skin	1 medium	2.0	1.0	1.0	**Nuts and Seeds**				
Pear, fresh, w/skin	1/2 large	2.9	1.1	1.8					
Plum, red, fresh	2 medium	2.4	1.1	1.3	Almonds	6 whole	0.6	0.1	0.5
Prunes, dried	3 medium	1.7	1.0	0.7	Flax seeds	1 tbsp	3.3	1.1	2.2
Raisins, dried	2 tbsp	0.4	0.2	0.2	Peanut butter, smooth	1 tbsp	1.0	0.3	0.7
Raspberries, fresh	1 cup	3.3	0.9	2.4	Peanuts, roasted	10 large	0.6	0.2	0.4
Strawberries, fresh	1 1/4 cup	2.8	1.1	1.7	Sesame seeds	1 tbsp	0.5	0.2	0.3
Watermelon	1 1/4 cup cubed	0.6	0.4	0.2	Sunflower seeds	1 tbsp	0.5	0.2	0.3
					Walnuts	2 whole	0.3	0.1	0.2

Adapted from Anderson *JW. Plant Fiber in Foods*. 2 nd ed. HCF Nutrition Research Foundation Inc, PO Box 22124, Lexington, KY 40522, 1990.
Nutrition Service -beb, Harvard University Health Services, May 2004.

Flax Seeds

Flax (*Linum usitatissimum*, also known as linseed) is one of the most versatile plants for human use.[30] Flax seeds should be considered food, but are included here because most individuals consume flax by intentional supplementation (though it is becoming more common in commercial baked goods). The stem fibers can be used for paper and linen and the seed is important for its omega-3 essential fatty acid (alpha-linolenic acid), its fiber content (25% soluble), and its lignan content. It is this combination that makes flax seeds one of the most versatile, although sometimes overlooked, healthy

foods. There are few people who would not benefit by adding flax, in one or more forms, to their daily diet. Its lignan components are currently being investigated for their role in the prevention of breast cancer, prostate cancer, blood sugar dysregulation, lipid dysregulation, and for their potential phytoestrogenic effects.[31]

Flax seeds ability to help in constipation is due to its combined fiber/mucilage and oil which adds both bulk and lubrication to the stool. Few clinical trials have been performed using flax seed powder in constipated subjects, though one small trial showed it performed similarly to psyllium when each were consumed at 15 g per day.[32] Several animal studies have also confirmed its laxative properties.[33,34] As flax seeds contain so much polyunsaturated oil, seeds are usually purchased and ground just prior to use, although freshly ground flax seeds can be purchased and kept refrigerated. Patients should experiment with different doses (1 to 3 tablespoons of ground flax seeds are usually adequate for most); adding the powder to smoothies, yogurt, juice or water. Flax seed powder can also be added to many cookies, muffins and breads, though some of the omega-3 benefits may be neutralized by the baking process.

Psyllium Seeds or Seed Husks

Seeds from psyllium (*Plantago psyllium*) or ispaghula (*Plantago ovata*) are perhaps the most widely used ingredients in natural bulk laxatives, and for good reason. The husk and whole seed powder of psyllium is very high in soluble fiber (mostly arabinoxylans) and it has extremely high water-holding capacity. As a bulk laxative, it increases both stool frequency as well as stool weight. The use of psyllium for the relief of constipation has been confirmed by randomized controlled clinical trials, several of which compared the use of psyllium with other laxatives and have found it superior in almost all cases.[35] In one such trial, compared to the stool softener/laxative docusate sodium, patients on psyllium (5 g bid) had significantly more frequent bowel movements and increased stool water output in two weeks.[36] In addition, psyllium seeds have proven useful in relieving constipation in patients with Parkinson's disease,[37] maintaining remission in patients with ulcerative colitis,[38] and reducing the potential for gallbladder disease.[39] Ironically, the water-holding capacity of psyllium that makes it so effective in treating constipation, is also capable of controlling both fecal incontinence and radiation-induced diarrhea.[40,41]

The long-term safety of psyllium-containing supplements is extremely high, with the exception of those individuals who are allergic to psyllium. These products, as with other bulk laxatives should not be used by individuals with bowel obstructions or narrowing of the esophagus or gastrointestinal tract. Psyllium is often a major ingredient in OTC fiber supplements as well as many combined fiber dietary supplements. Effective doses range from a few grams per day to well over 15 g psyllium fiber per day. Patients should be instructed to start with a lower dose, perhaps for several days or weeks, before slowly escalating to the target dose.

Glucomannan

Glucomannan is a highly viscous fiber derived commercially from the tuber root of *Amorphophallus konjac* (and related species) and is thus often called konjac mannan in the literature. While the body of research is smaller than with psyllium, glucomannan has much of the same chemical properties and therapeutic potential as a laxative. One study showed 4.5 g per day of konjac mannan given to constipated Chinese subjects consuming a low-fiber diet improved bowel movements by 30% after three weeks of supplementation.[42] Konjac mannan has also been used successfully to improve symptoms of constipation in children (maximum dose of 5 g per day).[43]

Other Fiber Supplement Ingredients

Many other soluble and insoluble fibers have been used as ingredients in foods and dietary supplements intended to help with constipation. Guar gum is derived from the seed of the East Asian guar bean (*Cyamopsis tetragonoloba)*. It is a galactomannon fiber, and has many of the same properties found in psyllium and glucomannon already mentioned.

For many years, partially hydrolyzed guar gum powder was the primary ingredient in one of the most popular over-the-counter fiber laxatives, though it has since been replaced with wheat dextrin.[44,45] Other ingredients that one is likely to see in addition to those mentioned already are: pectin (apple or citrus), wheat dextrins and oat bran (more common in foods), sugar-beet fiber, fenugreek fiber, other gums (locust bean, karaya), celluloses, and fructoligosacharides (FOS), each with varying levels of reported laxative activity.

Finally, while prunes (dried plums) and prune juice are foods or beverages (not supplements), they are often eaten specifically for therapeutic relief of constipation. Anecdotal evidence suggests that prunes and prune juice are likely to be of some benefit, and they are also known to have other health benefits.[46] In one small study comparing 6 g fiber per day from prunes (about 12 prunes) or psyllium seeds (two tablespoons) in subjects with idiopathic constipation (crossover design), prunes showed a statistically better improvement in stool frequency after just three weeks.[47] We encourage clinicians to recommend the consumption of prunes or prune juice as a dietary modification for those concerned with or experiencing symptoms of constipation.

Water Intake and Constipation

It would seem obvious that if constipation is often associated with hard, dry stools, then water intake would be beneficial for decreasing constipation. This is also one of the mechanisms attributed to fibers; their ability to hold water in the stool, increasing stool size, lubrication and stimulating peristaltic function. The function of water, in relation to fiber intake, was studied in a group of patients experiencing chronic constipation. One hundred and seventeen patients were put on a standard diet providing 25 g per day of dietary fiber. One half of the group was given no instructions on water consumption while the other group was instructed to drink 2 liters of mineral water per day. The second group drank, on average, double what the first group consumed (2.1 vs. 1.1 liters). In both stool frequency (p<0.001) and laxative use

(p=<0.001) there was a statistical improvement in the group with the higher intake of water.[48] One study even suggests carbonated water alone, as opposed to tap water, may have additional benefits for relieving constipation, as well as dyspepsia and gall bladder emptying.[49] In contrast to these studies, in non-constipated individuals, water seems to be important only when intake is very low, while additional water intake was not shown to statistically increase stool frequency in these subjects.[50,51] Water intake from all non-sweetened beverages, soups and foods should be included on diet diaries as part of the patient's history. All subjects, especially those concerned with constipation, should be advised to consume adequate non-sweetened water intake daily (especially fresh fruits and vegetables).

Natural Laxative Agents Beyond Fiber

For many subjects, dietary changes, increased water and fiber intake, and other lifestyle changes (see below) still do not provide adequate relief for their constipation or do not fully satisfy their desire for regularity. In those circumstances, there are some non-pharmacological options the clinician can recommend that are likely to be safe and effective in most individuals. These natural laxatives fall into three categories: bulking/hydrophilic laxatives (essentially fiber and water, already discussed), osmotic agents, and stimulant laxatives. Lubricating agents may make defecation easier, though they do not alter bowel transit time or stool frequency.

Osmotic Agents

Osmotic agents (or hyperosmotic agents) are essentially compounds that ionize or polymerize when ingested (or before ingestion when placed in liquid) that, when consumed in an amount that limits their gastrointestinal absorption, will force the retention of water in the colon, thereby providing a laxative effect. OTC laxatives containing polyethylene glycol (PEG) and lactulose are considered osmotic laxatives. Other common osmotic laxatives include poorly absorbed magnesium or phosphate salts such as magnesium sulfate (Epsom salts), magnesium hydroxide (milk of magnesia), and sodium phosphate. Other sugar alcohols such as sorbitol and mannitol also have this property, as does glycerin,

which is more often used as a suppository/stool softener. Ascorbic acid, in higher doses, also has the same effect on the stool. Made popular by Linus Pauling, it is commonly known that high doses of ascorbic acid will induce "bowel intolerance." These elevated doses of vitamin C may have other benefits, but such regimens should be used for short-term treatment only, unless the physician is familiar with high-dose vitamin C regimens.[52] Osmotic agents are dose-dependent and each person may have a different threshold for efficacy and tolerability. Caution should be taken to use the lowest dose necessary to induce laxation, as these compounds can absorb and create mineral imbalances when taken at high doses.

Botanical Stimulant Laxatives

There are several different botanically-derived stimulant laxatives currently available, though they each contain a similar class of compounds called anthraquinone glycosides (see Figure 14).[53] Once these anthranoid laxative compounds are ingested, they pass unabsorbed into the colon, where they are activated by microbes with specific enzymes. These enzymes remove the sugar moiety, forming the active aglycone form. These compounds then act on epithelial cells in the colon, causing changes in water absorption, mucosal secretions and motility and leading to laxation.[54,55]

Anthraquinone Glycosides

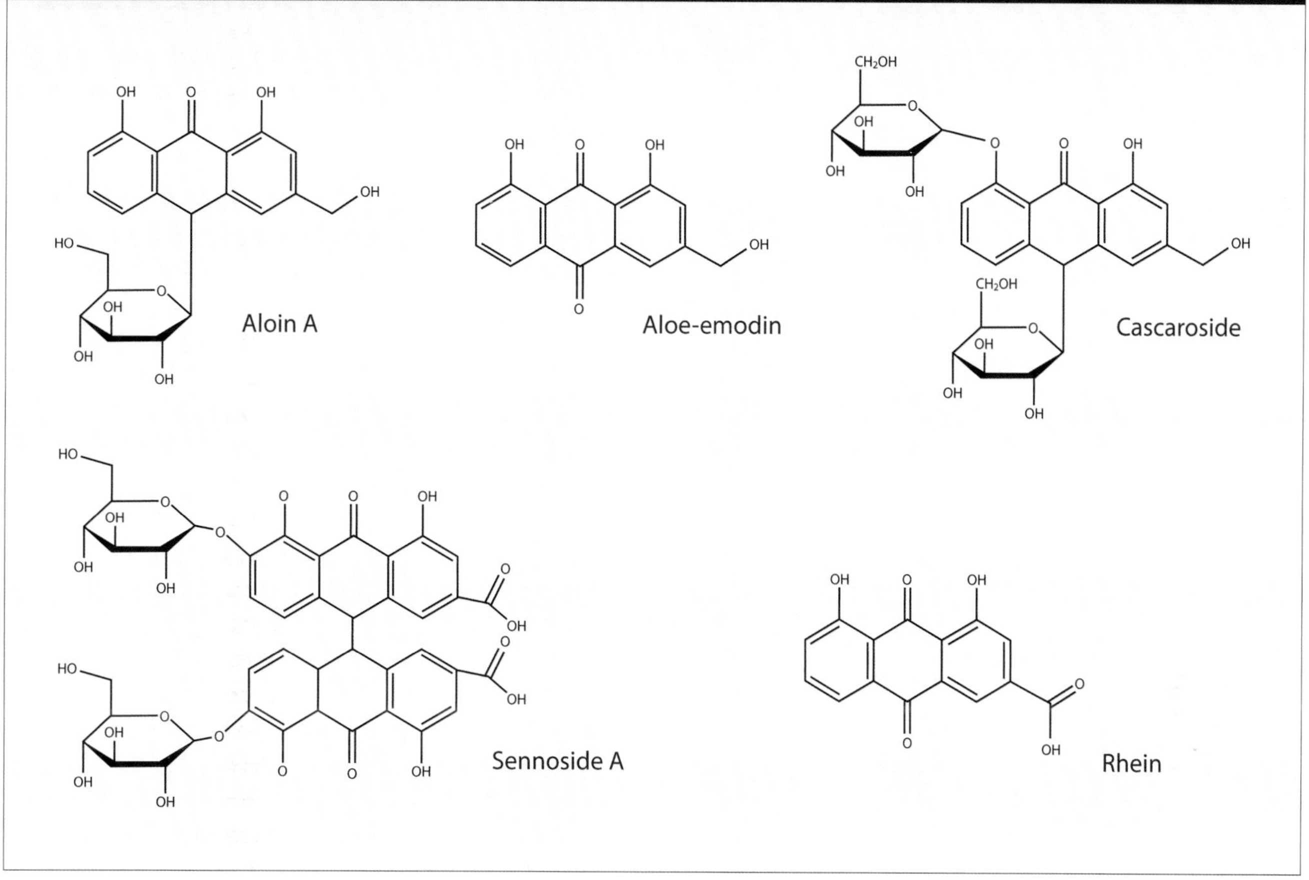

Figure 14: Common Anthroquinone compounds found in botanical laxatives.

Aloes

Aloes powder is the solid residue obtained by evaporating the liquid which drains from the transversely cut leaves of Cape Aloes (*Aloe ferox*) or other *Aloe spp*. The juice is then concentrated by boiling and allowed to solidify upon cooling. It is characteristically dark brown or greenish-brown. It has a sour odor and an extremely bitter taste. Cape Aloes is found primarily on the Cape Horn of South Africa, where it can grow between six and 10 feet tall.

The best-characterized constituents of this resin are the anthroquinone glycosides aloin A (barbaloin) and aloin B (isobarbaloin), though some aglycone compounds are present as well. Aloins A and B are converted into emodin-derivatives within the colon by the gut microbiota where they become potent purging laxatives.[56,57,58] The effect of aloes is primarily caused by its influence on the motility of the colon—an inhibition of stationary and stimulation of propulsive contractions.

This results in an accelerated intestinal passage and, because of the shortened contraction time, a reduction in liquid absorption. In addition, stimulation of active chloride secretion increases the water and electrolyte content in the stool. Various aloe-derived anthraquinone compounds have been tested in animal studies to confirm their efficacy.[59,60]

Despite the long-term use of aloes and its reputation as one of the most potent natural laxatives, few rigorous clinical trials have been performed in human subjects.[61] This may be partly due to the popularity of similar botanical ingredients derived from cascara sagrada and senna (see below) or the commonly held notion that aloes is more often associated with side-effects such as cramping and nausea. This, however, has not been the case when used in recent decades as a dietary supplement and likely is attributed to information passed on from the use of preparations nearly a century ago.[62] The preparations of aloes have been in the US Pharmacopoeia for over 100 years and has a positive Commission E monograph, where it is listed for short-term constipation.[63]

Dosing aloes is different depending on the individual. The optimum dose is the smallest dosage necessary to obtain a soft stool that passes without difficulty. For many individuals, this is between 250 and 900 mg taken in one or more capsules. Therefore, patients should be instructed to take a small dose (i.e., 250 mg capsule) and wait to see how they respond before increasing the dose. Twenty-four hours should be allowed to pass before the next dose is administered, as aloes and similar products should have a noticeable effect in six to 12 hours. Aloes should not be used during pregnancy because of its uterine stimulant potential. Anthroquinone compounds are thought to be secreted in breast milk of nursing mothers and this may negatively affect the taste of the milk or even purge the child along with the mother (some consider this an adverse reaction, others, an intentional effect). As with all stimulant laxatives, aloes should not be recommended as a long-term therapy and should be used primarily to relieve occasional constipation (see cautions below).

Cascara Sagrada

Cascara sagrada ("sacred bark" in Spanish) describes the small- to medium-sized buckthorn tree *Rhamnus purshiana* (syn. *Frangula purshiana*) and closely related species. The bark of cascara sagrada has a long history of medicinal use among Native Americans and Western herbalists, particularly as a laxative. The active compounds are considered to be the anthraquinone diglycosides termed cascarosides (A, B, C, D, see Figure 14).[64] Like aloes, there is little in the way of published clinical research on cascara sagrada preparations or concentrated cascarosides, though the German Commission E has a positive therapeutic monograph for laxative formulas with a dose corresponding to 20 to 30 mg cascaroside A (or equivalent).[65] A further note suggests the individually correct dosage is the smallest dosage necessary to maintain soft stool.

Senna

The dried leaflets and pods of *Cassia senna* (syn. *Senna alexandrina* or related species) are most often referred to medicinally as senna. These preparations contain the anthroquinone glycosides sennoside A and B, both of which are potent laxative compounds in humans and animals when hydrolyzed to form rhein by gut microbiota (see Figure 14).[66] The laxative preparation for senna has been used in medicinal teas in Europe, and powdered extracts have become very popular in OTC laxative products in the United States. Due to the larger commercial interest in sennosides, there has been more published literature on the mechanisms and actions of these compounds compared to similar compounds found in *Aloe spp*, *Rhamnus spp.* and rhubarb (similar compounds and activities are found in rhubarb root preparations [*Rheum officinale*], although rhubarb is a more commonly used starting material in Asia.).[67,68,69] The typical dose is 0.6 to 2 g leaf or seedpod preparation (equivalent to 20 to 30 mg sennoside B). As with other laxatives containing anthroquinone glycosides, the smallest effective dose should be considered adequate, increasing doses slowly over time to discover the appropriate dose for occasional constipation. Senna also has a positive Commission E monograph for use in laxative formulations.[70]

Cautions with Stimulant Laxatives

The use of botanical stimulant laxatives should be considered only after diet, lifestyle, and bulk laxatives have proven ineffective, and other causes of constipation have been ruled out. They are contraindicated in cases of bowel obstruction, acute intestinal inflammation and abdominal pain of unknown origin. They should not generally be used in children under 12 or in pregnant or nursing women. Overuse and abuse of laxatives is common, though published adverse events are relatively few.[71] Potential dangers include electrolyte imbalance, especially potassium deficiency which can lead to muscle weakness and heart function disorders. This potassium imbalance can be further exacerbated by the use of thiazide diuretics, corticosteroids or high doses of licorice root.

Chronic use of anthraquinone glycosides have been associated with an increased pigmentation of the intestinal mucosa called melanosis coli (or sometimes pseudomelanosis coli), a condition that was reported in JAMA as early as 1933.[72] Remarkable incidences of laxative-induced melanosis coli are still reported as case studies around the world.[73,74,75,76] While this altered physiology has been suspected of increasing the risk of carcinogenesis,[77] it is generally deemed to be a benign condition; though it is diagnostic for laxative abuse and often alters the ability to diagnose other colon diseases.[78,79,80,81] While the available evidence is divided on whether chronic use of stimulant laxatives will result in a condition of a "sluggish" colon (not studied since the 1960s), all attempts should be made to move patients to bulk-forming laxatives and refrain from chronic use of stimulant laxatives.

Other Lifestyle Risks and Remedies

Physical Activity

Associating constipation with other lifestyle factors has been problematic, at least in the published research. While constipation has often been related to sedentary lifestyles, no conclusive evidence exists for a positive effect of physical exercise as a treatment option for chronic constipation, though it is a common recommendation.[82,83] In one study of Japanese subjects, exercise (walking), as well as dietary fiber intake (from rice), were significantly associated with reduced symptoms of constipation.[84] Similarly, a group of middle-aged subjects from The Netherlands, all complaining of chronic constipation, were instructed to walk briskly for 30 minutes each day for 12 weeks[85] Compared to subjects given no instructions concerning physical activity, walkers realized a statistical decrease in constipation symptoms and objective measures of bowel transit time. Since this amount of walking generally fits with the recommendations we would give to sedentary patients (for cardiometabolic-related or other benefits), this seems to be a fitting place to begin with sedentary patients (even those not complaining of constipation).

Stress and HPA Axis Dysfunction

Regularity, by its very definition, implies a cyclical reliability. If civilized life can be accused of stripping the "regularity" from our foods, it can certainly be accused of stripping the regularity from our life. The lack of regular eating, sleeping, working, exercising and recreating is rampant in our culture. Meals are eaten in haste, and often at different times each day. Hormones intended to be rhythmic and regular are often irregular in many people due to chronic physical and emotional stress. Since the HPA axis and circadian control are closely tied together, both may be implicated in GI dysfunctions including constipation, especially IBS-C (see page 189 for IBS). For a complete discussion of the stress response, see our Standard Road map: *The Role of Stress and the HPA Axis in Chronic Disease Management* (Point Institute, 2015).

The Migrating Motor Complex

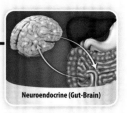

Neuroendocrine (Gut-Brain)

The migrating motor complex (MMC) is a cyclical "housekeeping" motility pattern that occurs in the stomach and small intestine during fasting in order to clear food or nonfood residue (e.g., secretions, microbes, debris) from the upper gastrointestinal tract.[1] Three distinct phases mark the MMC cycle:

Phase I
Marked by quiescence due to the absence of motility contractions, this phase is estimated to comprise about 55% of the total gastric cycle.[2]

Phase II
This phase is marked by irregular low-amplitude contractions that do not propel the luminal contents, and is estimated to comprise about 41% of the total gastric cycle.[2] GI "rumbling" may be associated with late Phase II, as the maximal sound index was estimated to occur at this time.[3]

Phase III
The most characteristic and active phase of the cycle, with a five to 10-minute period of intense, high-pressure, propagating contractions (marked by two to three contractions per minute for two minutes in the stomach, and 11 to 12 contractions per minute for three minutes in the duodenum).[2] Consequently, Phase III is also known as the activity front. This phase is estimated to contribute about 4% to the total gastric phase. Phase III contractions may begin in the stomach or the small intestine; it is estimated about 70% of measured spontaneous contractions in healthy subjects begin in the stomach antrum.[4] The contractions of Phase III act to "sweep" the luminal contents of either the stomach into the duodenum, or the contents of the small intestine into the colon. A secretory component of Phase III occurs in parallel with the increased motility, whereby Phase III in the stomach is associated with increased acid and pepsin secretion (and therefore a pH change), and Phase III in the small intestine is associated with intestinal and pancreatic secretion of water, bicarbonate and pancreatic enzymes.[5]

After the conclusion of Phase III, the cycle repeats again with Phase I until food is consumed; food consumption abolishes the MMC cycle.[2]

Note: Some describe a fourth phase marked by a transition of reduced motility back to the quiescence of Phase I.[6]

Dooley et al. performed early work studying the MMC across six healthy subjects, and found MMC cycling duration varied significantly across subjects (range 113 to 230 minutes, p<0.001), and within subjects (standard deviation range: 58 to 70 minutes).[4] Generally, it is noted that the duration of the MMC cycle is around 130 minutes.[2] The velocity of the MMC decreases as it migrates along the small intestine, and the complex generally dissipates and concludes at the distal ileum proximal to the ileocecal valve. The MMC has a circadian pattern, whereby reduced activity (propagation velocity and duration) of the cycle has been reported during sleep.[7]

Factors Affecting the Duration of the Cycle Include:
- **Origin of Phase III:** When MMC originates in the antrum, both Phase III and total MMC cycle duration was significantly longer than when Phase III was initiated in the duodenum.[8]
- **Stress:**[9] McRae et al. studied 11 healthy medical students in a stressful situation, seven subjects were found to be "responders" to stress as evaluated by an appreciable cardiovascular response to stress.[10] In these seven responders, the researchers observed that stress induced an inhibition of MMC during the first two hours of stress exposure.

The MMC is regulated under complex neurohormonal control by gastrointestinal hormones, the enteric nervous system, and the autonomic nervous system via the vagus nerve; the specific mechanisms are not well understood.[2] It appears that the gastric and the duodenal MMCs are controlled by different mechanisms. The best evidence for hormonal control of the gastric MMC is with the gut hormone motilin. Endogenous levels of motilin have been shown to fluctuate regularly with the gastric MMC phases, with the highest concentration of motilin present just before Phase III.[11] Also, exogenous administration of motilin has been shown to induce gastric Phase III contractions.[12] The precise mechanism surrounding motilin release has not yet been described.[2,6] Administration of the macrolide antibiotic erythromycin (a motilin receptor agonist) has been shown to induce phase III gastric motility.[13] Other hormones that may be involved in MMC regulation include ghrelin, somatostatin, pancreatic polypeptide, serotonin (5-hydroxytryptamine, 5-HT), and xenin.[2]

Dysfunction or absence of Phase III of the MMC is associated with bacterial overgrowth of the small intestine, and therefore is related to SIBO.[14,15] It has been shown that Phase III disruption in rats using opiates (i.e., morphine) caused duodenal bacterial overgrowth and translocation.[16] In a 2002 case-control study, Pimentel et al. found a reduced frequency (p < 0.000001) and duration of Phase III (p<0.001) in IBS subjects with a positive lactulose breath test (indicating SIBO) compared to healthy controls. Though SIBO eradication in a subgroup of these subjects improved motility compared to those with SIBO persistence (via positive breath test, p < 0.05), motility was still significantly less than that of the control group (p < 0.05).[17] Dysfunction of the MMC has been documented in other conditions, including IBS, functional dyspepsia,[18] diabetes,[19] obesity,[20] and anorexia nervosa.[1,2]

References

1. Deloose E, Tack J. Redefining the functional roles of the gastrointestinal migrating motor complex and motilin in small bacterial overgrowth and hunger signaling. *Am J Physiol Gastrointest Liver Physiol*. 2016 Feb 15;310(4):G228-33.
2. Deloose E, Janssen P, Depoortere I, Tack J. The migrating motor complex: control mechanisms and its role in health and disease. *Nat Rev Gastroenterol Hepatol*. 2012 Mar 27;9(5):271-85.
3. Tomomasa T, Morikawa A, Sandler RH, et al. Gastrointestinal sounds and migrating motor complex in fasted humans. *Am J Gastroenterol*. 1999 Feb;94(2):374-81.
4. Dooley CP, Di Lorenzo C, Valenzuela JE. Variability of migrating motor complex in humans. *Dig Dis Sci*. 1992 May;37(5):723-8.
5. Sjövall H. Meaningful or redundant complexity - mechanisms behind cyclic changes in gastroduodenal pH in the fasting state. *Acta Physiol (Oxf)*. 2011 Jan;201(1):127-31.
6. Takahashi T. Interdigestive migrating motor complex -its mechanism and clinical importance. *J Smooth Muscle Res*. 2013;49:99-111.
7. Gorard DA, Vesselinova-Jenkins CK, Libby GW, Farthing MJ. Migrating motor complex and sleep in health and irritable bowel syndrome. *Dig Dis Sci*. 1995 Nov;40(11):2383-9.
8. Luiking YC, van der Reijden AC, van Berge Henegouwen GP, Akkermans LM. Migrating motor complex cycle duration is determined by gastric or duodenal origin of phase III. *Am J Physiol*. 1998 Dec;275(6 Pt 1):G1246-51.
9. Plourde V. Stress-induced changes in the gastrointestinal motor system. *Can J Gastroenterol*. 1999 Mar;13 Suppl A:26A-31A.
10. McRae S, Younger K, Thompson DG, Wingate DL. Sustained mental stress alters human jejunal motor activity. *Gut*. 1982 May;23(5):404-9.
11. Vantrappen G, Janssens J, Peeters TL, Bloom SR, et al. Motilin and the interdigestive migrating motor complex in man. *Dig Dis Sci*. 1979 Jul;24(7):497-500.
12. Janssens J, Vantrappen G, Peeters TL. The activity front of the migrating motor complex of the human stomach but not of the small intestine is motilin-dependent. *Regul Pept*. 1983 Aug;6(4):363-9.
13. Coulie B, Tack J, Peeters T, Janssens J. Involvement of two different pathways in the motor effects of erythromycin on the gastric antrum in humans. *Gut*. 1998 Sep;43(3):395-400.
14. Husebye E. Gastrointestinal motility disorders and bacterial overgrowth. *J Intern Med*. 1995 Apr;237(4):419-27.
15. Husebye E. The patterns of small bowel motility: physiology and implications in organic disease and functional disorders. *Neurogastroenterol Motil*. 1999 Jun;11(3):141-61.
16. Nieuwenhuijs VB, Verheem A, van Duijvenbode-Beumer H, et al. The role of interdigestive small bowel motility in the regulation of gut microflora, bacterial overgrowth, and bacterial translocation in rats. *Ann Surg*. 1998 Aug;228(2):188-93.
17. Pimentel M, Soffer EE, Chow EJ, Kong Y, Lin HC. Lower frequency of MMC is found in IBS subjects with abnormal lactulose breath test, suggesting bacterial overgrowth. *Dig Dis Sci*. 2002 Dec;47(12):2639-43.
18. Wilmer A, Van Cutsem E, Andrioli A, et al. Ambulatory gastrojejunal manometry in severe motility-like dyspepsia: lack of correlation between dysmotility, symptoms, and gastric emptying. *Gut*. 1998 Feb;42(2):235-42.
19. Samsom M, Smout AJ. Abnormal gastric and small intestinal motor function in diabetes mellitus. *Dig Dis*. 1997 Jul-Oct;15(4-5):263-74.
20. Deloose E, Janssen P, Lannoo M, et al. Higher plasma motilin levels in obese patients decrease after Roux-en-Y gastric bypass surgery and regulate hunger. *Gut*. 2016 Jul;65(7):1110-8.

Elimination of Toxins and the Gut/Liver Axis

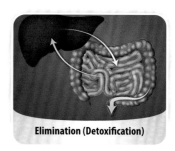

Elimination (Detoxification)

In the broader context of "elimination," one of the five core functions of the GI tract described in this Road map, it is important to expand this definition beyond simply the removal of undigested food particles, bile, and dead cells (mostly bacteria) that leave the GI tract in the feces. As we have already discussed above, regular bowel movements and adequate stool mass are indeed important foundations for the elimination process. However, they are also vital conduits for the elimination of other metabolites that cannot be easily visualized, as one might do by comparing each bowel movement with the Bristol Stool Scale (see page 52). In general, these metabolites result from a wide-range of enzymatic biotransformation reactions that are collectively termed "detoxification" since many of the pathways were first discovered in the context of toxin elimination.

While the detailed description of each of these reactions, enzymes, and the toxins or metabolites detoxified through these pathways is beyond the scope of this text, it is important for the clinician to understand the principles (and evidence) upon which a number of popular detoxification protocols are founded. As will become clear, since the laboratory measures of detoxification status or capacity are limited, the research on most detoxification protocols is also limited (beyond certain types of acute toxicity or metal toxicity). Also, since we believe the majority of the readers of this Road map need little convincing that chronic exposure to environmental toxins is harmful to human physiology (or have access to such information from other resources), we have included only a limited discussion of some of the more common toxins and their mechanisms, with some references for further study.

Common Exogenous Toxins

Bisphenol-A (BPA)

We start with BPA, not necessarily because it is the most harmful compound, but because of the attention it has received in the past decade or so.[86] Bisphenol-A (BPA) is a widespread plasticizer found in polycarbonate bottles (such as baby bottles and water bottles), thermal paper, food cans and in a variety of other common everyday products. Infants and children have often been the most highly exposed populations. Unsafe levels of BPA have been found in maternal and umbilical cord blood, placental tissue, amniotic fluid and the urine and tissues of infants. The international attention placed upon BPA lately has led to many changes in the manufacturing of certain items, especially those available for infants and children. It is quite common now to see "BPA-free" products being advertised, though this does not mean that they may not contain other potentially harmful BPA-analogs.[87,88]

As a toxin, BPA is classified as an endocrine disruptor, primarily affecting estrogen signaling.[89] This disruption of hormone signaling is thought to affect reproduction as well as a number of other hormone-related processes including changes in breast tissues leading to cancer and in adipocytes which may promote obesity.[90] Therefore, BPA is often considered to be "obesogenic" because of its ability to increase fat production and its association with obesity.[91] However, linking exposure to BPA (usually determined by urinary output of BPA metabolites) and specific outcomes is controversial since exposure limits are debated and there are many confounding factors.[92] Nonetheless, epidemiological studies (mostly cross-sectional) have clearly shown links between BPA exposure and increased risks for hypertension, diabetes and obesity, as well as a number of non-cardiometabolic outcomes.[93,94]

What is more alarming is the gathering research showing the epigenetic effects of BPA exposure in certain cells and tissues. Since we know that these effects can alter genetic expression, and even cell differentiation and development if exposure is early enough, epigenetic and toxicogenomics studies (animal and human cell culture studies) are leading the way to hint at how these compounds cause long-term human disease outcomes.[95,96,97,98] There is a silver lining in some of this research, however. The Agouti mouse model, one of the premier models for understanding epigenetic influence through DNA methylation, suggests that the hypomethylation induced by BPA can be ameliorated when the mouse is fed methyl-donors/inducers such as folate or genistein (from soy).[99] So, while it is true that avoidance of toxins is still the key to protecting ourselves and our future offspring, we may be able to decrease or even eliminate our susceptibility for these toxins by maintaining other healthy lifestyle inputs, especially through the diet.

Phthalates

Phthalates are compounds used in the production of most plastics to impart flexibility and resilience. They are also found in adhesives, glues, detergents, flooring, shower curtains, personal care products (shampoos, cosmetics, etc.), plastic bags, paints, pharmaceuticals, and building materials. Since they are not chemically bound to the plastics to which they are added, they are easily released into the environment and reach especially high levels in indoor air where they are thought to contribute to lung-related disorders.[100]

Like BPA, phthalates are known endocrine disruptors, and high doses have been shown to alter hormone levels and lead to birth defects, especially in the development of the male reproductive system.[101] In two national cross-sectional studies of men in the United States, an increased concentration of phthalate metabolites was significantly correlated with insulin resistance and abnormal obesity for which the authors suggest may be mediated through toxin-induced testosterone depletion.[102] In elderly women, specific phthalate metabolites have been recently linked to increased abdominal fat gain over just a two-year period.[103] Currently, there are limited epigenetic and toxicogenomic studies that have been conducted using phthalates; although it is likely that these two mechanisms are at least partly responsible for the outcomes related to phthalate exposure.[104,105]

Dioxins

Dioxins refer to the compound dioxin (2, 3, 7, 8-tetrachlorodibenzo para dioxin or TCDD) and related dioxin-like compounds. Dioxins are generally by-products of industrial processes and are commonly used in the paper bleaching process, chemical and pesticide manufacturing, and combustion activities (incineration of waste, burning of trash, etc.), though forest fires and volcanic activity account for some dioxin release. According to the World Health Organization, "Although formation of dioxins is local, environmental distribution is global. Dioxins are found throughout the world in the environment. The highest levels of these compounds are found in some soils, sediments and food, especially dairy products, meat, fish and shellfish. Very low levels are found in plants, water and air."[106] As far back as 1994, the United States EPA reported that dioxins at very low levels, are a probable carcinogen; but also reported that other effects of dioxins, such as their non-cancer causing effect (reproductive, sexual development, and immune system issues), may pose an even greater threat to human health. Epidemiological studies have shown that high levels of exposures to dioxins lead to an increased risk of tumors at all sites, though some have questioned the strength of these data.[107,108]

Dioxins are known to bind to a receptor known as the Aryl hydrocarbon receptor (AhR), which acts to alter the expression of a wide range of important genes managing cellular function and metabolism, including those expressing certain detoxification enzymes.[109] The alteration of these genes, and their subsequent proteins, can increase the level of toxic intermediates and is thought to be the main signaling pathway in dioxin-induced toxicity.[110] In cell culture, animal models and some human clinical studies, various phytonutrients have been shown to diminish some of the toxic effects related to AhR-receptor mediated dioxin interaction.[111,112,113,114,115]

Pesticides

Pesticides (such as DDT, DDE, DDD, aldrin, dieldrin, heptachlor, heptachlor epoxide, and PCBs) are not only sprayed onto growing foods (especially fruits and vegetables), but subsequently seep into soil and groundwater/drinking water, and the air.[116] Pesticides (such as chlorinated pesticides) have been found in the breast milk of women from all over the globe.[117] Furthermore, chlorinated pesticide residues have been detected in the adipose tissue from residents living in the United States, Europe, Israel, Africa and even Greenland.[118] Various studies have documented the presence of these pesticides in maternal umbilical cord blood.[119] Chronic exposure to pesticides has been shown to be associated with numerous adverse health effects from simple irritation of the skin and eyes[120] to hormonal disruption,[121] neurotoxicity[122] and potential carcinogenic activity.[123]

The use of pesticides and herbicides on foods generally considered "healthy" (i.e., fruits and vegetables) has led many consumers to purchase organically-grown produce, a trend that is growing rapidly in the United States and elsewhere. While there is great debate about the nutrient differences between organic and non-organic produce, it is clear that the consumption of organic produce significantly reduces a person's exposure to pesticides.[124]

Toxic Metals
Certain metals/minerals, often called "heavy metals" because of their molecular weight, are known to be toxic to humans. The most common of these are mercury, lead, cadmium, arsenic and aluminum. These metals are commonly found in cookware, dental fillings, antiperspirants, batteries, foods, fertilizers, water and tobacco smoke. Acute poisoning of high doses of heavy metals is well-documented and will not be discussed here. Instead, we will focus on the fact that chronic environmental exposures can cause heavy metals to accumulate in human tissues, which has been linked to the increased risk of various chronic diseases. The effect of metal compounds, both positive and negative, on human health has been called "metallomics."[125]

Mercury (Hg): Chronic exposure to mercury, arguably the most persistently harmful heavy metal in our environment, has been associated with numerous health consequences. The US population is primarily exposed to mercury in the form of methyl-mercury by consuming fish and seafood (which act as terminal bio-accumulators from the aquatic food chain). The guideline cautioning overconsumption of fish, including canned tuna, especially for pregnant women and children is designed to limit mercury ingestion during fetal and early child development. Other common sources of mercury are found in drugs for the eye, ear, nose, throat, and skin; in bleaching creams; as preservatives in cosmetics, toothpastes, lens solutions, vaccines, allergy test and immunotherapy solutions; in antiseptics, disinfectants, and contraceptives; in fungicides and herbicides; and in dental fillings and thermometers. While still very controversial, the preponderance of the evidence favors acceptance that mercury exposure, from multiple sources, is capable of causing some forms of autism.[126]

Several studies have shown a correlation between heart disease and chronic mercury exposure.[127] A study of European mercury miners found a significant relationship between mercury exposure and total mortality, hypertension, heart disease, renal disease, and stroke.[128] Mercury's mechanisms of toxicity are not well-understood, but appear to be based on four main processes leading to genotoxicity: the generation of free radicals and oxidative stress, action on microtubules (critical for the structural network within cells), altered DNA repair, and direct interaction with DNA molecules.[129] Mercury, in particular, depletes certain tissues of the important antioxidant glutathione, because it binds so tightly to other thiol groups. Substances that increase glutathione levels have been shown to reduce the toxic effects of mercury in some models, including N-acetyl cysteine, alpha-lipoic acid, lycopene, proanthocyanins, polyphenols from tea, quercetin and even garlic.[130,131,132,133,134,135] The minerals zinc and selenium have also been shown to inhibit some of the toxic effects of mercury.[136]

Lead (Pb): The harmful effects of lead have been well-known and documented for years. Even in antiquity, the mining and use of lead was known to cause toxicity. Today, while we have ceased using lead in gasoline and paint in the United States, according to the CDC, there are still approximately 24 million housing units (most built prior to 1978) with deteriorated lead paint and elevated levels of lead-contaminated house dust.[137] Likewise, environmental air, water and especially soil lead levels allow certain crops to concentrate lead levels (even many products that meet the definition of "organic"). Lead exposure is known to affect neuronal development and the function of a variety of organ systems including the cardiovascular, renal and reproductive systems.

The toxic mechanism of lead is not completely understood. Like mercury, lead also is a strong oxidant which depletes cell antioxidants, especially thiols like glutathione. Lead also interferes with calcium function and reduces nitric oxide signaling.[138,139] Since the depletion of antioxidants appears to be critical for the chronic effects caused by lead toxicity, some evidence suggests that antioxidants may be able to diminish the negative effects of lead toxicity.[140,141] Chelating agents, however, are the method of choice for therapeutic reduction of body lead levels (as it is also with mercury).[142,143]

Other Toxic Metals:

There are other toxic metals to consider, including **arsenic (As), cadmium (Cd), and aluminum (Al)**. Arsenic is a particularly toxic metal, and can still be found in drinking water in some locations in the United States. Arsenic can also be found in older "green-treated" lumber. Common sources of cadmium in the US include fossil fuel combustion, phosphate fertilizers, municipal solid waste incineration, and in iron, steel and cement production. However, smoking is the most important single source of cadmium exposure in the general population. While arsenic effectively inhibits cells from producing ATP, cadmium exerts its toxic effect by binding to the endoplasmic reticulum and mimicking estrogen.[144,145] Chronic exposure to arsenic manifests in many ways, but primarily through the production of reactive oxygen species, which places a burden on the antioxidant reserve of the cells and tissues. Links to metabolic diseases (especially insulin resistance and type 2 diabetes), as well as some cancers, are the most frequently cited with chronic low-dose arsenic exposure.[146,147,148]

The issue of aluminum is a bit more complex. Research appears to clearly link Al neurotoxicity with the risk for Alzheimer's disease.[149] A debate exists about the cause-effect relationship between Al exposure and Alzheimer's disease progression. Some studies, such as the PAQUID cohort, define aluminum exposure as a risk factor for Alzheimer's disease, and cell culture studies have found neuritic plaques contain increased levels of aluminum.[150,151] Other studies have shown increased population risks for Alzheimer's disease with elevated aluminum concentrations in public drinking water supplies.[152] Although the data are incomplete, an increasing number of researchers have expressed concern that aluminum found in certain deodorants may increase the risk of breast cancer, and have implicated such sources of aluminum as a factor in Alzheimer's disease.[153,154]

Managing the Exposome

Two related fields of study, both owing to the emerging science of genetics and genomics, are beginning to help us discover the role toxins play in human health and disease. The first is toxicogenetics, which describes how the genetic differences between certain individuals allow for varying susceptibility to different toxins.[155] Since there are hundreds of different enzymes involved in our detoxification pathways, many individuals carry gene variants (polymorphisms) that allow for more efficient conversion and removal of toxins than others. Those individuals with slower detoxification pathways for a given toxin will show signs of toxicity at much lower doses than those with normal detoxification capacity. These differences often complicate "cause-and-effect" studies in large populations that carry over into the clinic. That is, just because a large epidemiological trial does not find a statistically significant relationship between exposure to a particular toxin and a particular health outcome (the average of all genetic variants), does not mean that such a relationship does not exist in the genetically-susceptible patient.

The second field of study is based on how cells respond to the exposure to toxins as a consequence of both immediate and lifetime exposures. In essence, which genes, proteins and metabolites are altered under the influence of various toxins? The term toxicogenomics is used to describe these effects. Just as nutrigenomics tells us what genes are activated or repressed after the consumption of a nutrient, so toxicogenomic studies tell us what genes are activated or repressed when cells are exposed to a particular toxin. Another related term, the "exposome," has emerged to describe the total lifetime exposure to environmental agents which affect genomics (the mixed term for this is "exposomics").[156,157]

The reason this is so important, and why so many new terms need to be created, is that the impact of toxins is both cumulative (over time) and synergistic (between different substances), requiring the overlapping of numerous disciplines. High doses of some toxins over a very short period of time may have one type of negative outcome (usually well-understood acute toxicity syndromes), while smaller doses over a long period of time may have quite a different set of negative outcomes (difficult to study, chronic effects of long-term low exposures). Likewise, small doses of a particular toxin in a person with a strong detoxification capacity may have no discernible negative outcomes at all, while the same or even lower dose in another person might lead to a wide range of abnormalities which often go unexplained. This is why many clinicians consider detoxification protocols, those protocols designed to periodically increase the body's detoxification processes, to be part of a long-term strategy to maintain health in the modern world.

Detoxification (Biotransformation) Pathways: The Basics

The majority of the toxins that accumulate without rapid excretion are lipid-soluble compounds. In order for these toxins to be safely and efficiently removed from the body, they need to be transformed (i.e., biotransformation) into water-soluble compounds and eliminated via the bile or urine. In humans, this critical function occurs mostly in the liver, through a two-step process involving Phase I and II detoxification pathways (Figure 15). When these pathways are functioning sub-optimally, fat-soluble toxins pass through the liver unmodified or partially modified, and are deposited in various tissues (mostly adipocytes). A general discussion of these pathways is described below and in Figure 15.

Phase I (Bioactivation): The Phase I detoxification system, composed mostly of the cytochrome P450 enzyme system, contributes to the metabolism of a variety of exogenous and endogenous compounds such as pharmaceuticals, carcinogens, steroids and eicosanoids. This system is composed of a group of more than 50 enzymes. A vast amount of knowledge of the substrates, cofactors and genomic activation of Phase I detoxification enzymes in the liver has been derived from pharmacokinetic studies, the study of drug metabolism. While a bit of an oversimplification, the purpose of the Phase I enzymes is to form a reactive intermediate that is then ready for a Phase II enzymatic reaction. As is often the case, the intermediate metabolite may actually be more toxic, though it is rarely available for circulation due to the tight coupling of the Phase I and Phase II systems within the liver.

Phase I cytochrome P450 enzyme activities include oxidation, reduction, hydrolysis, hydration, and dehalogenation reactions (see Figure 15). Of these, the most well-known is oxidation, which has been explored in numerous pharmacokinetic studies of certain drugs. In this pathway, a cytochrome P450 enzyme uses oxygen and NADH (as a cofactor) to add a hydroxyl group to the lipid-soluble toxin. As an illustration, estrogens can be metabolized by one of three different CYP450 enzyme pathways, which differ in the reactive intermediate that is generated prior to phase II conjugation. These different

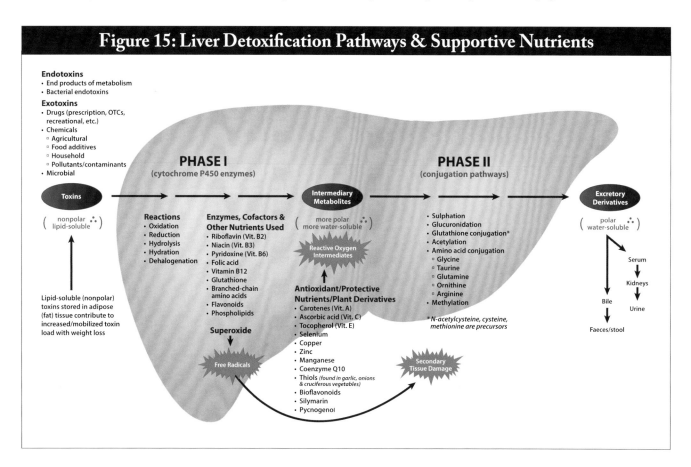

Figure 15: Liver Detoxification Pathways & Supportive Nutrients

intermediates involve hydroxylation at different sites of the estrogen molecule (positions 2, 4 or 16), performed by different cytochrome P450 enzymes (CYP 1A1, 1B1 and 2C/3A4-respectively); differences that have been shown to confer relatively different estrogenic effects in various tissues.[158]

All three estrogen molecules formed from Phase I (e.g., 2-OH, 4-OH, and 16-OH estrogens) must be further detoxified by Phase II reactions, prior to removal from the body. This occurs mainly through the methylation, sulfation and glucuronidation pathways (discussed in greater detail below). If these intermediate metabolites are not further metabolized by the Phase II enzymes (or are deconjugated by colonic bacterial enzymes and recirculated), they may have the potential to cause damage to proteins, DNA and RNA, leading to carcinogenesis.

Table 6: PHASE I ENZYMES	
CYP1A & B	Polycyclic Hydrocarbons, Nitrosoamines
CYP2A-H	Drugs, Alcohol, Steroids
CYP3A	Drugs, Antibiotics, Flavonoids
CYP4	⍵-oxidation Fatty Acids
CYP5	Thromboxane Synthase
CYP7A	7α-Hydroxylase, Bile Acids
CYP8A & B	Prostacyclin Synthase, Bile Acids
* CYP11A & B	Cholesterol Side-chain Cleavage, Aldosterone Synthesis
CYP51	Cholesterol Biosynthesis, 14-Demethylase
* CYP40	Vitamin D3 - 1α-Hydroxylase
* CYP27	Bile Acid Synthesis
CYP26	Retinoic Acid Hydroxylase
* CYP24	Vitamin D Degradation
CYP21	Progesterone 21-Hydroxylase
CYP19	Estrogen Biosynthesis, Aromatase
CYP17	Steroid 17α-Hydroxylase, Steroid C17/21 Lyase

Mitochondrial Enzyme

Phase II (Conjugation): The main goal of Phase II detoxification pathways is to conjugate, or attach, specific molecules to the intermediate metabolite formed from Phase I, so it can be excreted through the urine or bile as a water soluble non-toxic substance. Specifically, there are six Phase II conjugation pathways.[159,160] Reactions that occur in these pathways all rely on specific nutrient cofactors that must be replenished either through the diet or nutritional supplementation. In addition, large amounts of energy (i.e., ATP) are used in this process and must be replenished for optimal detoxification function.

The Six Phase II Detoxification Pathways:
- **Sulfation**: Sulfation is the conjugation of toxins with sulfur-containing compounds. Neurotransmitters, steroid hormones (such as cortisol), certain pharmaceuticals (such as acetaminophen), food additives, and many xenobiotic and phenolic compounds utilize this pathway as a primary route of detoxification.

- **Glucuronidation**: The UDP-glucuronosyltransferase (UGT) enzyme plays a critical role in this pathway. The reaction catalyzed by the UGT enzyme involves the conjugation of glucuronic acid to xenobiotics. This pathway is considered an important detoxification mechanism when sulfation or glycination activity is impaired or saturated, and is upregulated in obese patients.[161] In particular, glucuronidation helps to detoxify certain medications (aspirin), food additives (benzoates), preservatives, reproductive and adrenal hormones (esp. estrogen), and bilirubin. It is also known that this reaction can be reversed by beta-glucuronidase enzyme activity by certain species of the gut microbiota. It is speculated that increased beta-glucuronidase activity may be partly responsible for the development of estrogen-dominant conditions such as fibrocystic breast disease, breast cancer, and prostate cancer, though the evidence for such influence is limited.

- **Glutathione conjugation**: The attachment of glutathione to toxins helps to detoxify and eliminate many harmful electrophilic compounds (either xenobiotics or their metabolites). This conjugation step is mediated by the enzyme glutathione transferase (GST). Glutathione is an important nutrient with powerful antioxidant and detoxification properties. Since glutathione is composed of the amino acids cysteine, glutamic acid and glycine, it is important that these nutrients are in adequate supply.

- **Acetylation**: The conjugation of acetyl Co-A to toxins occurs via the N-acetyl transferase enzymes. This, in turn, helps to detoxify xenobiotics, such as tobacco smoke. Individuals with slow acetylation activity have a higher toxic burden, while rapid acetylators add acetyl groups rapidly, which may result in increased levels of toxic intermediate metabolites. Both slow and rapid acetylators are at increased risk for toxic overload if they are exposed to environmental toxins. While not much is known about how to directly improve the detoxification activity of this system, it is known that acetylation is dependent on thiamin, pantothenic acid and vitamin C.

- **Amino acid conjugation**: Conjugation of toxins to amino acids such as glycine, taurine, glutamine, arginine, and ornithine are additional means to prepare intermediate metabolites for excretion. Of these amino acids, glycine is the most common. In normal adults, there is a wide range in the measures of activity through the glycine conjugation pathways due to known genetic variation of the enzymes catalyzing these reactions and bioavailability of glycine in the liver.

- **Methylation**: Methylation consists of conjugating methyl groups to active intermediates through one of several methyl transferase enzymes. Magnesium, SAMe, vitamin B12, folates and choline are required as co-factors in this pathway.

Supporting Detoxification: Principles and Protocols

Even in the absence of overt signs and symptoms from harmful exogenous toxins, the human body is tasked with enormous biochemical and physiological challenges. When we consider the need to perform these functions while buffering and neutralizing a vast amount of toxins encountered within the environment, the cells performing these important functions are quickly challenged. Unfortunately, the combined burden of our environment, diet, lifestyle, and metabolic processes upon these processes each day can overwhelm the detoxification capacity of many individuals, leading to a wide range of dysfunctions. Additionally, nutritional deficiencies can reduce the liver's capacity to transform and eliminate toxins, exacerbating nutrigenomic and toxicogenomic susceptibilities.

The Clinician's Dilemma
Patients experiencing elevated levels of toxic burden often present with a complex clinical picture. Ironically, these patients will seldom present with a history of overt toxic exposure, and will experience symptoms that manifest from different organ systems. For the conventionally trained clinician, toxin exposure can be difficult to detect since most conventional laboratory tests are designed to discover extreme measures of toxin exposure. For this reason, many clinicians overlook the possibility of toxic burden unless patients present with overt signs of toxicity, or have a specific health history involving a known toxic environment. Currently, the use of detoxification therapy and testing (among conventional medical practitioners) is largely limited to patients who have drug and/or alcohol dependency. Once a clinician understands how even small accumulation of toxins can burden the health of patients in diverse ways, the benefit of removing these toxins will increase in priority. In addition, several specialized laboratories now offer a variety of testing options that can help determine levels of a particular stored toxin (such as solvents, pesticides, heavy metals, etc.).

While any subject with a chronic disease is a candidate for toxin exposure testing and detoxification, certain patients are commonly considered to have a higher likelihood of toxic burden or sensitivity. Such patients may present with the following "cardinal" signs and symptoms related to toxicity:
- Chronic fatigue syndrome
- Multiple chemical sensitivities
- Fibromyalgia and similar pain-type syndromes
- Immune disorders
- Neuropsychiatric disorders and cognitive disturbances

Conditions or Lifestyles That May Benefit from Detoxification
- **Exposure to tobacco products, alcohol, caffeine, pharmaceutical medications and industrial chemicals:** Patients who are frequently exposed to these substances are at an increased risk for an imbalanced Phase I/Phase II liver detoxification. These substances can induce or up-regulate Phase I liver detoxification, causing an inability for Phase II pathways to conjugate and neutralize the increase in intermediary metabolites formed from Phase I pathways. The activated intermediates and free radicals react with and damage cellular proteins, RNA, and DNA, leading to poor cell signaling.

- **Obesity/overweight:** Since most exogenous (and some endogenous) toxins are fat-soluble, the volume of fat mass has been related (either as a cause or effect) of toxic burden. A buildup of toxins is also commonly thought to affect a patient's ability to lose more weight after shedding a few pounds due to their obesogenic effects.[162] Patients with a higher fat mass have increased toxin-storage capacity. The role of toxic burden and detoxification should be considered as a helpful adjunct therapy for patients undergoing fat mass or weight loss therapies.

- **Hormone-related imbalances:** Patients who have conditions with links to estrogen-dominance (prostate cancer, fibrocystic breast disease, breast cancer, etc.) or other types of hormonal imbalances may benefit from a protocol that promotes detoxification capacity, given that all hormones must be properly detoxified through the liver. This is also true of subjects using hormone therapies of any kind, including pharmaceutical estrogens or progestins, bio-identical hormone therapies, oral contraceptives and corticosteroids.

- **Increased measures of intestinal permeability:** When the intestinal tract becomes permeable to bacterial toxins or other compounds that require detoxification, this additional burden can tax the liver's capacity to metabolize the total toxic burden. Endotoxemia appears to reduce the activity of many Phase 1 enzymes and depletes liver glutathione.[163,164,165] This might include subjects with food allergies, dysbiosis, celiac disease, IBD or IBS.[166,167]

- **Increased HPA axis stress:** The HPA axis can trigger alterations in GI function, including changes in gut permeability. Some of these HPA axis-induced permeability changes can lead to endotoxemia.[168] In addition, HPA axis stress is known to alter steroid metabolism, requiring additional detoxification capacity.

- **Digestion or elimination issues:** Maldigestion or absorption issues can often result in lower nutrient availability. As a result, these patients may not have adequate levels of the vitamins, minerals and other nutrients that are required cofactors needed for optimal liver detoxification.

Avoidance/Removal: The Starting Point for All
While not technically a detoxification therapy, it is clear that intentionally avoiding or limiting toxin exposure should be a high priority in any subject that wants to maintain their long-term health. Using a detailed patient history, a comprehensive physical exam and

laboratory testing, clinicians should help to discover potential sources of toxin exposure in their patients. As many clinicians know, low levels of exposure that may be discovered via laboratory analysis of hair, urine or other tissues (e.g., fat biopsy) often requires some lengthy detective work and historical relationship to symptom onset. In the case of immunogenic toxins such as allergens, this may require a combination of allergy testing and elimination/rotation diets. Once the toxin or toxins have been identified, patients should work diligently to avoid exposure as quickly as possible. The removal of toxins and allergens is a critical first step in the 4R program, commonly taught as a foundational way to treat complex GI-related dysfunctions (see page 22 for more details on the 4R program).

Testing a Patient's Detoxification Capacity

Testing Phase I and II liver detoxification activity
One of the only ways to evaluate an individual's ability to detoxify both endogenous and exogenous toxins is by provocation. Certain laboratories provide test kits intended to measure efficiency of these pathways by having the subject ingest specific amounts of compounds with very predictable detoxification outcomes. For example, caffeine detoxification/clearance can be calculated following the ingestion of a caffeine caplet (usually 150 to 300 mg), in the morning, followed by specimens collected at various time points afterward (serum, urine, saliva).[169] Low caffeine clearance can indicate reduced function of the Phase I CYP450 enzyme activity (CYP1A2 particularly), either caused by genetic factors or other lifestyle factors. Conversely, a high caffeine clearance can reflect an excessive CYP450 enzyme induction due to high toxin exposure. High clearance also implies greater production of free radicals. Other tests, such as the erythromycin breath test (CYP3A4/midazolam clearance) or antipyrine clearance test (general CYP-P450/predominant CYP3A4) have been used to test the activities of various CYP450 enzymes.[170,171]

Several other compounds, such as aspirin or acetaminophen can be used to test the activity of Phase II conjugation reactions. Usually aspirin or acetaminophen is ingested in the evening, and the metabolic by-products from detoxification are assessed in a 10-hour overnight urine specimen. The challenge dose may consist of two capsules of aspirin (650 mg total) or two capsules of acetaminophen (650 mg total). If low levels of acetaminophen or salicylate conjugates (such as acetaminophen sulfate or salicyluric acid) are present, it may indicate inadequate Phase II conjugation activity. This may be due to the depletion of particular amino acids or nutrient cofactors used in the reactions. Some tests include several different compounds for testing multiple pathways.

Other available tests

There are other assays that some laboratories may include and interpret as measuring one or more aspects of detoxification. Some of these tests may include:

- **Glutathione levels:** If low, this represents reduced glutathione reserve available for removal of toxic intermediates, generation of sulfate and cysteine reserves, and antioxidant activity.

- **Stool Metabolites:** These tests may include stool microbial analysis (for yeast and parasites), markers of digestive efficiency, metabolites of healthy gut microbes and markers of immune function. This is an important test to identify any GI-related condition that can contribute to an increased toxic load. (for discussion of CSA/CDSA™, see page 51).

- **Glutathione peroxidase:** If low, this implies inadequate defense against accumulation of oxidized lipids

in cell membranes. Low levels may be found in those with Down syndrome, Alzheimer's dementia and beta-thalassemia minor, and may indicate insufficient nutrient cofactors.

- **Genetic polymorphisms:** Several labs now provide genetic testing that evaluates single nucleotide polymorphisms (SNPs) within the CYP450 enzyme genes or other genes related to detoxification. While this information can be very helpful in predicting or explaining a toxic sensitivity in a given individual, genetic information alone should not be used to treat a patient with no phenotypic symptoms.

- **Beta glucuronidase activity:** As mentioned previously, the glucuronidation pathway in Phase II conjugates glucuronic acid with estrogen (or drugs and carcinogens). However, elevated levels of beta glucuronidase activity in the gut (microbiota) facilitates the cleavage of the glucuronide moiety from the "toxin," allowing the toxin to be reabsorbed via the enterohepatic circulation as a more reactive compound. This test may be available as part of some comprehensive stool analyses.

- **Provoked or passive measures of toxins in bodily fluids, tissue biopsies, or hair:** These types of tests can be useful for measuring pesticides, solvents, industrial chemicals, household chemicals, and heavy metals.

Enhancing the Detoxification Process

Detoxification protocols are designed to help an individual minimize their exposure to toxins and immunologically reactive agents, while also attempting to increase access to agents that increase their detoxification capacity.

The following are commonly part of a comprehensive detoxification protocol (see more details in Tables on pages 77-80):

- **Providing conjugation precursors:** This may include the increased intake of amino acids needed for conjugation (glycine, taurine, glutamine, arginine, and ornithine), sulfur groups (N-acetyl cysteine, lipoic acid, methionine, cysteine) or methyl groups (SAMe, folates, choline).

- **Increasing glutathione levels:** This can be accomplished quite well by the use of NAC, lipoic acid and the availability of the amino acids glycine, glutamic acid and cysteine. Since glutathione is used directly in Phase II detoxification and as a key cellular antioxidant, the importance of glutathione cannot be overemphasized.

- **Providing co-factors:** As Figure 15 shows, there are a number of known co-factors for both the Phase I and Phase II detoxification enzymes, most of which are familiar vitamins and minerals. It is critical to ensure subjects have a robust reserve of these nutrients to ensure no detoxification enzyme has diminished activity due to depletion in an available cofactor.

- **Providing genomic enhancers of detoxification:** As we will outline further below, there are many compounds in nature known to enhance the process of detoxification by upregulating various detoxification enzyme genes. These can be helpful when used appropriately to enhance the detoxification process, though some (e.g., grapefruit juice) are also problematic when combined with pharmaceutical drugs as the activation of detoxification can reduce the serum levels of certain drugs leading to reduced efficacy of those drugs.

- **Building antioxidant reserve:** Since a tremendous amount of oxygen radicals are formed during the process of detoxification, it is important that subjects be given compounds to help quench these free radicals. These can be classic redox antioxidants (e.g., vitamin C, E), co-factors for enzyme antioxidants (e.g., Se, Mn), glutathione precursors, and genomic antioxidants (e.g., Nrf2-modulators, see page 75).

- **Supporting cellular energy:** The process of detoxification is considered one the most energy-intense activities of the body; especially when faced with constant toxic burden. The process of detoxification should be accompanied with available ingredients that help to sustain efficient ATP production by the mitochondria. This might include supplementation with ingredients such as carnitine, acetyl-L-carnitine, lipoic acid, N-acetyl cysteine, or CoQ-10.

- **Ensuring removal (binding/moving fat and fecal matter/fiber, urine/water):** It is always important to ensure toxic metabolites moved into the bowels or kidney are actually removed from the body. Detoxification protocols will usually include gentle laxatives and bile-sequestering fibers to ensure removal of feces with minimal enterohepatic recirculation of bile/fat as well as water to ensure the dilution of toxins and the excretion through the urine. Also, bile-stimulating herbs (choleretics/cholagogues) may also be helpful. These might include extracts of milk thistle seed, dandelion root or artichoke leaf (see page 42 for more details).

- **Ensuring a healthy microbiota:** See page 74 for role of gut microbiota and detoxification and page 104 for ways to support microbiome.

Comprehensive Detoxification Protocols (The Detox Kit Approach)

Clinicians who have been practicing within the functional medicine/integrative medicine area for some time are aware that numerous detoxification protocols (kits) are available through practitioner channel supplement suppliers and many direct-to-consumer supplement manufacturers. Clinicians should evaluate these programs, realizing some are designed on sound detoxification principles with ingredients designed (and dosed) to carry out those ends, while other products are simply laxative ingredients with slick marketing.

Most of these programs are designed to be accomplished in seven to 28 days and are commonly recommended to patients on an annual or even biannual basis. They include instructions for specific dietary restrictions to be maintained throughout the length of the program and usually include a ready-to-mix blend of ingredients in a protein-base, along with capsules or tablets to provide additional vitamins, minerals and phytonutrients to enhance the detoxification process and provide necessary co-factors.

Detox Diets and Fasting

At minimum, well-designed detoxification programs will instruct subjects to avoid common allergens and avoid all processed foods, though some recommend a more comprehensive elimination diet. In many cases, the use of an elimination diet as part of a detoxification protocol can be used by the clinician as an empirical way to test sensitivity to various foods or food groups. This can be accomplished when the patient abstains from various food groups (e.g., dairy, soy, eggs, etc.) for approximately two weeks before adding these foods back one category at a time (with several days separating the reintroduction of food categories). Reactions to the reintroduced foods can then be noted as a potential allergy or insensitivity that can be followed with additional testing or a recommendation for further abstinence.

The role of fasting, in general, or in the context of detoxification is controversial. While it is almost universally agreed that subjects with blood sugar control issues, extremely poor nutrition or previous history of fainting when fasting should avoid fasting during a detoxification protocol, many clinicians believe a fast or modified fast can be a helpful way to quickly reduce and control the number of compounds the intestines and liver need to absorb and metabolize.

For the most part, these protocols often include a ready-to-mix product that provides several hundred calories and is intended to be consumed two or more times per day for the first few days before adding back allowable foods for the rest of the protocol. Hence, many protocols initiate their detoxification process with a modified/low calorie fast.

Some clinicians believe that since detoxification is an intense energy-requiring process, fasting is contraindicated during a detoxification protocol. Others believe fasting (or in this case, modified fasting) can be helpful to reduce the input of potential toxins that can offset the burden of low calorie intake. Short-term fasting is known to increase detoxification through some Phase I pathways, while slowing others.[172] Needless to say, there are no well-designed studies to test the specific merits of calorie-reduction during the first days of a detoxification protocol and, therefore, the recommendation of fasting should be done based on the experience of the clinician and desire of the patient.

Phase II Support First

Clinicians should evaluate their recommended protocols to ensure they are designed to promote Phase II detoxification and elimination (water, fiber, etc.) in the initial stages of the protocol, prior to aggressive stimulation of Phase I detoxification. In many cases, ingredients are known to promote both enzyme systems, so some crossover is inevitable. The obvious reason for this step-wise process is to ensure there is adequate conjugation capacity within the Phase II system prior to up-regulating the conversion of toxins to their reactive intermediate metabolites.

Detoxification and the Gut Microbiota

For many years, the role of detoxification, as with much of human physiology in general, was understood with little regard to the gut microbiota. However, the past few decades have radically altered our understanding of the host-microbiome relationship, which includes the role of detoxification (see pages 85-113 for a complete discussion of the gut microbiome). However, research performed in germ-free animals and subjects given antibiotics have revealed the gut microbiota is critically involved in the biotransformation of a wide range of endogenous and exogenous bioactive compounds. In fact, the activation or de-activation of many compounds (drugs, phytochemicals, bile acids, conjugated compounds from liver detoxification, etc.) depends on the unique metabolic capacity of specific species of bacteria in the gut, the absence of which can alter (for good or bad) important health outcomes.[173,174,175,176]

Though we do cover some of the ramifications of these metabolic functions in the next section of this Standard Road map, the information detailing these microbial enzymes and their specific metabolic outcomes is beyond the scope of this project, and is not yet ready to be leveraged in the clinic. Nonetheless, clinicians should be aware that the gut microbiome is significantly involved in the ability to utilize many phytonutrients, synthesize secondary bile acids, activate certain drugs and help detoxify a host of endogenous and exogenous toxins. The use of antibiotics can severely alter these metabolic functions, leaving the patient at a deficit in these critical areas. Efficacy of some therapies may depend on a healthy, balanced gut microbiome.

Unfortunately, there is not enough evidence to tell the clinician which species or which enzymatic activities are necessary to create an ideal microbiome for these functions, and therefore no specific therapeutic recommendation that can be given at this time. Clinicians should consider gut dysbiosis a risk factor for poor detoxification and use appropriate means to help bring the gut microbiome into balance (see recommendations on page 104).

Nrf2 Activation: A Key Regulator of Detoxification

The Nrf2 pathway is one of the important genomic regulators protecting the cell from environmental stressors and managing the antioxidant and detoxification processes within many cells.[1] Like most complex genomic regulatory systems, Nrf2 (Nuclear factor erythroid 2-related factor 2) is sequestered in the cytoplasm until it is able to translocate into the nucleus, where it forms a heterodimer with MAF (another transcription factor) and binds to the promoter region of genes with an antioxidant response element (ARE) sequence. Nrf2 regulates important genes such as heme-oxygenase 1(HO-1), glutathione S-transferase (GST), glutathione reductase (GR), glutamate-cysteine ligase subunits (GCLc and GCLm), NAD(P)H quinone oxidoreductase-1 (NQO1), and thioredoxins (TrxR1), among others.[2,3] Nrf2 stays sequestered in the cytoplasm by its interaction with the Keap1 protein complex (Keap1-Kelch-like ECH-associated protein 1). When an oxidative stressor or electrophile interacts with the Keap1-Nrf2 complex, it allows for the release and subsequent nuclear accumulation of Nrf2 through a complex process of ubiquitination-inhibition, thus triggering an anti-stress response by the cell.[4] In some circumstances, Nrf2-activation can mitigate some of the effects of the NF-κb inflammatory signaling pathway.[5]

There has been a wealth of research looking at agents (naturally occurring and synthetic) that can upregulate this global antioxidant and detoxification

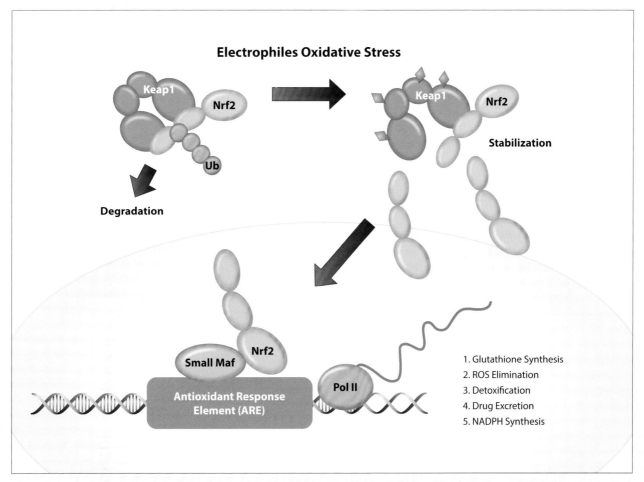

The Keap1–Nrf2 system. Under normal conditions, Nrf2 is constantly ubiquitinated through Keap1 and degraded in the proteasome. Following exposure to electrophiles or oxidative stress, Keap1 is inactivated. Stabilized Nrf2 accumulates in the nucleus and activates many cytoprotective genes. Ub, ubiquitin. Figure modified from Mitsuishi et al.[6]

system. Sulforaphane (a glucosinolate compound found in some cruciferous vegetables like broccoli) is one of the most commonly cited natural Nrf2 activators, though there are many others shown to have similar effects on Nrf2-induced enzymatic activities and metabolites. There are well over 100 different nutrients, phytonutrients, and related dietary supplement ingredients thought to function as antioxidants or detoxification enhancing agents, at least in part, because of their ability to up-regulate Nrf2 activation. A small portion of these have been confirmed to alter such responses when consumed at reasonable oral doses in human or animals and are listed below[7]:

- Cruciferous glucosinolates (broccoli, Brussels sprouts, etc.)[8,9,10]
- Sulforaphane (as a concentrate)[11,12]
- Curcuminoids (Turmeric), Quercetin[13,14,15,16]
- Resveratrol[17,18]
- Phenethyl isothiocyanate (PEITC, from watercress)[19,20]
- Diallyl sulfide (garlic)[21,22]

The list of natural compounds shown to modulate Nrf2 pathways or ARE-containing genes is too numerous to list in this text,[7,23] though common ingredients for which the reader might be familiar include all those listed above and also, baicalein (*Scutellaria baicalensis*), catechins (tea, cocoa), genistein (soy), carnosol and carnosic acid (*Rosmarinus officinalis*), andrographolide (*Andrographis paniculata*), ginsenoside Rb1 (*Panax ginseng*), schisandrin B (*Schisandra chinensis*), quercetin and related flavonoids, indole-3-carbinol (I3C) and diindolylmethane (DIM), hydroxytyrosol (*Olea europaea*-olive), Pterostilbene, Xanthohumol (*Humulus lupulus*), berberine, [6]-gingerol (*Zingiber officinale*), vitamin D,[24] and even exercise (though it decreases with age).[25]

Dose recommendations for these ingredients for detoxification is not possible, though it is likely there is a dose-response and even a dose at which some inhibition of Nrf2 activation occurs. This information is intended to strengthen the recommendation to encounter a wide range of phytonutrients in the diet and consider some of these (low-dose, but persistent intake) to combat the constant low-dose, but persistent intake of environmental toxins.

References

1. Suzuki T, Yamamoto M. Molecular basis of the Keap1-Nrf2 system. *Free Radic Biol Med*. 2015 Nov;88(Pt B):93-100.
2. Buendia I, Michalska P, Navarro E, et al. Nrf2-ARE pathway: An emerging target against oxidative stress and neuroinflammation in neurodegenerative diseases. *Pharmacol Ther*. 2016 Jan;157:84-104.
3. Lu SC. Glutathione synthesis. *Biochim Biophys Acta*. 2013 May;1830(5):3143-53.
4. Huang Y, Li W1, Su ZY, Kong AN. The complexity of the Nrf2 pathway: beyond the antioxidant response. *J Nutr Biochem*. 2015 Dec;26(12):1401-13.
5. Li W, Khor TO, Xu C, Shen G, Jeong WS, Yu S, Kong AN. Activation of Nrf2-antioxidant signaling attenuates NFkappaB-inflammatory response and elicits apoptosis. *Biochem Pharmacol*. 2008 Dec 1;76(11):1485-9.
6. Mitsuishi Y, Motohashi H, Yamamoto M. The Keap1-Nrf2 system in cancers: stress response and anabolic metabolism. *Front Oncol*. 2012 Dec 26;2:200.
7. Qin S, Hou DX. Multiple regulations of Keap1/Nrf2 system by dietary phytochemicals. *Mol Nutr Food Res*. 2016 Aug;60(8):1731-55.
8. Dinkova-Kostova AT, Kostov RV. Glucosinolates and isothiocyanates in health and disease. *Trends Mol Med*. 2012 Jun;18(6):337-47.
9. Yang L, Palliyaguru DL, Kensler TW. Frugal chemoprevention: targeting Nrf2 with foods rich in sulforaphane. *Semin Oncol*. 2016 Feb;43(1):146-53.
10. Gasper AV, Al-Janobi A, Smith JA, et al. Glutathione S-transferase M1 polymorphism and metabolism of sulforaphane from standard and high-glucosinolate broccoli. *Am J Clin Nutr*. 2005 Dec;82(6):1283-91.
11. Kensler TW, Egner PA, Agyeman AS, et al. Keap1-nrf2 signaling: a target for cancer prevention by sulforaphane. *Top Curr Chem*. 2013;329:163-77.
12. Houghton CA, Fassett RG, Coombes JS. Sulforaphane and Other Nutrigenomic Nrf2 Activators: Can the Clinician's Expectation Be Matched by the Reality? *Oxid Med Cell Longev*. 2016;2016:7857186.
13. Scapagnini G, Vasto S, Abraham NG, Caruso C, Zella D, Fabio G. Modulation of Nrf2/ARE pathway by food polyphenols: a nutritional neuroprotective strategy for cognitive and neurodegenerative disorders. *Mol Neurobiol*. 2011 Oct;44(2):192-201.
14. Shehzad A, Ha T, Subhan F, Lee YS. New mechanisms and the anti-inflammatory role of curcumin in obesity and obesity-related metabolic diseases. *Eur J Nutr*. 2011 Apr;50(3):151-61.
15. Shoskes D, Lapierre C, Cruz-Correa M, et al. Beneficial effects of the bioflavonoids curcumin and quercetin on early function in cadaveric renal transplantation: a randomized placebo controlled trial. *Transplantation*. 2005 Dec 15;80(11):1556-9.
16. Li C, Zhang WJ, Frei B. Quercetin inhibits LPS-induced adhesion molecule expression and oxidant production in human aortic endothelial cells by p38-mediated Nrf2 activation and antioxidant enzyme induction. *Redox Biol*. 2016 Jun 28;9:104-113.
17. Chow HH, Garland LL, Hsu CH, et al. Resveratrol modulates drug- and carcinogen-metabolizing enzymes in a healthy volunteer study. *Cancer Prev Res (Phila)*. 2010 Sep;3(9):1168-75.
18. Kumar A, Negi G, Sharma SS. Neuroprotection by resveratrol in diabetic neuropathy: concepts & mechanisms. *Curr Med Chem*. 2013;20(36):4640-5.
19. Fuentes F, Paredes-Gonzalez X, Kong AT. Dietary Glucosinolates Sulforaphane, Phenethyl Isothiocyanate, Indole-3-Carbinol/3,3'-Diindolylmethane: Anti-Oxidative Stress/Inflammation, Nrf2, Epigenetics/Epigenomics and In Vivo Cancer Chemopreventive Efficacy. *Curr Pharmacol Rep*. 2015 May;1(3):179-196.
20. Konsue N, Kirkpatrick J, Kuhnert N, King LJ, Ioannides C. Repeated oral administration modulates the pharmacokinetic behavior of the chemopreventive agent phenethyl isothiocyanate in rats. *Mol Nutr Food Res*. 2010 Mar;54(3):426-32.
21. Ho CY, Cheng YT, Chau CF, Yen GC. Effect of diallyl sulfide on in vitro and in vivo Nrf2-mediated pulmonic antioxidant enzyme expression via activation ERK/p38 signaling pathway. *J Agric Food Chem*. 2012 Jan 11;60(1):100-7.
22. Colín-González AL, Santana RA, Silva-Islas CA, et al. The antioxidant mechanisms underlying the aged garlic extract- and S-allylcysteine-induced protection. *Oxid Med Cell Longev*. 2012;2012:907162.
23. Kumar H, Kim IS, More SV, Kim BW, Choi DK. Natural product-derived pharmacological modulators of Nrf2/ARE pathway for chronic diseases. *Nat Prod Rep*. 2014 Jan;31(1):109-39.
24. Nakai K, Fujii H, Kono K, et al. Vitamin D activates the Nrf2-Keap1 antioxidant pathway and ameliorates nephropathy in diabetic rats. *Am J Hypertens*. 2014 Apr;27(4):586-95.
25. Done AJ, Gage MJ, Nieto NC, Traustadóttir T. Exercise-induced Nrf2-signaling is impaired in aging. *Free Radic Biol Med*. 2016 Jul;96:130-8.

Foods and Nutrient Modulators of Detoxification Enzymes

The number of foods, food nutrients, phytonutrients and other compounds used as dietary supplements that have been reported to have some modulatory effect on one or more of the enzymes involved in detoxification is vast. In many cases, this evidence is based on cell culture experiments, though many are based on animal studies. In some cases, there are human clinical trial data to confirm these data. As with many biological responses to nutrients, these actions can be dose-dependent and often the same compound that acts as an inducer of an enzyme at one dose, can exhibit inhibitory effects at a different (often higher) dose. The following tables summarize the inducing or inhibitory actions of

a number of foods and food components on Phase I and Phase II detoxification enzymes. These tables have been modified from an excellent review of this topic by Romilly Hodges and Deanna Minich entitled "Modulation of Metabolic Detoxification Pathways Using Foods and Food-Derived Components: A Scientific Review with Clinical Application" (*J Nutr Metab.* 2015;2015:760689. doi: 10.1155/2015/760689). Their article is an excellent review of this topic and includes over 200 references (which we do not provide here). It is published in an open access journal and is available free online; we encourage clinicians interested in this topic to find the complete article for more details.

Food, beverage, or bioactive compounds (Food sources in italics)	Type of study	Dosages used
TABLE A: CYTOCHROME P450 PHASE I INDUCERS		
CYP1A1		
Cruciferous vegetables	Clinical	500 mg/d indole-3-carbinol
Resveratrol (Grapes, wine, peanuts, soy, and itadori tea)	Clinical	1 g/d resveratrol (note high dose used)
Green tea	In vivo	45 mL/d/rat (avg. 150 g animal weight) green tea
Black tea	In vivo	54 mL/d/rat (avg. 150 g animal weight) black tea
Curcumin (Tumeric, curry powder)	In vivo	1,000 mg/kg/d/rat curcumin (or about 150 mg per rat per day)
Soybean	In vivo	100 mg/kg soybean extract
Garlic	In vivo	30 to 200 mg/kg garlic oil
Fish oil	In vivo	20.5 g/kg fish oil (note: high dose used)
Rosemary	In vivo	Diet of 0.5% rosemary extract
Astaxanthin (Algae, yeast, salmon, trout, krill, shrimp, and crayfish)	In vivo	Diets of 0.001–0.03% astaxanthin for 15 days
CYP1A2		
Cruciferous vegetables	Clinical	7–14 g/kg cruciferous vegetables including frozen broccoli and cauliflower, fresh daikon radish sprouts and raw shredded cabbage, and red and green; 500 g/d broccoli; 250 g/d each of Brussel sprouts and broccoli
Green tea	In vivo	45 mL/d/rat (avg. 150 g animal weight) green tea; Green tea (2.5% w/v) as sole beverage
Black tea	In vivo	54 mL/d/rat (avg. 150 g animal weight) black tea
Chicory root	In vivo	Diet of 10% dried chicory root
Astaxanthin (Algae, yeast, salmon, trout, krill, shrimp, and crayfish)	In vivo	Diets of 0.001–0.03% astaxanthin for 15 days
CYP1B1		
Curcumin (Tumeric, curry powder)	In vivo	Diet of 0.1% curcumin
Cruciferous vegtables	In vivo	25–250 mg/kg indole-3-carbinol
CYP2A		
Chicory root	In vivo	Diet of 10% dried chicory root
CYP2A6		
Quercetin (Apple, apricot, blueberries, yellow onion, kale, alfalfa sprouts, green beans, broccoli, black tea, and chili powder)	Clinical	500 mg/d quercetin
Broccoli	Clinical	500 g/d broccoli
CYP2B1		
Rosemary	In vivo	Diet of 0.5% rosemary extract
Garlic	In vivo	0.5 and 2.0 mmol/kg diallyl sulfide, or about 75 and 300 mg, respectively

TABLE A, CONTINUED: CYTOCHROME P450 PHASE I INDUCERS

Food, beverage, or bioactive compounds (Food sources in italics)	Type of study	Dosages used
CYP2B2		
Rosemary	In vivo	Diet of 0.5% rosemary extract
CYP2E1		
Fish oil	In vivo	20.5 g/kg fish oil (note: high dose used)
Chicory root	In vivo	Diet of 10% dried chicory root
CYP3A		
Rooibos tea	In vivo	Rooibos tea, 4 g/L simmered for 5 minutes, as sole beverage
CYP3A1		
Garlic	In vivo	30 to 200 mg/kg garlic oil; 80 and 200 mg/kg garlic oil 3 times weekly
Fish oil	In vivo	20.5 g/kg fish oil (note: high dose used)
CYP3A2		
Garlic	In vivo	200 mg/kg diallyl sulfide
Cruciferous vegetables	In vivo	50 mg/kg/d indole-3-carbinol
CYP3A4		
Curcumin (Tumeric, curry powder)	In vivo	50 and 100 mg/kg curcumin
CYP4A1		
Green tea	In vivo	Green tea (2.5% w/v) as sole beverage
CYP4B1		
Caffeic acid (Coffee)	In vivo	179 mg/kg caffeic acid

TABLE B: CYTOCHROME P450 PHASE I INHIBITORS

Food, beverage, or bioactive compounds (Food sources in italics)	Type of study	Dosages used
CYP1A1		
Black raspberry	In vivo	Diet of 2.5% black raspberry
Blueberry	In vivo	Diet of 2.5% blueberry
Ellagic acid (Berries, pomegranate, grapes, walnuts, and blackcurrants)	In vivo	30 mg/kg/d ellagic acid; 400 ppm ellagic acid
Black soybean	In vivo	1 g/kg black soybean seed coat extract (note: high dose used)
Black tea	In vivo	20 mg/kg theaflavins
Turmeric	In vivo	Diet of 1% turmeric
CYP1A2		
Apiaceous vegetables	Clinical	4 g/kg apiaceous vegetables, including frozen carrots and fresh celery, dill, parsley, and parsnips
Quercetin (Apple, apricot, blueberries, yellow onion, kale, alfalfa sprouts, green beans, broccoli, black tea, and chili powder)	Clinical	500 mg/d quercetin
Daidzein (Soybean)	Clinical	200 mg twice daily dosing of daidzein
Grapefruit	Clinical	300 mL grapefruit juice
Kale	In vivo	2 g/kg/d kale, as freeze-dried kale drink
Garlic	In vivo	100 mg/kg garlic oil
Chamomile	In vivo	Free access to 2% chamomile tea solution
Peppermint	In vivo	Free access to 2% peppermint tea solution
Dandelion	In vivo	Free access to 2% dandelion tea solution
Turmeric	In vivo	Diet of 1% turmeric
CYP2B		
Ellagic acid (Berries, pomegranate, grapes, walnuts, and blackcurrants)	In vivo	10 and 30 mg/kg/d ellagic acid
Green tea	In vivo	100 mg/kg/d green tea extract
Cruciferous vegetables	In vivo	3 and 12 mg/kg/d sulforaphane
CYP2B1		
Turmeric	In vivo	Diet of 1% turmeric

TABLE B, CONTINUED: CYTOCHROME P450 PHASE I INHIBITORS		
Food, beverage, or bioactive compounds (Food sources in italics)	**Type of study**	**Dosages used**
CYP2C		
Green tea	In vivo	45 mL/d/rat (avg. 150 g animal weight) green tea
Black tea	In vivo	54 mL/d/rat (avg. 150 g animal weight) black tea
Ellagic acid (Berries, pomegranate, grapes, walnuts, and blackcurrants)	In vivo	30 mg/kg/d ellagic acid
CYP2C6		
Ellagic acid (Berries, pomegranate, grapes, walnuts, and blackcurrants)	In vivo	30 mg/kg/d ellagic acid
CYP2C9		
Resveratrol (Grapes, wine, peanuts, soy, and itadori tea)	Clinical	1 g/d resveratrol (note high dose used)
Myricetin (Onions, berries, grapes, and red wine)	In vivo	2 and 8 mg/kg myricetin
CYP2C19		
Kale	In vivo	2 g/kg/d kale, as freeze-dried kale drink
CYP2D6		
Resveratrol (Grapes, wine, peanuts, soy, and itadori tea)	Clinical	1 g/d resveratrol (note high dose used)
Garden cress	Clinical	7.5 g twice daily intake of garden cress seed powder
Kale	In vivo	2 g/kg/d kale, as freeze-dried kale drink
Watercress	Clinical	50 g watercress homogenate
Garlic	Clinical and In vivo	0.2 mg/kg diallyl sulfide, equivalent to high human garlic consumption; 100 mg/kg garlic oil; 200 mg/kg diallyl sulfide; 30 to 200 mg/kg garlic oil; Diet of 2% and 5% garlic powder
N-acetyl cysteine (Allium vegetables)	In vivo	25 mg/kg and 50 mg/kg N-acetyl cysteine
CYP2E1		
Ellagic acid (Berries, pomegranate, grapes, walnuts, and blackcurrants)	In vivo	10 and 30 mg/kg/d ellagic acid
Green tea	In vivo	45 mL/d/rat (avg. 150 g animal weight) green tea
Black tea	In vivo	54 mL/d/rat (avg. 150 g animal weight) black tea
Dandelion	In vivo	0.5 and 2 g/kg dandelion leaf water extract
Chrysin (Honey, honeycomb)	In vivo	20 and 40 mg/kg/d chrysin
Medium-chain triglycerides (MCTs) (Coconut and coconut oil)	In vivo	32% calories as MCTs
CYP3A		
Green tea	In vivo	45 mL/d/rat (avg. 150 g animal weight) green tea; 400 mg/kg green tea extract; 100 mg/kg/d green tea extract
Black tea	In vivo	54 mL/d/rat (avg. 150 g animal weight) black tea
Quercetin (Apple, apricot, blueberries, yellow onion, kale, alfalfa sprouts, green beans, broccoli, black tea, and chili powder)	In vivo	10 and 20 mg/kg
CYP3A2		
Cruciferous vegetables	In vivo	12 mg/kg/d sulforaphane
CYP3A4		
Grapefruit	Clinical	200 mL grapefruit juice 3 times daily
Resveratrol (Grapes, wine, peanuts, soy, and itadori tea)	Clinical	1 g/d resveratrol (note high dose used)
Garden cress	Clinical	7.5 g twice daily dose of garden cress seed powder
Soybean	In vivo	100 mg/kg soybean extract
Kale	In vivo	2 g/kg/d kale, as freeze-dried kale drink
Myricetin (Onions, berries, grapes, and red wine)	In vivo	0.4, 2, and 8 mg/kg myricetin

TABLE C: PHASE II: SULFATION		
Food, beverage, or bioactive compounds (Food sources in italics)	**Type of study**	**Dosages used**
Inducers of Sulfation Activity		
Caffeine (Coffee, cocoa, black tea, and green tea)	In vivo	2, 10, and 50 mg/kg caffeine
Retinoic acid (bioactive form of vitamin A) (Meat (especially liver), fish, egg, and dairy products contain retinol; apple, apricot, artichokes, arugula, asparagus, and other plant foods contain provitamin A carotenes)	In vivo	2, 10, and 50 mg/kg/d retinoic acid suspension in corn oil

TABLE D: PHASE II: GLUCURONIDATION (UGT)		
Food, beverage, or bioactive compounds (Food sources in italics)	**Type of study**	**Dosages used**
Inducers UGT Activity		
Cruciferous vegetables	Clinical	Approximately 5 and 10 servings/d of cruciferous vegetables including frozen broccoli, cauliflower, fresh cabbage (red and green), and fresh radish sprouts; 250 g/d each of Brussel sprouts and broccoli; 2 oz (56.8 g) watercress three times daily
Resveratrol (Grapes, wine, peanuts, soy, and itadori tea)	Clinical	1 g/d resveratrol (note high dose used)
Citrus	Observational	0.5+ servings/day of citrus fruits or foods
Dandelion	In vivo	Free access to 2% dandelion tea solution
Rooibos tea	In vivo	Rooibos tea as sole beverage; concentration 2 g tea leaves/100 mL water steeped for 30 minutes
Honeybush tea	In vivo	Honeybush tea as sole beverage; concentration 4 g tea leaves/100 mL water steeped for 30 minutes
Rosemary	In vivo	Diet of 0.5% rosemary extract
Soy	In vivo	150 and 500 mg/kg soy extract
Ellagic acid (Berries, pomegranate, grapes, walnuts, and blackcurrants)	In vivo	Diet of 1% ellagic acid
Ferulic acid (Whole grains, roasted coffee, tomatoes, asparagus, olives, berries, peas, vegetables, and citrus)	In vivo	Diet of 1% ferulic acid
Curcumin (Turmeric, curry powder)	In vivo	Diet of 1% curcumin
Astaxanthin (Algae, yeast, salmon, trout, krill, shrimp, and crayfish)	In vivo	Diets of 0.001–0.03% astaxanthin for 15 days

TABLE E: PHASE II: GLUTATHIONE S-TRANFERASES (GST)		
Food, beverage, or bioactive compounds (Food sources in italics)	**Type of study**	**Dosages used**
Inducers of GST Activity		
Cruciferous vegetables	Clinical, observational	Approximately 5 and 10 servings/d of cruciferous vegetables including frozen broccoli, cauliflower, fresh cabbage (red and green), and fresh radish sprouts; >31.2 g/d cruciferous vegetables; 4.5 cups of cruciferous vegetables/d, including 0.5 cups of radish sprouts, 1 cup of frozen cauliflower, 2 cups of frozen broccoli, and 1 cup of fresh cabbage; 300 g/d cooked Brussels sprouts
Allium vegetables	Clinical	3 tbsp fresh chives, 1.33 cups of fresh leeks, 1 tsp garlic, and 0.5 cups of fresh onion
Resveratrol (Grapes, wine, peanuts, soy, and itadori tea)	Clinical	1 g/d resveratrol (note high dose used)
Citrus	Observational, in vivo	> 76 g/d citrus; 20 mg limonoid mixture every 2 days
Garlic	In vivo	30 to 200 mg/kg garlic oil; 80 and 200 mg/kg garlic oil 3 times weekly
Fish oil	In vivo	20.5 g/kg fish oil (note high dose used)
Black soybean	In vivo	1 g/kg black soybean seed coat extract
Purple sweet potato	In vivo	100 and 200 mg/kg anthocyanin extract from purple sweet potato
Curcumin	In vivo	Diet of 2% curcumin
Green tea	In vivo	Equivalent of 4 cups/d (200 mL each) of green tea
Rooibos tea	In vivo	Rooibos tea as sole beverage; concentration 2 g tea leaves/100 mL water steeped for 30 minutes
Honeybush tea	In vivo	Honeybush tea as sole beverage; concentration 4 g tea leaves/100 mL water steeped for 30 minutes
Ellagic acid (Berries, pomegranate, grapes, walnuts, and blackcurrants)	In vivo	30 mg/kg/d ellagic acid
Rosemary	In vivo	20 mg/kg carnosic acid 3 times weekly
Ghee (clarified butter)	In vivo	19.5 mg CLA (conjugated linoleic acid)/g fat
Genistein (kidney GSTs) (Fermented soy (e.g., miso, tempeh) contains up to 40% bioavailable genistein versus 1% or less in other soy products)	In vivo	1.5 g/kg genistein (note: high dose used)
Inhibitors of GST Activity		
Apiaceous vegetables	Clinical	1 tsp fresh dill weed, 0.5 cups of fresh celery, 3 tbsp. fresh parsley, 1.25 cups of grated parsnips, and 0.75 cups of frozen carrots
Quercetin (Apple, apricot, blueberries, yellow onion, kale, alfalfa sprouts, green beans, broccoli, black tea, and chili powder)	In vivo	2 g/kg quercetin (note: high dose used)
Genistein (liver GSTs) (Fermented soy (e.g., miso, tempeh) contains up to 40% bioavailable genistein versus 1% or less in other soy products)	In vivo	1.5 g/kg genistein (note: high dose used)

References

1. Lewis SJ, Heaton KW. Stool form scale as a useful guide to intestinal transit time. *Scand J Gastroenterol*. 1997 Sep;32(9):920-4.
2. Longstreth GF, Thompson WG, Chey WD, et al. Functional bowel disorders. *Gastroenterology*. 2006 Apr;130(5):1480-91.
3. Lane MM, Czyzewski DI, Chumpitazi BP, Shulman RJ. Reliability and validity of a modified Bristol Stool Form Scale for children. *J Pediatr*. 2011 Sep;159(3):437-441.e1.
4. Ghanma A, Puttemans K, Deneyer M, et al. Amsterdam infant stool scale is more useful for assessing children who have not been toilet trained than Bristol stool scale. *Acta Paediatr*. 2014 Feb;103(2):e91-2.
5. Sanchez MI, Bercik P. Epidemiology and burden of chronic constipation. *Can J Gastroenterol*. 2011 Oct;25 Suppl B:11B-15B.
6. Sommers T, Corban C, Sengupta N, et al. Emergency department burden of constipation in the United States from 2006 to 2011. *Am J Gastroenterol*. 2015 Apr;110(4):572-9.
7. Choung RS, Locke GR 3rd, Rey E, et al. Factors associated with persistent and nonpersistent chronic constipation, over 20 years. *Clin Gastroenterol Hepatol*. 2012 May;10(5):494-500.
8. Roerig JL, Steffen KJ, Mitchell JE, Zunker C. Laxative abuse: epidemiology, diagnosis and management. *Drugs*. 2010 Aug 20;70(12):1487-503.
9. Mearin F, Lacy BE, Chang L, et al. Bowel Disorders. *Gastroenterology*. 2016 Feb; 150: 1393-1407.
10. Whitehead WE, Palsson OS, Simrén M. Biomarkers to distinguish functional constipation from irritable bowel syndrome with constipation. *Neurogastroenterol Motil*. 2016 Jun;28(6):783-92.
11. Siah KT, Wong RK, Whitehead WE. Chronic Constipation and Constipation-Predominant IBS: Separate and Distinct Disorders or a Spectrum of Disease? *Gastroenterol Hepatol (N Y)*. 2016 Mar;12(3):171-8.
12. Costilla VC, Foxx-Orenstein AE. Constipation: understanding mechanisms and management. *Clin Geriatr Med*. 2014 Feb;30(1):107-15.
13. Vandeputte D, Falony G, et al. Stool consistency is strongly associated with gut microbiota richness and composition, enterotypes and bacterial growth rates. *Gut*. 2016 Jan;65(1):57-62.
14. Parthasarathy G, Chen J, Chen X, et al. Relationship Between Microbiota of the Colonic Mucosa vs Feces and Symptoms, Colonic Transit, and Methane Production in Female Patients With Chronic Constipation. *Gastroenterology*. 2016 Feb;150(2):367-79.
15. Roager H, Hansen L, Bahl M, et al. Colonic transit time is related to bacterial metabolism and mucosal turnover in the gut. *Nature Microbiology* 2016: 1, Article number: 16093.
16. Tian H, Ding C, Gong J, Ge X, et al. Treatment of Slow Transit Constipation With Fecal Microbiota Transplantation: A Pilot Study. *J Clin Gastroenterol*. 2016 Jan 8. [Epub ahead of print]
17. Dimidi E, Christodoulides S, Fragkos KC, et al. The effect of probiotics on functional constipation in adults: a systematic review and meta-analysis of randomized controlled trials. *Am J Clin Nutr*. 2014 Oct;100(4):1075-84.
18. Miller LE, Zimmermann AK, Ouwehand AC. Contemporary meta-analysis of short-term probiotic consumption on gastrointestinal transit. *World J Gastroenterol*. 2016 Jun 7;22(21):5122-31.
19. As quoted by: Whorton, James C. Inner Hygeine: Constipation and the pursuit of health in modern society. 2000 Oxford University Press (New York)- page 217.
20. Bae SH. Diets for constipation. *Pediatr Gastroenterol Hepatol Nutr*. 2014 Dec;17(4):203-8.
21. Mobley AR, Jones JM, Rodriguez J, et al. Identifying practical solutions to meet America's fiber needs: proceedings from the Food & Fiber Summit. *Nutrients*. 2014 Jul 8;6(7):2540-51.
22. Lewis SJ, Heaton KW. Roughage revisited: the effect on intestinal function of inert plastic particles of different sizes and shape. *Dig Dis Sci*. 1999 Apr;44(4):744-8.
23. Anderson JW, Baird P, Davis RH Jr, et al. Health benefits of dietary fiber. *Nutr Rev*. 2009 Apr;67(4):188-205.
24. Salmean YA, Zello GA, Dahl WJ. Foods with added fiber improve stool frequency in individuals with chronic kidney disease with no impact on appetite or overall quality of life. *BMC Res Notes*. 2013 Dec 5;6:510.
25. Morais MB, Vitolo MR, Aguirre AN, Fagundes-Neto U. Measurement of low dietary fiber intake as a risk factor for chronic constipation in children. *J Pediatr Gastroenterol Nutr*. 1999 Aug;29(2):132-5
26. Roma E, Adamidis D, Nikolara R, Constantopoulos A, Messaritakis J. Diet and chronic constipation in children: the role of fiber. *J Pediatr Gastroenterol Nutr*. 1999 Feb;28(2):169-74.
27. McClung HJ, Boyne L, Heitlinger L. Constipation and dietary fiber intake in children. *Pediatrics*. 1995 Nov;96(5 Pt 2):999-1000.
28. Howard LV, West D, Ossip-Klein DJ. Chronic constipation management for institutionalized older adults. *Geriatr Nurs*. 2000 Mar-Apr;21(2):78-82.
29. Tse PW, Leung SS, Chan T, Sien A, Chan AK. Dietary fibre intake and constipation in children with severe developmental disabilities. *J Paediatr Child Health*. 2000 Jun;36(3):236-9.
30. Goyal A, Sharma V, Upadhyay N, Gill S, Sihag M. Flax and flaxseed oil: an ancient medicine & modern functional food. *J Food Sci Technol*. 2014 Sep;51(9):1633-53.
31. Adolphe JL, Whiting SJ, Juurlink BH, Thorpe LU, Alcorn J. Health effects with consumption of the flax lignan secoisolariciresinol diglucoside. *Br J Nutr*. 2010 Apr;103(7):929-38.
32. Dahl WJ, Lockert EA, Cammer AL, Whiting SJ. Effects of flax fiber on laxation and glycemic response in healthy volunteers. *J Med Food*. 2005 Winter;8(4):508-11.
33. Hanif Palla A, Gilani AH. Dual effectiveness of Flaxseed in constipation and diarrhea: Possible mechanism. J *Ethnopharmacol*. 2015 Jul 1;169:60-8.
34. Xu J, Zhou X, Chen C, et al. Laxative effects of partially defatted flaxseed meal on normal and experimental constipated mice. *BMC Complement Altern Med*. 2012 Mar 9;12:14.
35. Dettmar PW, Sykes J. A multi-centre, general practice comparison of ispaghula husk with lactulose and other laxatives in the treatment of simple constipation. *Curr Med Res Opin*. 1998;14(4):227-33.
36. McRorie JW, Daggy BP, Morel JG, Diersing PS, Miner PB, Robinson M. Psyllium is superior to docusate sodium for treatment of chronic constipation. *Aliment Pharmacol Ther*. 1998 May;12(5):491-7.
37. Ashraf W, Pfeiffer RF, Park F, Lof J, Quigley EM. Constipation in Parkinson's disease: objective assessment and response to psyllium. *Mov Disord*. 1997 Nov;12(6):946-51.
38. Fernandez-Banares F et al. Randomized clinical trial of Plantago ovata seeds (dietary fiber) as compared with mesalamine in maintaining remission in ulcerative colitis. Spanish Group for the Study of Crohn's Disease and Ulcerative Colitis (GETECCU). *Am J Gastroenterol*. 1999 Feb;94(2):427-33.
39. Moran S, Uribe M, Prado ME, de la Mora G, Munoz RM, Perez MF, Milke P, Blancas JM, Dehesa M. [Effects of fiber administration in the prevention of gallstones in obese patients on a reducing diet. A clinical trial] *Rev Gastroenterol Mex*. 1997 Oct-Dec;62(4):266-72. Spanish.
40. Markland AD, Burgio KL, Whitehead WE, et al. Loperamide Versus Psyllium Fiber for Treatment of Fecal Incontinence: The Fecal Incontinence Prescription (Rx) Management (FIRM) Randomized Clinical Trial. *Dis Colon Rectum*. 2015 Oct;58(10):983-93.
41. Murphy J, Stacey D, Crook J, Thompson B, Panetta D. Testing control of radiation-induced diarrhea with a psyllium bulking agent: a pilot study. *Can Oncol Nurs J*. 2000 Summer;10(3):96-100.
42. Chen HL, Cheng HC, Wu WT, Liu YJ, Liu SY. Supplementation of konjac glucomannan into a low-fiber Chinese diet promoted bowel movement and improved colonic ecology in constipated adults: a placebo-controlled, diet-controlled trial. *J Am Coll Nutr*. 2008 Feb;27(1):102-8.
43. Loening-Baucke V, Miele E, Staiano A. Fiber (glucomannan) is beneficial in the treatment of childhood constipation. *Pediatrics*. 2004 Mar;113(3 Pt 1):e259-64.
44. Yoon SJ, Chu DC, Raj Juneja L. Chemical and physical properties, safety and application of partially hydrolized guar gum as dietary fiber. *J Clin Biochem Nutr*. 2008 Jan;42:1-7.
45. Quartarone G. Role of PHGG as a dietary fiber: a review article. *Minerva Gastroenterol Dietol*. 2013 Dec;59(4):329-40.
46. Stacewicz-Sapuntzakis M, Bowen PE, Hussain EA, et al. Chemical composition and potential health effects of prunes: a functional food? *Crit Rev Food Sci Nutr*. 2001 May;41(4):251-86.
47. Attaluri A, Donahoe R, Valestin J, Brown K, Rao SS. Randomised clinical trial: dried plums (prunes) vs. psyllium for constipation. *Aliment Pharmacol Ther*. 2011 Apr;33(7):822-8.
48. Anti M, Pignataro G, Armuzzi A, Valenti A, Iascone E, Marmo R, Lamazza A, Pretaroli AR, Pace V, Leo P, Castelli A, Gasbarrini G. Water supplementation enhances the effect of high-fiber diet on stool frequency and laxative consumption in adult patients with functional constipation. *Hepatogastroenterology*. 1998 May-Jun;45(21):727-32.

49. Cuomo R, Grasso R, Sarnelli G, Capuano G, Nicolai E, Nardone G, Pomponi D, Budillon G, Ierardi E. Effects of carbonated water on functional dyspepsia and constipation. *Eur J Gastroenterol Hepatol.* 2002 Sep;14(9):991-9.

50. Klauser AG, Beck A, Schindlbeck NE, Muller-Lissner SA. Low fluid intake lowers stool output in healthy male volunteers. *Z Gastroenterol.* 1990 Nov;28(11):606-9.

51. Chung BD, Parekh U, Sellin JH. Effect of increased fluid intake on stool output in normal healthy volunteers. *J Clin Gastroenterol.* 1999 Jan;28(1):29-32.

52. To see the complete vitamin C monograph published by the Linus Pauling Institute, see their website page here: http://lpi.oregonstate.edu/mic/vitamins/vitamin-C

53. Cirillo C, Capasso R. Constipation and Botanical Medicines: An Overview. *Phytother Res.* 2015 Oct;29(10):1488-93.

54. Malik EM, Müller CE. Anthraquinones as Pharmacological Tools and Drugs. *Med Res Rev.* 2016 Jul;36(4):705-48

55. Yang H, Xu LN, He CY, Liu X, Fang RY, Ma TH. CFTR chloride channel as a molecular target of anthraquinone compounds in herbal laxatives. *Acta Pharmacol Sin.* 2011 Jun;32(6):834-9.

56. Ishii Y et al. Studies of aloe. VI. Cathartic effect of isobarbaloin. *Biol Pharm Bull* 1998; 21(11):1226-7.

57. Yagi T et al. The synergistic purgative action of aloe-emodin anthrone and rhein anthrone in mice: synergism in large intestinal propulsion and water secretion. J Pharm Pharmacol 1997; 49(1):22-5

58. Akao T et al. A purgative action of barbaloin is induced by Eubacterium sp. Strain BAR, a human intestinal anaerobe, capable of transforming barbaloin to aloe-emodin anthrone. Biol Pharm Bull. 1996 Jan;19(1):136-8.

59. Wintola OA, Sunmonu TO, Afolayan AJ. The effect of Aloe ferox Mill. in the treatment of loperamide-induced constipation in Wistar rats. *BMC Gastroenterol.* 2010 Aug 19;10:95.

60. Zheng YF, Liu CF, Lai WF, et al. The laxative effect of emodin is attributable to increased aquaporin 3 expression in the colon of mice and HT-29 cells. *Fitoterapia.* 2014 Jul;96:25-32.

61. Ulbricht C, Chao W, Clark A, Ernst E, et al. An evidence-based systematic review of Aloe vera by the natural standard research collaboration. *J Herb Pharmacother* 2011;17(1):279–323.

62. I have been associated with the distribution of over 5 million daily doses of cape aloes preparation through healthcare professionals over the past 20 years and have received few reported cases of side-effects; and many personal communications of the mild nature of cape aloes compared to other laxatives.

63. Blumenthal et al. The Complete German Commission E Monographs. American Botanical Council.1998. pp80-81

64. van den Berg AJ, Labadie RP. Anthraquinones, Anthrones and Dianthrones in Callus Cultures of Rhamnus frangula and Rhamnus purshiana. *Planta Med.* 1984 Oct;50(5):449-51.

65. Blumenthal et al. The Complete German Commission E Monographs. American Botanical Council.1998. pp104-105.

66. Mehta N, Laddha KS. A modified method for isolation of rhein from senna. *Indian J Pharm Sci.* 2009 Mar;71(2):128-9.

67. Kobayashi M, Yamaguchi T, Odaka T, et al. Regionally differential effects of sennoside A on spontaneous contractions of colon in mice. *Basic Clin Pharmacol Toxicol.* 2007 Aug;101(2):121-6.

68. Tajima Y, Ishida H, Yamamoto A, et al. Comparison of the risk of surgical site infection and feasibility of surgery between sennoside versus polyethylene glycol as a mechanical bowel preparation of elective colon cancer surgery: a randomized controlled trial. *Surg Today.* 2016 Jun;46(6):735-40.

69. Ishibashi K, Kumamoto K, Kuwabara K, et al. Usefulness of sennoside as an agent for mechanical bowel preparation prior to elective colon cancer surgery. *Asian J Surg.* 2012 Apr;35(2):81-7.

70. Blumenthal et al. The Complete German Commission E Monographs. American Botanical Council.1998. pp206-208.

71. Vitalone A, Menniti-Ippolito F, Raschetti R, et al. Surveillance of suspected adverse reactions to herbal products used as laxatives. *Eur J Clin Pharmacol.* 2012 Mar;68(3):231-8.

72. Bockus H, Willard J, Banks J. Melanosis coli. The ethiologic significance of the anthracene laxatives: a report of forty-one cases. *J Am Med Assoc* 1933: 101:1-6.

73. Cowley K, Jennings HW, Passarella M. Who Turned Out the Lights? An Impressive Case of Melanosis Coli. *ACG Case Rep J.* 2015 Oct 9;3(1):13-4.

74. Fleischer I, Bryant D. Melanosis coli or mucosa ischemia? A case report. *Ostomy Wound Manage.* 1995 May;41(4):44, 46-7.

75. Mellouki I, Meyiz H. Melanosis coli: a rarity in digestive endoscopy. *Pan Afr Med J.* 2013 Nov 9;16:86.

76. Willems M, van Buuren HR, de Krijger R. Anthranoid self-medication causing rapid development of melanosis coli. *Neth J Med.* 2003 Jan;61(1):22-4.

77. van Gorkom BA, de Vries EG, Karrenbeld A, Kleibeuker JH. Review article: anthranoid laxatives and their potential carcinogenic effects. *Aliment Pharmacol Ther.* 1999 Apr;13(4):443-52.

78. Morales MA, Hernández D, Bustamante S, Bachiller I, Rojas A. Is senna laxative use associated to cathartic colon, genotoxicity, or carcinogenicity? *J Toxicol.* 2009;2009:287247.

79. Nascimbeni R, Donato F, Ghirardi M, Mariani P, Villanacci V, Salerni B. Constipation, anthranoid laxatives, melanosis coli, and colon cancer: a risk assessment using aberrant crypt foci. *Cancer Epidemiol Biomarkers Prev.* 2002 Aug;11(8):753-7.

80. Nusko G, Schneider B, Ernst H, Wittekind C, Hahn EG. Melanosis coli--a harmless pigmentation or a precancerous condition? *Z Gastroenterol.* 1997 May;35(5):313-8.

81. Nusko G, Schneider B, Schneider I, Wittekind C, Hahn EG. Anthranoid laxative use is not a risk factor for colorectal neoplasia: results of a prospective case control study. *Gut.* 2000 May;46(5):651-5.

82. Iovino P, Chiarioni G, Bilancio G, et al. New onset of constipation during long-term physical inactivity: a proof-of-concept study on the immobility-induced bowel changes. *PLoS One.* 2013 Aug 20;8(8):e72608.

83. Tuteja AK, Talley NJ, Joos SK, et al. Is constipation associated with decreased physical activity in normally active subjects? *Am J Gastroenterol.* 2005 Jan;100(1):124-9.

84. Nakaji S, Tokunaga S, Sakamoto J, Todate M, Shimoyama T, Umeda T, Sugawara K. Relationship between lifestyle factors and defecation in a Japanese population. *Eur J Nutr.* 2002 Dec;41(6):244-8.

85. De Schryver AM, Keulemans YC, Peters HP, et al. Effects of regular physical activity on defecation pattern in middle-aged patients complaining of chronic constipation. *Scand J Gastroenterol.* 2005 Apr;40(4):422-9.

86. Rochester JR. Bisphenol A and human health: a review of the literature. *Reprod Toxicol.* 2013 Dec;42:132-55.

87. Sartain CV, Hunt PA. An old culprit but a new story: bisphenol A and "NextGen" bisphenols. *Fertil Steril.* 2016 Aug 6. pii: S0015-0282(16)62552-9.

88. Usman A, Ahmad M. From BPA to its analogues: Is it a safe journey? *Chemosphere.* 2016 Sep;158:131-42.

89. Khan D, Ahmed SA. Epigenetic Regulation of Non-Lymphoid Cells by Bisphenol A, a Model Endocrine Disrupter: Potential Implications for Immunoregulation. *Front Endocrinol (Lausanne).* 2015 Jun 5;6:91.

90. Giulivo M, Lopez de Alda M, Capri E, Barceló D. Human exposure to endocrine disrupting compounds: Their role in reproductive systems, metabolic syndrome and breast cancer. A review. *Environ Res.* 2016 Aug 6;151:251-264.

91. Trasande L, Attina TM, Blustein J. Association between urinary bisphenol A concentration and obesity prevalence in children and adolescents. *JAMA.* 2012 Sep 19;308(11):1113-21.

92. Beronius A, Ruden C, Hakansson H, Hanberg A. Risk to all or none? A comparative analysis of controversies in the health risk assessment of Bisphenol A. *Reprod Toxicol.* Apr 2010;29(2):132-146.

93. Chevalier N, Fénichel P. Bisphenol A: Targeting metabolic tissues. *Rev Endocr Metab Disord.* 2015 Dec;16(4):299-309.

94. Han C, Hong YC. Bisphenol A, Hypertension, and Cardiovascular Diseases: Epidemiological, Laboratory, and Clinical Trial Evidence. *Curr Hypertens Rep.* 2016 Feb;18(2):11.

95. Xin F, Susiarjo M, Bartolomei MS. Multigenerational and transgenerational effects of endocrine disrupting chemicals: A role for altered epigenetic regulation? *Semin Cell Dev Biol.* 2015 Jul;43:66-75.

96. Kundakovic M, Champagne FA. Epigenetic perspective on the developmental effects of bisphenol A. *Brain Behav Immun.* Aug 2011;25(6):1084-1093.

97. Ferreira LL, Couto R, Oliveira PJ. Bisphenol A as epigenetic modulator: setting the stage for carcinogenesis? *Eur J Clin Invest.* 2015 Jan;45 Suppl 1:32-6.

98. Anderson OS, Nahar MS, Faulk C, et al. Epigenetic responses following maternal dietary exposure to physiologically relevant levels of bisphenol A. *Environ Mol Mutagen.* 2012 Jun;53(5):334-42.

99. Dolinoy DC, Huang D, Jirtle RL. Maternal nutrient supplementation counteracts bisphenol A-induced DNA hypomethylation in early development. *Proc Natl Acad Sci U S A.* Aug 7 2007;104(32):13056-13061.

100. Jaakkola JJ, Knight TL. The role of exposure to phthalates from polyvinyl chloride products in the development of asthma and allergies: a systematic review and meta-analysis. *Environmental health perspectives.* Jul 2008;116(7):845-853.

101. Sedha S, Kumar S, Shukla S. Role of Oxidative Stress in Male Reproductive Dysfunctions with Reference to Phthalate Compounds. *Urol J.* 2015 Nov 14;12(5):2304-16.

102. Stahlhut RW, van Wijngaarden E, Dye TD, Cook S, Swan SH. Concentrations of urinary phthalate metabolites are associated with increased waist circumference and insulin resistance in adult U.S. males. *Environmental health perspectives.* Jun 2007;115(6):876-882.

103. Lind PM, Roos V, Ronn M, et al. Serum concentrations of phthalate metabolites related to abdominal fat distribution two years later in elderly women. *Environ Health.* Apr 2 2012;11(1):21.

104. Martinez-Arguelles DB, Papadopoulos V. Prenatal phthalate exposure: epigenetic changes leading to lifelong impact on steroid formation. *Andrology.* 2016 Jul;4(4):573-84.

105. Singh S, Li SS. Epigenetic effects of environmental chemicals bisphenol A and phthalates. *Int J Mol Sci.* 2012;13(8):10143-53.

106. http://www.who.int/mediacentre/factsheets/fs225/en/ Last updated 2014.

107. Crump KS, Canady R, Kogevinas M. Meta-analysis of dioxin cancer dose response for three occupational cohorts. *Environ Health Perspect.* 2003 May;111(5):681-7.

108. Boffetta P, Mundt KA, Adami HO, Cole P, Mandel JS. TCDD and cancer: a critical review of epidemiologic studies. *Crit Rev Toxicol.* 2011 Aug;41(7):622-36.

109. Mulero-Navarro S, Fernandez-Salguero PM. New Trends in Aryl Hydrocarbon Receptor Biology. *Front Cell Dev Biol.* 2016 May 11;4:45.

110. Bradshaw TD, Bell DR. Relevance of the aryl hydrocarbon receptor (AhR) for clinical toxicology. *Clin Toxicol (Phila).* Aug 2009;47(7):632-642.

111. Ishida T, Takeda T, Koga T, et al. Attenuation of 2,3,7,8-tetrachlorodibenzo-p-dioxin toxicity by resveratrol: a comparative study with different routes of administration. *Biol Pharm Bull.* May 2009;32(5):876-881.

112. Singh NP, Singh US, Nagarkatti M, Nagarkatti PS. Resveratrol (3,5,4'-trihydroxystilbene) protects pregnant mother and fetus from the immunotoxic effects of 2,3,7,8-tetrachlorodibenzo-p-dioxin. *Mol Nutr Food Res.* 2011 Feb;55(2):209-19.

113. Megna BW, Carney PR, Nukaya M, et al. Indole-3-carbinol induces tumor cell death: function follows form. *J Surg Res.* 2016 Jul;204(1):47-54.

114. Tutel'yan VA, Gapparov MM, Telegin LY, et al. Flavonoids and resveratrol as regulators of Ah-receptor activity: protection from dioxin toxicity. *Bull Exp Biol Med.* 2003 Dec;136(6):533-9.

115. Izawa H, Watanabe G, Taya K, Sagai M. Inhibitory effects of foods and polyphenols on activation of aryl hydrocarbon receptor induced by diesel exhaust particles. *Environ Sci.* 2007;14(3):149-56.

116. Rizzati V, Briand O, Guillou H, Gamet-Payrastre L. Effects of pesticide mixtures in human and animal models: An update of the recent literature. *Chem Biol Interact.* 2016 Jul 25;254:231-46.

117. Kuhnlein HV, Receveur O, Muir DC, Chan HM, Soueida R. Arctic indigenous women consume greater than acceptable levels of organochlorines. *J Nutr.* Oct 1995;125(10):2501-2510.

118. Jensen GE, Clausen J. Organochlorine compounds in adipose tissue of Greenlanders and southern Danes. *Journal of toxicology and environmental health.* Jul 1979;5(4):617-629.

119. Sagiv SK, Thurston SW, Bellinger DC, Tolbert PE, Altshul LM, Korrick SA. Prenatal organochlorine exposure and behaviors associated with attention deficit hyperactivity disorder in school-aged children. *Am J Epidemiol.* Vol 171. 2010:593-601.

120. Adams RD, Lupton D, Good AM, Bateman DN. UK childhood exposures to pesticides 2004-2007: a TOXBASE toxicovigilance study. *Arch Dis Child.* Jun 2009;94(6):417-420.

121. Ewence A, Brescia S, Johnson I, Rumsby PC. An approach to the identification and regulation of endocrine disrupting pesticides. *Food Chem Toxicol.* 2015 Apr;78:214-20.

122. Franco R, Li S, Rodriguez-Rocha H, Burns M, Panayiotidis MI. Molecular mechanisms of pesticide-induced neurotoxicity: Relevance to Parkinson's disease. *Chem Biol Interact.* Vol 188. Ireland: 2010 Elsevier Ireland Ltd; 2010:289-300.

123. Choi S. Critical review on the carcinogenic potential of pesticides used in Korea. *Asian Pac J Cancer Prev.* 2014;15(15):5999-6003.

124. Smith-Spangler C, Brandeau ML, Hunter GE, et al. Are organic foods safer or healthier than conventional alternatives?: a systematic review. *Ann Intern Med.* 2012 Sep 4;157(5):348-66.

125. Mounicou S, Szpunar J, Lobinski R. Metallomics: the concept and methodology. *Chem Soc Rev.* 2009 Apr;38(4):1119-38.

126. Kern JK, Geier DA, Sykes LK, et al. The relationship between mercury and autism: A comprehensive review and discussion. *J Trace Elem Med Biol.* 2016 Sep;37:8-24.

127. Houston MC. Role of mercury toxicity in hypertension, cardiovascular disease, and stroke. *J Clin Hypertens (Greenwich).* Aug 2011;13(8):621-627.

128. Boffetta P, Sallsten G, Garcia-Gomez M, et al. Mortality from cardiovascular diseases and exposure to inorganic mercury. *Occup Environ Med.* Jul 2001;58(7):461-466.

129. Crespo-Lopez ME, Macedo GL, Pereira SI, et al. Mercury and human genotoxicity: critical considerations and possible molecular mechanisms. *Pharmacol Res.* Oct 2009;60(4):212-220.

130. Falluel-Morel A, Lin L, Sokolowski K, McCandlish E, Buckley B, DiCicco-Bloom E. N-acetyl cysteine treatment reduces mercury-induced neurotoxicity in the developing rat hippocampus. *J Neurosci Res.* Apr 2012;90(4):743-750.

131. Anuradha B, Varalakshmi P. Protective role of DL-alpha-lipoic acid against mercury-induced neural lipid peroxidation. *Pharmacol Res.* Jan 1999;39(1):67-80.

132. Deng Y, Xu Z, Liu W, Yang H, Xu B, Wei Y. Effects of lycopene and proanthocyanidins on hepatotoxicity induced by mercuric chloride in rats. *Biol Trace Elem Res.* May 2012;146(2):213-223.

133. Liu W, Xu Z, Yang H, Deng Y, Xu B, Wei Y. The protective effects of tea polyphenols and schisandrin B on nephrotoxicity of mercury. *Biol Trace Elem Res.* Dec 2011;143(3):1651-1665.

134. Barcelos GR, Angeli JP, Serpeloni JM, et al. Quercetin protects human-derived liver cells against mercury-induced DNA-damage and alterations of the redox status. *Mutat Res.* Dec 24 2011;726(2):109-115.

135. El-Shenawy SM, Hassan NS. Comparative evaluation of the protective effect of selenium and garlic against liver and kidney damage induced by mercury chloride in the rats. *Pharmacol Rep.* Mar-Apr 2008;60(2):199-208.

136. Joshi D, Mittal D, Shrivastav S, Shukla S, Srivastav AK. Combined effect of N-acetyl cysteine, zinc, and selenium against chronic dimethylmercury-induced oxidative stress: a biochemical and histopathological approach. *Archives of environmental contamination and toxicology.* Nov 2011;61(4):558-567.

137. CDC. Lead- Prevention Tips. 2014; http://www.cdc.gov/nceh/lead/tips.htm.

138. Nemsadze K, Sanikidze T, Ratiani L, Gabunia L, Sharashenidze T. Mechanisms of lead-induced poisoning. *Georgian Med News.* Jul-Aug 2009(172-173):92-96.

139. Vaziri ND. Mechanisms of lead-induced hypertension and cardiovascular disease. *Am J Physiol Heart Circ Physiol.* Aug 2008;295(2):H454-465.

140. Hsu PC, Guo YL. Antioxidant nutrients and lead toxicity. *Toxicology.* Oct 30 2002;180(1):33-44.

141. Sharma V, Shrivastava S, Shukla S. Reversal of lead-induced toxicity due to the effect of antioxidants. *J Environ Pathol Toxicol Oncol.* 2013;32(2):177-87.

142. Cao Y, Skaug MA, Andersen O, Aaseth J. Chelation therapy in intoxications with mercury, lead and copper. *J Trace Elem Med Biol.* 2015;31:188-92.

143. Flora SJ, Pachauri V. Chelation in metal intoxication. *Int J Environ Res Public Health.* 2010 Jul;7(7):2745-88.

144. Jomova K, Jenisova Z, Feszterova M, et al. Arsenic: toxicity, oxidative stress and human disease. *J Appl Toxicol.* Mar 2011;31(2):95-107.

145. Jana K, Jana S, Samanta PK. Effects of chronic exposure to sodium arsenite on hypothalamo-pituitary-testicular activities in adult rats: possible an estrogenic mode of action. *Reprod Biol Endocrinol.* 2006 Feb 16;4:9.

146. Rossman TG. Mechanism of arsenic carcinogenesis: an integrated approach. *Mutat Res.* Dec 10 2003;533(1-2):37-65.

147. Navas-Acien A, Silbergeld EK, Pastor-Barriuso R, Guallar E. Arsenic exposure and prevalence of type 2 diabetes in US adults. *JAMA.* Aug 20 2008;300(7):814-822.

148. Celik I, Gallicchio L, Boyd K, et al. Arsenic in drinking water and lung cancer: a systematic review. *Environ Res.* Sep 2008;108(1):48-55.

149. Tomljenovic L. Aluminum and Alzheimer's disease: after a century of controversy, is there a plausible link? *Journal of Alzheimer's disease : JAD.* 2011;23(4):567-598.

150. Rondeau V, Jacqmin-Gadda H, Commenges D, Helmer C, Dartigues JF. Aluminum and silica in drinking water and the risk of Alzheimer's disease or cognitive decline: findings from 15-year follow-up of the PAQUID cohort. *Am J Epidemiol.* Vol 169. United States2009:489-496.

151. Yumoto S, Kakimi S, Ohsaki A, Ishikawa A. Demonstration of aluminum in amyloid fibers in the cores of senile plaques in the brains of patients with Alzheimer's disease. *J Inorg Biochem.* Vol 103. United States2009:1579-1584.

152. McLachlan DR, Bergeron C, Smith JE, Boomer D, Rifat SL. Risk for neuropathologically confirmed Alzheimer's disease and residual aluminum in municipal drinking water employing weighted residential histories. *Neurology.* Feb 1996;46(2):401-405.

153. Exley C, Charles LM, Barr L, Martin C, Polwart A, Darbre PD. Aluminium in human breast tissue. *J Inorg Biochem.* Vol 101. United States2007:1344-1346.

154. Ferreira PC, Piai Kde A, Takayanagui AM, Segura-Munoz SI. Aluminum as a risk factor for Alzheimer's disease. *Rev Lat Am Enfermagem.* Vol 16. Brazil2008:151-157.

155. Alam G, Jones BC. Toxicogenetics: in search of host susceptibility to environmental toxicants. *Front Genet.* 2014 Sep 22;5:327.

156. Lioy PJ, Rappaport SM. Exposure science and the exposome: an opportunity for coherence in the environmental health sciences. *Environmental health perspectives.* Nov 2011;119(11):A466-467.
157. Rappaport SM. Discovering environmental causes of disease. *J Epidemiol Community Health.* Feb 2012;66(2):99-102.
158. Cavalieri EL, Rogan EG. Unbalanced metabolism of endogenous estrogens in the etiology and prevention of human cancer. *J Steroid Biochem Mol Biol.* 2011 Jul;125(3-5):169-80.
159. Iyanagi T. Molecular mechanism of phase I and phase II drug-metabolizing enzymes: implications for detoxification. *Int Rev Cytol.* 2007;260:35-112.
160. Jancova P, Anzenbacher P, Anzenbacherova E. Phase II drug metabolizing enzymes. *Biomed Pap Med Fac Univ Palacky Olomouc Czech Repub.* 2010 Jun;154(2):103-16.
161. Brill MJ, Diepstraten J, van Rongen A, et al. Impact of obesity on drug metabolism and elimination in adults and children. *Clin Pharmacokinet.* 2012 May 1;51(5):277-304.
162. Tremblay A, Pelletier C, Doucet E, Imbeault P. Thermogenesis and weight loss in obese individuals: a primary association with organochlorine pollution. *Int J Obes Relat Metab Disord.* 2004 Jul;28(7):936-9.
163. Roe AL1, Warren G, et al. The effect of high dose endotoxin on CYP3A2 expression in the rat. *Pharm Res.* 1998 Oct;15(10):1603-8.
164. Cheng PY, Wang M, Morgan ET. Rapid transcriptional suppression of rat cytochrome P450 genes by endotoxin treatment and its inhibition by curcumin. *J Pharmacol Exp Ther.* 2003 Dec;307(3):1205-12.
165. Tomasi ML, Ryoo M, Yang H, et al. Molecular mechanisms of lipopolysaccharide-mediated inhibition of glutathione synthesis in mice. *Free Radic Biol Med.* 2014 Mar;68:148-58.
166. Fukui H. Gut-liver axis in liver cirrhosis: How to manage leaky gut and endotoxemia. *World J Hepatol.* 2015 Mar 27;7(3):425-42.
167. de Punder K, Pruimboom L. Stress induces endotoxemia and low-grade inflammation by increasing barrier permeability. *Front Immunol.* 2015 May 15;6:223.
168. Glaros TG, Chang S, Gilliam EA, et al. Causes and consequences of low grade endotoxemia and inflammatory diseases. *Front Biosci (Schol Ed).* 2013 Jan 1;5:754-65.
169. Hakooz NM. Caffeine metabolic ratios for the in vivo evaluation of CYP1A2, N-acetyltransferase 2, xanthine oxidase and CYP2A6 enzymatic activities. *Curr Drug Metab.* 2009 May;10(4):329-38.
170. Lown KS, Thummel KE, Benedict PE, et al. The erythromycin breath test predicts the clearance of midazolam. *Clin Pharmacol Ther.* 1995 Jan;57(1):16-24.
171. Michael M, Cullinane C, Hatzimihalis A, et al. Docetaxel pharmacokinetics and its correlation with two in vivo probes for cytochrome P450 enzymes: the C(14)-erythromycin breath test and the antipyrine clearance test. *Cancer Chemother Pharmacol.* 2012 Jan;69(1):125-35.
172. Lammers LA, Achterbergh R, de Vries EM, et al. Short-term fasting alters cytochrome P450-mediated drug metabolism in humans. *Drug Metab Dispos.* 2015 Jun;43(6):819-28.
173. Kim DH. Gut Microbiota-Mediated Drug-Antibiotic Interactions. *Drug Metab Dispos.* 2015 Oct;43(10):1581-9.
174. Swanson HI. Drug Metabolism by the Host and Gut Microbiota: A Partnership or Rivalry? *Drug Metab Dispos.* 2015 Oct;43(10):1499-504.
175. Kang MJ, Kim HG, Kim JS, et al. The effect of gut microbiota on drug metabolism. *Expert Opin Drug Metab Toxicol.* 2013 Oct;9(10):1295-308.
176. Klaassen CD, Cui JY. Review: Mechanisms of How the Intestinal Microbiota Alters the Effects of Drugs and Bile Acids. *Drug Metab Dispos.* 2015 Oct;43(10):1505-21.

Supporting the Microbial Ecosystems in the Gut

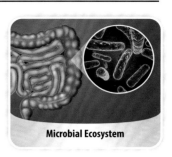

Microbial Ecosystem

One of the greatest paradigm shifts in medicine over the past few decades has been the unfolding discoveries revealing the metabolic influence of the human microbiome, especially that which resides within the gastrointestinal tract. Indeed, it is difficult to find a medical discipline that is not actively investigating the potential role played by the gut microbiome in human health and disease. This explosion of knowledge has been welcome news for many healthcare providers, though keeping up with the published research, changing nomenclature and therapeutic ramification of this information has been a difficult task. Our goal in this chapter is not to provide a comprehensive review of all the current literature (though we provide updated references for those who want to investigate this further[†]); instead, we will overview the fundamental and clinically-relevant aspects of the human GI microbiota, focusing our attention on modifiable behaviors and therapies that have been shown to alter these organisms, their environment and influence (good or bad). In addition, we have specifically attempted to answer, with the best available evidence, the most frequently asked questions clinicians have posed to us related to these issues.

Nomenclature Related to GI Microbes

Basic definitions and common terms used to describe features of the gastrointestinal microbial community. As indicated, many of these terms are interchangeable (practically), even if they represent different features (technically).

Microbiota: The total microbial organisms within the gut (or other defined ecosystem). This generally includes friendly and unfriendly organisms: bacteria (bacteriome), fungi (mycobiome) and virus (virome). To date, with the exception of a few fungal species, our study of the microbiota is almost entirely focused on bacteria.

Microflora: Considered (and favored) by many to be equivalent to "microbiota" (i.e., "microbial flora"), though others consider it to be an incorrect term remnant of the days when bacteria and fungi were considered part of the plant kingdom. Nonetheless, the term is still common in both scientific and popular writings.

Microbiome: This term is considered by many to be interchangeable with "microbiota," though it is often used to describe the total microbial community with its environment (i.e., biome). Others use this term exclusively to describe the total genomic information

contained in these microbes (i.e., microbial genome). We prefer and will use the first definition throughout this chapter, and use "metagenome" to describe the second.

Metagenome: This term refers to the total non-human genetic material (bacterial, fungal, viral) that can be isolated from humans (e.g., identifiable genomic material from GI bacteria, etc.). Additional "omic" terms such as metatranscriptome, metaproteome, metametabolome are equivalent terms used to describe non-human transcripts, protein expression and metabolites found in or on humans.

Operational Taxonomic Unit (OTU): This operational definition of species is used when only genetic material (DNA or RNA) is analyzed to distinguish one species from another. Since many bacteria within the gut microbiome cannot be isolated, grown and investigated in a laboratory

---

† A growing list of references related to the microbiome can also be found at http://americangut.org/publications/

Nomenclature Related to GI Microbes, continued

setting, they are identified by their genetic sequences and classified into OTUs. Diversity is often described as the number of OTUs. For the clinician, this is functionally identical to the number of species.

Enterotypes: A term used to define distinct clusters of species found within the human microbiome across different populations. Some have proposed that one of three enterotypes can be described for most human subjects.

Shannon (or Simpson) Index: Diversity indexes commonly used in microbial community ecology studies and reported sometimes in patients as a measure of microbiota diversity. The measured value of diversity increases as the number of species increases, and also as the relative abundance becomes more even. Simpson and Shannon Indexes have assumptions that affect the resultant diversity value. The Shannon index assumes all species are represented in the sample and assumes random sampling; such assumptions may skew actual diversity measures in the case of rare species with only a few individuals in a given community. The Simpson index, known as a dominance index, takes into account the weight of dominant species in a community. Rare species with few individuals likely will not affect the Simpson index.

Commensal: Generically, this means an organism that provides a benefit to the host (symbiotic, mutualistic, etc.) and has also come to mean the totality of non-pathogenic bacteria that are "natural" residents of the gut (supplied through the environment or diet). This term can also be used to distinguish these "natural" organisms from "supplemented" organisms that are generally incapable of long-term GI residence (e.g., probiotics).

Pathobiont: This is a commensal organism with the potential for pathogenic activity that, in some circumstances, can trigger negative outcomes for the host (e.g., antibiotics and *C. difficile*). These might require the presence of other microorganisms, host immune system dysfunctions or other unknown factors to become pathogenic.

Biofilm: This describes a microbial community embedded in an extracellular matrix that allows it to strongly adhere to a surface like an implanted medical device or the gut mucosa. While many commensal organisms thrive in a gut biofilm microenvironment, many pathogenic organisms produce a biofilm community as a response to antimicrobial activities, making them difficult to inhibit.

Quorum-Sensing: This describes the means by which bacteria coordinate their activities with adjacent bacteria for (mostly) cooperative functions. This is best understood as modulation of microbial functions and signaling based on population density and cell-to-cell proximity.

Probiotic: A microorganism that, when intentionally consumed (or applied), confers a benefit to the host. Foodborne microbes are typically not referred to as probiotics, nor are microbes added during the fermentation of certain foods (e.g., cheese, sauerkraut, etc.). Some functional foods such as yogurt and kefir are specially designed to deliver live probiotic strains and fit the definition of a probiotic, though most do not. While most definitions include the need for the microbe to be "live" or viable, research now shows that some of the known benefits attributed to probiotics remain even when the microbe is no longer viable.

Prebiotic: A substance that, when consumed by the host, provides a substrate upon which commensal organisms can thrive and subsequently benefit the host. Practically speaking, these are mostly non-digestible carbohydrates that can be fermented by colonic bacteria (e.g., inulin, FOS, etc.).

Synbiotic: A product designed to deliver both a probiotic and prebiotic at the same time.

Bacteriophage: A virus that infects bacteria (sometimes called "phages"). Considered part of the microbiome, certain bacteriophages are being explored as therapeutic antimicrobial or anti-biofilm agents while others may promote the growth of certain commensal organisms (commercially, these latter bacteriophages have been marketed as "prebiotics").

The Human Gut Microbiome: The Basics

As most are now aware, the human GI tract is a host to countless microbes (some estimate 100 trillion bacteria alone) that have a powerful impact on human health. This impact extends well beyond the gut lumen, and has been implicated in nearly every facet of human physiology and metabolism.[1,2,3] In fact, the gut microbiome is now commonly viewed by many as a semi-autonomous symbiotic organ or organ-like system within the GI tract. However, while our knowledge of the microbiome within the human gut has greatly expanded in just the past few years, there is much we still do not know about this complex ecosystem, especially as it pertains to modifying its structure and metabolic functions to favor a healthy outcome for the host.

Our knowledge of the commensal gut microbiota is heavily weighted toward bacterial species, though there is a growing base of knowledge on GI-resident viruses, bacteriophages (viruses that infect bacteria), fungi, and protozoa. Recent technological advances that allow for the recovery, amplification and sequencing of genetic material from the gut have given us exponentially more information than the plating/growth technologies of the past, allowing for the identification of more than 1,300 different bacterial species in humans worldwide (identified primarily by ribosomal RNA sequences).[†4,5]

Acknowledging that the human GI tract is a highly complex network of microbes is one thing, understanding the important features within this complexity has been much more daunting. This is partly due to the fact that the primary tool used to study the gut microbiome in humans is the analysis of fecal microbiota (from stool samples), which we now know is only a rough approximation of the many microbial niches found within the GI tract. However, since this is how most of the data is generated, we will start our discussion there.

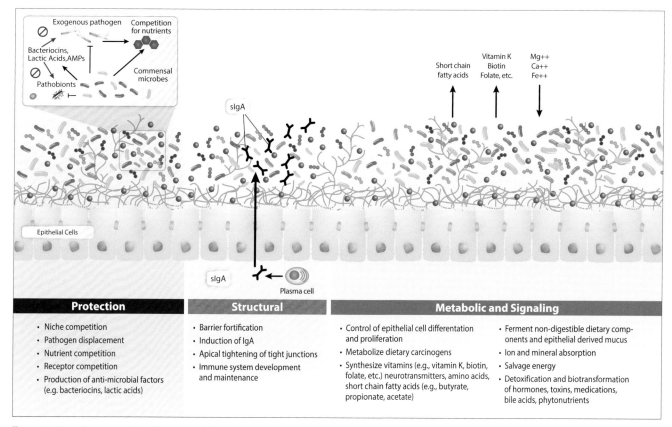

Figure 16: Basic Function of the Commensal Gut Microbiota. From the perspective of the host, this figure illustrates the three basic functional categories performed by the commensal gut microbiota. Some of these activities are also provided by certain probiotic organisms. See text for more details.

---

† There is some debate about the number of species identified with the global human microbiome based on the definition of a species and the techniques used to identify genetic differences. This number continues to expand as better genetic tools become available and larger populations are sampled.

Phylum-Level Differences

Of the more than 1,300 or so different subspecies of bacteria that have been associated with the human microbiome, each person may only have a few hundred of these subspecies residing within their GI tract at any given time, the ratio and diversity of which can be approximated by examining their feces (though fecal microbiota is, understandably, over-represented by species from the colon). The enumeration of human fecal microbiota is often reported by large groupings or classifications based on genetics or function; one of the largest of which is phylum-level classification (see Figure 17). Five phyla of bacteria are commonly reported, as they make up the vast majority of the gut bacterial microbiota: Firmicutes, Bacteroidetes,

Actinobacteria, Verricumicrobia, and Proteobacteria. Each is represented by dozens of species in any given individual (more than 10 phyla of bacteria, as well as archaea, have been isolated from within the human gut microbiome).

Based on these rudimentary phylum-level distinctions, certain gut microbiome patterns have emerged amongst different groups of individuals based on other health or lifestyle parameters. One of the most well-known distinctions is in obese Western subjects, who are more likely to show increased ratios of Firmicutes-to-Bacteroidetes compared to lean subjects.[6] Some suggest that this association is related to a more efficient extraction of calories

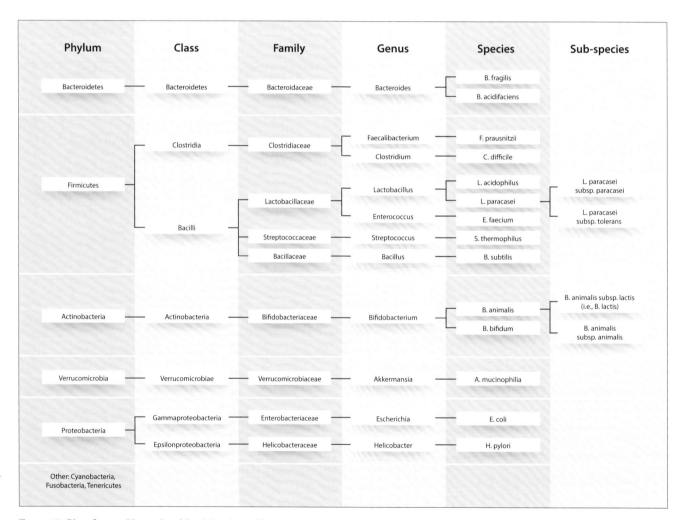

Figure 17: Classification Hierarchy of Gut Microbiota. This figure shows some of the major groups of bacteria that are resident in the human gut, showing key species and sub-species in the five major phyla.

from the diet by certain bacteria, though many other factors have been implicated.[7,8] However, the cause-effect relationship between phylum-level microbiota analysis and specific outcomes can obscure many details, including the fact that many bacterial species may increase (or decrease) in certain situations even while the total number of bacteria within the phylum to which they belong decreases (or increases). In addition, not all species within these two phyla have similar functions or potential benefits. For instance, all the *Lactobacilli* species, many with proven health benefits, are part of the Firmicutes phylum, while the Bacteroidetes phylum contain species that can be pathogenic. Beyond that, there are many important bacterial species found in other phyla altogether (*Bifidobacterium* are Actinobacteria; *Akkermansia* are Verrucomicrobiota, etc.). So while phylum-level analysis is a potential way to understand the microbiota, one that we will discuss when commonly linked to specific GI-related function or dysfunction, it can be misleading when viewed as a diagnosis or therapeutic goal.

Enterotypes and Microbiota Diversity

Categorizing an individual's or population's gut microbiota based on phylum-level ratios has many limitations. Instead, some researchers have used fecal metagenomics to propose that there are a limited number of clusters, or enterotypes, of microbiota within human populations across the globe. In a landmark paper published in *Nature* (2011), a collaboration from around the world defined one of three different enterotypes in most studied subjects, independent of their geography.[9] These enterotypes were named based on the genera of bacteria that are most abundant in each by Genus (Phylum): *Bacteroides* (Bacteroidetes), *Prevotella* (Bacteroidetes) and *Ruminococcus* (Firmicutes).

However, there is now considerable debate about whether such distinct enterotypes are broadly distributed across most human populations. Other researchers, instead, describe a continuum or gradient of species based on diet, geography and other factors.[10,11,12] Furthermore, as we shall see throughout this guidebook, the presence or absence (or change in abundance) of even one or two species, regardless of their overall abundance within the total microbiota, can often be an important feature associated with a specific gastrointestinal dysfunction. This is certainly true of many pathogenic organisms that, even when present at extremely low levels, can have profound physiological effects. This is also likely true of many other commensal organisms present at low overall abundance. Some, as we will note, may be a dominant species within a small niche of the gut, though they remain relatively difficult to quantify in fecal samples. Therefore, we will highlight genera or species-level differences as they relate to GI dysfunction below and in other chapters related to specific dysfunctions, mindful that these distinctions may not be the most important diagnostic feature of the microbiome in every patient.

Some Key Commensal and Pathobiont Species

While there are hundreds of sub-species of commensal bacterial organisms within the GI tract, here we select a few to highlight that are of historical or research interest. See the main text for discussions of other commensal or pathogenic species.

Escherichia coli   **Phylum:** Proteobacterium   **Family:** Enterobacteriaceae

---

E.coli is perhaps the most well-known, and certainly the most studied bacterium on the planet. It is a facultative anaerobe first discovered in the feces of healthy individuals by Theodor Escherich in 1885 (he called it *Bacterium coli commune*). Numerous strains of *E.coli* have been described, including both helpful and harmful strains. Because *E. coli* can grow in feces under aerobic conditions, it is considered a marker species for fecal contamination (i.e., coliform) and several virulent strains have been the cause of contamination in food-borne illnesses. *E. coli* are generally benign commensal strains that reside in the colon of healthy individuals, though they often trigger a potent inflammatory response when they infect the urinary tract. The K12 strain, having been adapted for growth in the laboratory, has been the workhorse of much of the recombinant DNA research done over the past three decades. One particular strain, *E. coli* Nissle 1917, was also used as one of the first probiotics.

  E. coli Nissle 1917 is a non-pathogenic strain first isolated in 1917 by Professor Nissle from the feces of a WWI soldier that, unlike his comrades, did not suffer from diarrhea.[1] It has since been a well-known probiotic strain. Genomic analysis has shown *E. coli* Nissle 1917 expresses fitness factors such as proteases and adhesins; and unlike some other *E. coli* strains, Nissle 1917 does not produce virulence factors, all of which contributes to the potential probiotic properties of this strain.[2] An *in vitro* study using Caco-2 intestinal epithelial cells has shown *E. coli* Nissle, like some *Lactobacilli* probiotic bacteria, is able to stimulate the expression of the antimicrobial peptide β-defensin-2 in a time and dose-dependent manner, which may protect the mucosal barrier against pathogenic bacteria.[3] Other protective mechanisms that have been researched for *E. coli* Nissle 1917 include maintenance of tight junctions through protein expression of zonula occludin-2, and an alteration of cytokine profiles with increased levels of IL-10, IL-12, MCP-1, MIP-2α and MIP-2β measured *in vitro*.[4,5,6] A recent systematic review and meta-analysis found *E. coli* Nissle 1917 equivalent to mesalazine in preventing disease relapse in ulcerative colitis.[7]

Faecalibacterium prausnitzii   **Phylum:** Firmicutes   **Family:** Clostridiaceae

---

F. prausnitzii is a highly abundant, anaerobic bacterium within the healthy human gut microbiome, and a commensal member of the Firmicutes phylum.[8] Studies suggest *F. prausnitzii* is highly sensitive to its environment; it is an extremely oxygen-sensitive bacterium and sensitive to acute or moderate intestinal inflammation. This sensitivity has made laboratory cultivation difficult, even under strict anaerobic conditions; however, techniques using culture medium supplemented with flavins and cysteine or glutathione may support the growth of *F. prausnitzii* under micro-aerobic conditions.[9] *F. prausnitzii* is one of the most abundant butyrate-producing bacterium in the gastrointestinal tract. Research surrounding *F. prausnitzii* greatly increased in the past decade since Sokol and colleagues found an association between low levels of *F. prausnitzii* in patients with Crohn's disease; research that suggests the potential of *F. prausnitzii* to be used as an indicator species of intestinal health.[10,11]

  Considerable research has evaluated the abundance of *F. prausnitzii* in diverse gastrointestinal disorders including: IBD, IBS, celiac disease, chronic idiopathic diarrhea, and colorectal cancer, amongst others.[8,12,13,14,15,16,17,18] Generally, these studies have shown a positive correlation between good intestinal health and an abundance of *F. prausnitzii* levels. Therefore, given the suggested anti-inflammatory properties of *F. prausnitzii* and its association with GI health, evaluating levels of *F. prausnitzii* has been suggested to be clinically relevant as a biomarker for intestinal inflammation.

Akkermansia muciniphila   **Phylum:** Verrucomicrobia   **Family:** Verrucomicrobiaceae

---

As of February 2016, eight species of *Akkermansia* have been identified, but only one has been cultured – *Akkermansia muciniphila*.[19] Furthermore, only one strain of *A. muciniphila*, type strain (Muc1), is available in public culture collections. Therefore, although this microbe has been the subject of intense study, much is left to be discovered about this commensal organism.

A. muciniphila is an important commensal organism in the mucosal layer of the human gastrointestinal tract, where the bacterium degrades the amino acids and oligosaccharides in mucus for energy, nitrogen and carbon.[20] *A. muciniphila* is a major component of the human gut microbiota in healthy subjects. While some contradictory studies exist, most published research generally correlates reduced abundance of *A. muciniphila* with greater incidence of inflammatory bowel and metabolic disorders.[21,22]

Perhaps the most interesting data centers on *A. muciniphila* in metabolic-related disorders. A seminal study, published in 2013, showed daily administration of *A. muciniphila* at a dosage of 10^8 CFU/day for four weeks could ameliorate many of the metabolic features of a high fat diet in mice, reversing fat-mass gain, metabolic endotoxemia, adipose tissue inflammation, insulin resistance, and restoring epithelial mucus integrity.[23] In an animal model of diabetes, Roux-en-Y gastric bypass surgery was shown to significantly increase *A. muciniphila* levels compared to levels before surgery and to control animals ($p < 0.05$).[24]

The modulation of *A. muciniphila* levels by diet, medication and antibiotic use have been studied, though many of these studies are complicated by the fact that they were completed in animal models which may not be directly applicable to human subjects. Many diet-related factors have been shown to increase levels of *A. muciniphila*, including polyphenols, prebiotic fibers, conjugated linolenic acid, oat bran, and caloric restriction (see review for comprehensive list).[19] Surprisingly, some antibiotics and metformin have been associated with increased relative abundance of *A. muciniphila*.[25,26,27]

Bacteroides Fragilis (Pathobiont)   **Phylum:** Bacteroidetes   **Family:** Bacteroidaceae

B. fragilis are obligate anaerobes and the most common pathobionts of the genus Bacteroides causing serious anaerobic infection (e.g., sepsis, peritonitis and abscesses).[28,29] Infection occurs as *B. fragilis* translocates endogenously from the patient's own gut microbiome to the blood or the peritoneum.[28,30] A triggering event is necessary for translocation as there is no evidence indicating that *B. fragilis* is invasive on its own. Triggering events include bowel surgery, trauma, or other chronic diseases.[28,30] The course and severity of illness is strongly influenced by the translocation of other anaerobic bacteria from the gut.[28] *B. fragilis* are exceptionally hardy and one of the most easily cultivated anaerobic bacteria via plating on blood agar under anaerobic conditions.[28] Perhaps a testament to their resiliency, *B. fragilis* are relatively oxygen-tolerant and able to grow in the presence of nano-molar oxygen via an oxidative stress response mediated by detoxifying enzymes like catalase and superoxide dismutase.[28,31] This stress response likely plays a vital role in the virulence of *B. fragilis,* as it aids in the survival of the bacteria in oxygenated tissues while translocating from the gut. In fact, it has been shown that *B. fragilis* can survive up to three days' exposure to atmospheric oxygen.[28,31]

Treatment of *B. fragilis* infection and other anaerobic infections more broadly includes drainage of abscesses, debridement of necrotic tissue, and administration of a combination of antibiotics.[28] *B. fragilis* produces a beta-lactamase, and is commonly resistant to tetracycline.[28]

Clostridium difficile (Pathobiont)   **Phylum:** Firmicutes   **Family:** Clostridiaceae

C. difficile are medically important anaerobic, gram-positive, exotoxin-producing bacteria responsible for many cases of acute diarrhea and pseudomembranous colitis (PMC) associated with the use of antimicrobial agents.[32] A few unique features of this bacterium allow it to flourish under conditions of antibiotic administration. First, *C. difficile* is resistant to most antibiotics, allowing it to dominate the gut microbiota as other commensals are destroyed by the antibiotic agent. Secondly, *C. difficile* can form protective spores, triggered by the bile salt taurocholate, further promoting its dominance. The exotoxins produced by *C. difficile*, termed toxin A (TcdA) and toxin B (TcdB), are released during the late growth phase of the vegetative cells. A hypervirulent strain has emerged, which produces another toxin termed *C. difficile* transferase (CDT) in addition to TcdA and TcdB. *C. difficile* is transmitted endogenously, or through the environment when spores are released via the fecal-oral route (common in hospital settings). Potential treatment for *C. difficile* infection is discussed further on page 165.

Helicobacter pylori (Pathobiont)   **Phylum:** Proteobacteria   **Family:** Helicobacteraceae

H. pylori are motile, gram-negative, spiral-shaped pathogens that take up residence in the stomach upon ingestion.[33,34] Infection with *H. pylori* is linked to gastritis, hypochlorhydria, peptic ulcer, duodenal ulcer, MALT lymphomas and gastric adenocarcinoma.[35] The bacterium grows optimally at a pH of 6.0-7.0, and has two key characteristics that allow colonization within the stomach (luminal pH 1.0-2.0).[33] First, the bacterium is urease positive and therefore able to produce ammonia, a feature that confers protection for *H. pylori* by neutralizing stomach acid. Secondly, *H. pylori* have multiple flagella at one pole, which allow the bacteria to move through the gastric mucosa epithelium layer to the basal layer where physiological pH is present.[33,35] Additionally, *H. pylori* produce a protease that modifies gastric mucus. *H. pylori* is discussed further on page 205.

References

1.   Jacobi CA, Malfertheiner P. Escherichia coli Nissle 1917 (Mutaflor): New insights into an old probiotic bacterium. *Dig Dis*. 2011;29(6):600-7.
2.   Grozdanov L, Raasch C, Schulze J, et al. Analysis of the genome structure of the nonpathogenic probiotic Escherichia coli strain Nissle 1917. *J Bacteriol*. 2004 Aug;186(16):5432-41.
3.   Wehkamp J, Harder J, Wehkamp K, et al. NF-kappaB- and AP-1-mediated induction of human beta defensin-2 in intestinal epithelial cells by Escherichia coli Nissle 1917: a novel effect of a probiotic bacterium. *Infect Immun*. 2004 Oct;72(10):5750-8.
4.   Zyrek AA, Cichon C, Helms S, et al. Molecular mechanisms underlying the probiotic effects of Escherichia coli Nissle 1917 involve ZO-2 and PKCzeta redistribution resulting in tight junction and epithelial barrier repair. *Cell Microbiol*. 2007 Mar;9(3):804-16.
5.   Ukena SN, Westendorf AM, Hansen W, et al. The host response to the probiotic Escherichia coli strain Nissle 1917: specific up-regulation of the proinflammatory chemokine MCP-1. *BMC Med Genet*. 2005 Dec 13;6:43.
6.   Gad M, Ravn P, Søborg DA, et al. Regulation of the IL-10/IL-12 axis in human dendritic cells with probiotic bacteria. *FEMS Immunol Med Microbiol*. 2011 Oct;63(1):93-107.
7.   Losurdo G, Iannone A, Contaldo A, et al. Escherichia coli Nissle 1917 in Ulcerative Colitis Treatment: Systematic Review and Meta-analysis. *J Gastrointestin Liver Dis*. 2015 Dec;24(4):499-505.
8.   Miquel S, Martín R, Rossi O, et al. Faecalibacterium prausnitzii and human intestinal health. *Curr Opin Microbiol*. 2013 Jun;16(3):255-61.
9.   Khan MT, Duncan SH, Stams AJ, et al. The gut anaerobe Faecalibacterium prausnitzii uses an extracellular electron shuttle to grow at oxic-anoxic interphases. *ISME J*. 2012 Aug;6(8):1578-85.
10. Sokol H, Pigneur B, Watterlot L, et al. Faecalibacterium prausnitzii is an anti-inflammatory commensal bacterium identified by gut microbiota analysis of Crohn disease patients. *Proc Natl Acad Sci U S A*. 2008 Oct 28;105(43):16731-6.
11. http://www.scientificamerican.com/article/among-trillions-of-microbes-in-the-gut-a-few-are-special/?print=true
12. Cao Y, Shen J, Ran ZH. Association between Faecalibacterium prausnitzii Reduction and Inflammatory Bowel Disease: A Meta-Analysis and Systematic Review of the Literature. *Gastroenterol Res Pract*. 2014;2014:872725.
13. Fujimoto T, Imaeda H, Takahashi K, et al. Decreased abundance of Faecalibacterium prausnitzii in the gut microbiota of Crohn's disease. *J Gastroenterol Hepatol*. 2013 Apr;28(4):613-9.
14. Sokol H, Pigneur B, Watterlot L, et al. Faecalibacterium prausnitzii is an anti-inflammatory commensal bacterium identified by gut microbiota analysis of Crohn disease patients. *Proc Natl Acad Sci U S A*. 2008 Oct 28;105(43):16731-6.
15. Rajilić-Stojanović M, Biagi E, Heilig HG, et al. Global and deep molecular analysis of microbiota signatures in fecal samples from patients with irritable bowel syndrome. *Gastroenterology*. 2011 Nov;141(5):1792-801.
16. De Palma G, Nadal I, Medina M, et al. Intestinal dysbiosis and reduced immunoglobulin-coated bacteria associated with coeliac disease in children. *BMC Microbiol*. 2010 Feb 24;10:63.
17. Swidsinski A, Loening-Baucke V, Verstraelen H, et al. Biostructure of fecal microbiota in healthy subjects and patients with chronic idiopathic diarrhea. *Gastroenterology*. 2008 Aug;135(2):568-79.
18. Lopez-Siles M, Martinez-Medina M, Surís-Valls R, et al. Changes in the Abundance of Faecalibacterium prausnitzii Phylogroups I and II in the Intestinal Mucosa of Inflammatory Bowel Disease and Patients with Colorectal Cancer. *Inflamm Bowel Dis*. 2016 Jan;22(1):28-41.
19. Derrien M, Belzer C, de Vos WM. Akkermansia muciniphila and its role in regulating host functions. *Microb Pathog*. 2016 Feb 11. pii: S0882-4010(15)30178-9.
20. Belzer C, de Vos WM. Microbes inside--from diversity to function: the case of Akkermansia. *ISME J*. 2012 Aug;6(8):1449-58.
21. Berry D, Reinisch W. Intestinal microbiota: a source of novel biomarkers in inflammatory bowel diseases? *Best Pract Res Clin Gastroenterol*. 2013 Feb;27(1):47-58.
22. Woting A, Blaut M. The Intestinal Microbiota in Metabolic Disease. *Nutrients*. 2016 Apr 6;8(4). pii: E202.
23. Everard A, Belzer C, Geurts L, et al. Cross-talk between Akkermansia muciniphila and intestinal epithelium controls diet-induced obesity. *Proc Natl Acad Sci U S A*. 2013 May 28;110(22):9066-71.
24. Yan M, Song MM, Bai RX, et al. Effect of Roux-en-Y gastric bypass surgery on intestinal Akkermansia muciniphila. *World J Gastrointest Surg*. 2016 Apr 27;8(4):301-7.
25. Shin NR, Lee JC, Lee HY, et al. An increase in the Akkermansia spp. population induced by metformin treatment improves glucose homeostasis in diet-induced obese mice. *Gut*. 2014 May;63(5):727-35.
26. Zhou ZY, Ren LW, Zhan P, et al. Metformin exerts glucose-lowering action in high-fat fed mice via attenuating endotoxemia and enhancing insulin signaling. *Acta Pharmacol Sin*. 2016 May 16. doi: 10.1038/aps.2016.21.
27. Hansen CH, Krych L, Nielsen DS, et al. Early life treatment with vancomycin propagates Akkermansia muciniphila and reduces diabetes incidence in the NOD mouse. *Diabetologia*. 2012 Aug;55(8):2285-94.
28. Ryan KJ, Ray C. Clostridium, Peptostreptococcus, Bacteroides, and Other Anaerobes. In: Ryan KJ, Ray C. eds. Sherris Medical Microbiology, 6e. New York, NY: McGraw-Hill; 2014.
29. Levinson W. Gram-Negative Rods Related to the Enteric Tract. In: Levinson W. eds. Review of Medical Microbiology and Immunology, 13e. New York, NY: McGraw-Hill; 2014.
30. Levinson W. Brief Summaries of Medically Important Organisms: Introduction. In: Levinson W. eds. Review of Medical Microbiology and Immunology, 14e. New York, NY: McGraw-Hill; 2016.
31. Sears CL, Geis AL, Housseau F. Bacteroides fragilis subverts mucosal biology: from symbiont to colon carcinogenesis. *J Clin Invest*. 2014 Oct;124(10):4166-72.
32. Ryan KJ, Ray C. Clostridium, Peptostreptococcus, Bacteroides, and Other Anaerobes. In: Ryan KJ, Ray C. eds. Sherris Medical Microbiology, 6e. New York, NY: McGraw-Hill; 2014.
33. Carroll KC, Hobden JA, Miller S, et al. Vibrio, Campylobacter, and Helicobacter. In: Carroll KC, Hobden JA, Miller S, Morse SA, Mietzner TA, Detrick B, Mitchell TG, McKerrow JH, Sakanari JA. eds. Jawetz, Melnick, & Adelberg's Medical Microbiology, 27e. New York, NY: McGraw-Hill; 2015.
34. Levinson W. Brief Summaries of Medically Important Organisms. In: Levinson W. eds. Review of Medical Microbiology and Immunology, 13e. New York, NY: McGraw-Hill; 2014.
35. Kao CY, Sheu BS, Wu JJ. Helicobacter pylori infection: An overview of bacterial virulence factors and pathogenesis. *Biomed J*. 2016 Feb;39(1):14-23.

Distribution: Diversity and Heterogeneity

Since most of the information gathered about the human microbiome is derived from fecal sampling, it may give the impression that the GI microbiome is a homogenous mixture of species. However, it is abundantly clear that there is not one *single* GI microbial environment, but many. As shown in Figure 18, the relative abundance and species distribution of the microbiota are radically different at each major section between the stomach and the colon of an adult GI tract.[†] The stomach is the least populated, while the colon houses the vast majority of microorganisms. Aerobic and facultative anaerobic bacteria are found in the stomach and much of the small bowel, while the distal ileum and colon are colonized almost exclusively by anaerobic species. A variety of factors, including available oxygen, pH, bile acids, nutrient availability and host immune functions all affect these differences.

Furthermore, along the intact GI tract, researchers have recognized numerous micro-

habitats. They have identified some organisms that preferentially associate closely with the inner mucus-layer and enterocytes, some with the outer mucus layer, some found in the crypt, and others loosely attached or in the lumen only (see Figure 19).[13]

Studies have shown that, when sampled by biopsy, significant variability in species exist in some colon sample locations that are only a centimeter apart.[14,15] Indeed, this emerging area of "biogeography" research simply confirms that there is still much we do not know about the intricate and dynamic architecture of the human gut microbiome; including many features that are hard to assess using fecal sampling alone. In addition to the mini ecosystems created by the architecture of the gut itself, many species of bacteria exist within a biofilm, a microbe-secreted extracellular matrix that permits many different bacteria to bind to the gut and function within a protected "capsule."

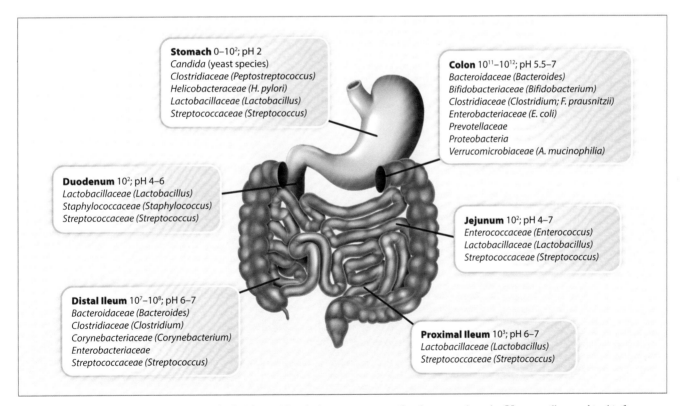

Stomach $0–10^2$; pH 2
Candida (yeast species)
Clostridiaceae (Peptostreptococcus)
Helicobacteraceae (H. pylori)
Lactobacillaceae (Lactobacillus)
Streptococcaceae (Streptococcus)

Colon $10^{11}–10^{12}$; pH 5.5–7
Bacteroidaceae (Bacteroides)
Bifidobacteriaceae (Bifidobacterium)
Clostridiaceae (Clostridium; F. prausnitzii)
Enterobacteriaceae (E. coli)
Prevotellaceae
Proteobacteria
Verrucomicrobiaceae (A. mucinophilia)

Duodenum 10^2; pH 4–6
Lactobacillaceae (Lactobacillus)
Staphylococcaceae (Staphylococcus)
Streptococcaceae (Streptococcus)

Jejunum 10^2; pH 4–7
Enterococcaceae (Enterococcus)
Lactobacillaceae (Lactobacillus)
Streptococcaceae (Streptococcus)

Distal Ileum $10^7–10^8$; pH 6–7
Bacteroidaceae (Bacteroides)
Clostridiaceae (Clostridium)
Corynebacteriaceae (Corynebacterium)
Enterobacteriaceae
Streptococcaceae (Streptococcus)

Proximal Ileum 10^3; pH 6–7
Lactobacillaceae (Lactobacillus)
Streptococcaceae (Streptococcus)

Figure 18: General Heterogeneity of GI Microbial Habitats. Microbial species are not uniformly present along the GI tract as illustrated in this figure. Differences in nutrient availability, lumen pH and a number of other factors (see Figure 19) contribute to the large heterogeneity of microbial species.

[†] The oral microbiome is not discussed in this Standard Road map, though it is very well-studied and important for maintaining human health. Esophageal microbiome information is more limited, though noticeably changed in conditions such as Barrett's esophagus.

Testing the Microbiome—What are the Options?

There are several different laboratory tests that can be performed to help the clinician evaluate the structure and function of a patient's gut microbiome. While a few of these tests are diagnostic (e.g., presence of a pathogenic organism), most of these biomarkers are merely indicative of an association with particular gastrointestinal imbalances or dysfunctions. Since the structure and function of the microbiome is easily altered by diet and other factors, it is important to realize that most biomarkers reflect the patient's diet and lifestyle influences in the previous days before sampling. Also, since most individuals have an aversion to handling feces, fecal samples are often non-uniform and are modified by the way they are handled and shipped to the laboratory. Several of the tests used to analyze the microbiome are included as part of a comprehensive stool analysis (CDA, CDSA™) offered by different labs. Clinicians should become familiar with the test they intend to use to analyze the microbiome's influence on their patients and what, if any, diagnostic benefit such tests will have on the therapies recommended. Most labs provide information about the analytes they measure, their reference ranges and potential interpretation of test results. Clinicians should be familiar with the information related to the particular lab providing the test results, as different reference ranges and testing methods may be employed by each.

Cultures

Culturing stool bacteria is a classic technique to identify and roughly estimate the presence of particular bacteria within the microbiome. This technique is obviously limited to identifying those organisms that are still alive in the feces after shipping to the laboratory and are capable of being cultured on one of several different growth media available. Culturing is widely available and primarily used to identify specific pathogenic organisms, but can also be used to provide a semi-quantitative abundance of certain beneficial commensal organisms. Interpreting these results can be straightforward, as in the identification of known pathogens (e.g., food poisoning with *Camplobacter* or *Salmonella*); or more nuanced when estimating commensal organisms (may suggest the need for prebiotics or probiotics with low *Bifidobacterium* or

Lactobacilli, though little evidence exists for connecting probiotics with cultured fecal samples). Enumeration of small intestinal aspirates is also used as the gold standard to define small intestinal bacterial overgrowth (SIBO- see page 231). When the enumeration exceeds $1x10^5$ CFU/ml, regardless of the type of bacteria cultured, this is considered a positive SIBO finding.

Microscopic Analysis (Parasites and Ova)

Examining fecal samples for parasitic organisms or their ova is best done using direct microscopic analysis by a trained technician. This can be done with a single fecal sample, though the CDC recommends examination of at least three samples taken on different days for conclusive results. This technique, along with immunoassay results, is used to help diagnose parasitic infections such as *Cryptosporidium spp.*, *Entamoeba spp.*, *Blastocystis hominis* and *Giardia lamblia*.

Immunoassays

Antibodies can be used to identify or quantify a variety of parasites, bacteria, or toxins in a stool sample. Often, these immunoassay tests are combined with other culture or microscopic techniques to enhance the detection or specificity of these tests.

Metabolites (Fecal and Urine)

Measuring certain metabolites in stool or urine samples can give some clue as to the types of microbial species present in the GI tract. For instance, the amounts or types of short chain fatty acids (SCFAs) detected in the stool gives some evidence of the fermentation activity in the colon, and can act as a surrogate marker for the presence and activity of certain commensal and pathobiont organisms (e.g., *Bifidobacterium spp.*, *Clostridium spp.*). Direct measure of bacterial enzyme activity (e.g., beta-glucuronidase) may also suggest the presence of certain bacteria. However, in many cases the metabolite measured can be influenced by other factors, especially diet and bowel transit time. In the case of SCFAs, the levels measured in the stool may be influenced by the availability of undigested fibers and amino acids more so than the specific levels of various species in the gut. In addition to stool testing, metabolites produced by gut microbiota can also be measured in the urine. In many cases, certain metabolites that are only produced by bacteria or yeast can be used as surrogate markers for the amounts or types of metabolic activities of specific species within the gut microbiota. While measuring such metabolites is rarely diagnostic for any particular GI dysfunction, they may help clinicians confirm the relationship between certain symptoms and a specific type of dysbiotic condition.

Finally, some reports of metagenomic analysis (discussed below) describe the likely metabolic profile of the microbiome. These profiles are not based upon measures of biological activity within the fecal sample, but are a theoretical calculation of the types of activities that are present based on the relative abundance of certain species and their metabolic capabilities. Since many of these metabolic functions are under genomic control and are not expressed at all times in each host (often being dependent of the substrates presence in the diet); these metabolic profiles should be used with extreme caution.

Genetics (Metagenomics)

The emerging standard for gut microbiome testing is a complete analysis of the metagenome within a fecal sample. Depending on the technique(s) used, this can identify hundreds of species of bacteria or usually what is referred to as operational taxonomic units (sometimes grouping similar species together). Several laboratories have made such tests directly available to the public, though a few are available for clinicians only. As the main text details, the analysis of the gut microbiome can be reported by phylum, family, class, genus or species of bacteria found in the stool sample; or by the types of metabolic functions that are capable of being expressed by certain types of bacteria. Often, the phylum ratios (primarily Firmicutes-to-Bacteroides) or the relative quantity of specific genera (e.g., *Akkermansia* or *Lactobacilli*) are shown in comparison to the general population or groups with particular dysfunctions (e.g., obesity or IBD).

While we generally believe such analysis will be the future of microbiome analysis, there are a few precautions that must be understood when interpreting these data. First, it should be reiterated that many species can increase or decrease within only a few days of dietary changes and therefore this should always be viewed as a snapshot of those potential changes. Also, there is evidence that fecal microbiota is not uniform throughout the whole feces and poor sampling technique could cause an over-representation or under-representation of a number of species. In addition, some species are known to rapidly multiply after the sample is taken and during shipping to the lab. While several labs attempt to account for this in the algorithm they use to calculate the enumeration of species, these adjustments are based on poorly tested assumptions.

Finally, and perhaps most importantly, these metagenomics tests are not uniform between different labs or genetic techniques; and perhaps even between different days or technicians in the same lab. A number of well-known social media sites have reported dramatically different results when sending the same fecal sample to different labs. Since each laboratory must perform various techniques (DNA/RNA extraction, amplification, hybridization, sequencing, computer algorithm analysis etc.), and each technique has a range of repeatability and reliability, the overall reproducibility of gut microbiome metagenomics testing is still a "work in progress." In fact, the issue of poor reproducibility has spawned the start of the Microbiome Quality Control Project, a collaboration of over a dozen universities, laboratories and hospitals, to create standards for sampling, handling, storing, analyzing and reporting microbiome information (www.mbqc.org).

For these reasons, clinicians using gut microbiome metagenomics data (whether ordered through the physician's clinic or helping a patient understand results from a test they did on their own) should interpret them with caution. Also, clinicians should keep a close watch on the rapid advances in this area of testing and the emerging techniques used in clinical research. As these techniques become more reliable, they are likely to help the clinician follow a person's gut microbiome changes through significant points along their life (or healing) journey. Currently, the information may be helpful to confirm things that are already suspected (dysbiosis, gut inflammation, obesity-prone microbiota, etc.), but metagenomics analysis is not considered to be a gold-standard diagnostic technique for any current condition. Many laboratories will offer associative data as part of their report when certain species are higher/lower than their "reference range;" suggesting this may be correlated to a particular disorder. Clinicians should be cautious to use these associates for the reasons mentioned above.

Microbial Biofilms: Their Structure and Function

We have already discussed quite a bit about microbes living in the gut, mostly focusing on different species of bacteria and their preferred location(s) within one or more of the many micro-ecosystems located along the GI tract (see Figures 18 and 19). Here, we want to summarize the importance of microbial biofilm communities and how they function to form the unique mucosal biofilm that helps define the function of much of the gut microbiome.

First, let us describe the basic structure and function of a biofilm formed by a generic bacterium (fungi biofilm form in a similar manner; some viral particles are also thought to control a biofilm-like matrix).[16,17,18] When a planktonic (free-floating) cell becomes attached to an inert or living surface, it alters its genetic expression to secrete extracellular polymeric substances (EPS), mostly polysaccharides and proteins, which form a kind of extracellular matrix. When examined, biofilms are made mostly of water (>95%), flowing in channels formed by the EPS. The architecture of the biofilm allows the resident bacteria to control this very local ecosystem, managing such things as cell density, nutrient availability, pH, temperature, and osmolarity. Hence, microbes living within a biofilm are less likely to become casualties of nutrient depletion, pH changes and other factors that would affect planktonic organisms of the same species. If the location of the attached biofilm becomes less hospitable for the microbes within, their genetic expression will be altered to dissolve the biofilm and allow cells to be released to find another suitable place to reform a biofilm.

Perhaps the most well-known feature of biofilms is that they provide resident bacteria more protection from harmful agents such as antibiotics, a characteristic trait of infectious biofilms.[19] Biofilms are commonly described in dental caries, otitis media, biliary tract infections, bacterial prostatitis, urinary tract infections and a wide-range of infections associated with foreign body materials such as contact lens, sutures, mechanical heart valves, medical implants, urinary catheters, and IUDs.[20] The need for higher doses of antibiotics over a longer period of time to treat biofilm-related infections has, unfortunately, led to the selection of bacterial strains that are resistant to many (if not most) antibiotics, as well as promoting the transfer of antibacterial genes to formerly non-resistant strains. Some species of bacteria require 1,000 times higher antibiotic concentrations to eradicate from biofilm, as compared to the same species in a free-living environment.[21]

Depending on the biofilm, many different species of bacteria may be present. Different bacterial species form and interact within the biofilm through a process called quorum sensing.[22] This process involves the production and secretion of small signaling molecules called autoinducers, which accumulate to a higher concentration as more cells cluster together (allowing the cells to gauge cell density or "a quorum" through various receptors). Some of these signaling molecules are shared across a wide range of different species, while some are very specific to a particular strain of bacteria (often accounting for the virulence of those strains).

Natural and synthetic agents that inhibit quorum sensing or promote biofilm dispersal (in one or more tested species) are being explored as promising ways to combat antibiotic-resistant biofilm-mediated infections (usually in combination with antibiotics).[23] Some of these compounds are found in traditional foods and medicines such as eugenol (cloves), curcumin (turmeric), ajoene (garlic), cinnamic acid (cinnamon), resveratrol (red wine), asiatic acid (*Centella asiatica* L.), and ursolic acid (variety of sources).[24,25,26,27,28,29,30] In fact, a wide variety of plant compounds known for being antimicrobial have some measurable level of biofilm-disrupting activity in laboratory settings.[31] Bacteriophages that inhibit biofilm formation have also been explored as a way to combat certain antibiotic-resistant organisms.[32]

Mucosal Biofilms in the GI Tract

In general, we know relatively little about "normal" biofilm communities along most of the human gastrointestinal tract because obtaining tissue from healthy human GI tracts (through biopsies) is not a common practice. Therefore, what we know has been conjectured from animal studies, fecal analysis and observations of mucosal biopsies in subjects with a GI disorder. However, most of these biopsies are done in patients treated prophylactically with antibiotics or anti-inflammatory drugs (i.e., steroids), or when the bowel has been purged before colonoscopy, all of which severely limit the assessment of an intact mucosal biofilm community.[33] Also, much of the complex biofilm architecture and lifecycle that is common among other non-GI biofilm structures (described above) has not been observed in the mucosal biofilm communities within the gut; and these mucosal biofilm communities have been referred to as immature biofilm structures.[34]

Consequently, most of what is known and described about non-GI biofilms and their microbes may not directly apply to biofilm formation and structure within the GI tract. One of the reasons these biofilm communities differ from those in other tissues, or those attached to inserted medical devises, is the presence of mucus and the proximity to gut epithelial and immune system cells (and their signals). In essence, the extracellular matrix of gut mucosal biofilms is a complex network of microbes and their secretions along with the secretions and signals from the host (primarily mucus/mucin). Mucin is a glycosylated protein secreted by goblet cells along the GI tract, and this, along with bacterial polysaccharides and protein (and mostly water), creates a unique mucosal biofilm that is home to a variety of commensal, pathobiont and pathogenic organisms in the host.[35]

Regardless, it is still known that within the same area of the GI tract, the microbiota inside the mucosal biofilm differs significantly (in type, concentrations and genetic expression) from the microbiota in the adjacent lumen; the total GI mucosal biofilm microbiome also differs significantly from the fecal microbiome.[36] It is important to note that most bacteria have the ability to form (or become resident) in biofilms, and both commensal and pathogenic organisms likely benefit from such structures. In fact, research has shown many of the beneficial functions of *Bifidobacteria* are related to their ability to produce exopolysaccharides (i.e., biofilm

precursors),[37] and such abilities have been noted for many successful probiotic strains.[38,39]

While the relationship between biofilm formation and specific infections have been described outside the GI tract, there is limited evidence for specific biofilm-related gastrointestinal infections or disorders. A recent review of this topic suggests the best examples of biofilm-related gastrointestinal disorders are *Helicobacter pylori* infections in the gastric mucosa (see page 207 for more details) and biofilm growth on feeding tubes placed into the GI tract; while limited data also suggest biofilm-related activities in ulcerative colitis, Barrett's esophagus and Crohn's disease.[33] This does not mean that biofilm formation is not involved in other GI disorders, only that confirmation of such involvement has been difficult to obtain or mostly studied in pathogenic organisms in a laboratory setting. For instance, it is generally assumed that certain virulent bacteria or fungi infecting the GI tract, especially those that are difficult to treat using antimicrobial or antifungal agents, are protected in some way by their ability to produce biofilm (confirmed in non-GI environments). This feature, however, is rarely documented in the clinic setting.

This begs the question: "Should we treat patients with agents intended to disrupt the GI biofilm in order to treat an infectious or other gastrointestinal condition?" This implies there are proven agents known to disrupt GI biofilms in a manner that has been shown to improve one or more gastrointestinal outcomes. For the most part, we are not aware of any such data. As we mentioned above, several natural agents (and synthetic analogs) are known to disturb biofilm formation or inhibit quorum sensing in laboratory tests, but we are not aware of any research specific to mucosal biofilms generally, or gastrointestinal outcomes specifically.

Therefore, we are very cautious on recommending GI biofilm-disrupting therapies because biofilm communities within the GI mucosa contain heterogeneous mixtures of mostly beneficial organisms along with those that are potentially harmful; and biofilm disruption is unlikely to discriminate between the good and the bad. Furthermore, virtually no evidence exists to guide the clinician in the selection of agents, doses and length of treatment for GI biofilm disrupting therapies related to GI-related clinical outcomes. The use of ingredients that perform well in *in vitro* tests of biofilm disruption of monocultures, have yet to be shown effective or beneficial for GI-related outcomes (though some are marketed as if they have).

With that said, we realize some agents have been shown to display anti-biofilm activity (in non-GI, *in vitro* systems) for specific organisms that may be present or show signs of overgrowth in the GI tract (e.g., *Candida albicans, Helicobacter pylori*). Where these agents have been shown to be safe at the recommended dose, they may be helpful when attempting to eliminate or reduce the target organism until the signs and symptoms (or test result) suggest the organism is no longer problematic (see page 239 for *Candida* and page 205 for *H. pylori*). The use of a multi-species probiotic formula should always accompany such a strategy, to help promote new beneficial mucosal biofilm communities. Also, while GI-related data are lacking, the use of natural or synthetic antibiotic or antifungal agents have been more effective in the presence of biofilm disrupting agents when tested in other non-GI biofilm-related infectious conditions and therefore may be helpful when eradicating a harmful GI organism.[40,41]

Micro-Environmental Factors that Shape and Determine Colonic Mucosal Biofilm Formation and Stability: A Highly Structured and Unique Gut Environment

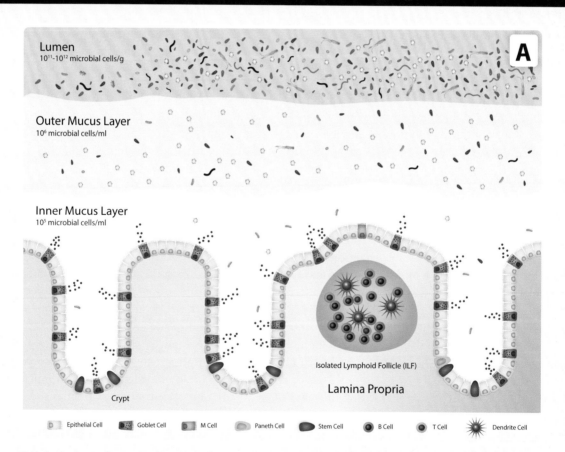

Figure 19: The majority of microbes are found in the lumen of the colon (10^{11}-10^{12} microbial cells/ml), with fewer microbes present in the outer mucus layer (10^6 microbial cells/ml) and fewer yet in the inner mucus layer covering the epithelial cells (10^5 microbial cells/ml). The luminal microbes (eventually make up the feces) not only differ by the mucosal microbes in terms of abundance, but also in terms of the types of microbes present (see Panel A). As the figure shows in panels B-G, the differences in the physiochemical properties of each distinct layer likely drive the differences in microbes across the lumen, inner mucus layer and outer mucus layer – which is the basis behind niche-specific communities within the gut microbiota. Mucosal microbes interact with the gut epithelium and gut-associated lymphoid tissue and are important modulators of human health. These images have been adapted from De Weirdt R, Van de Wiele T. Micromanagement in the gut: microenvironmental factors govern colon mucosal biofilm structure and functionality. *npj Biofilms and Microbiomes* (2015) 1, 15026. Licensed under a Creative Commons Attribution 4.0 International License.

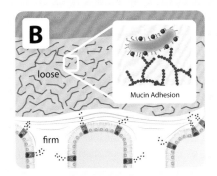

Mucus Rigidity

Within the colon, there is a gradient of rigidity of the mucus layer from the lumen, to the inner mucus layer. The lumen is most loose and fluid compared to the more firm inner mucus layer. This gradient effect has shown the ability to select for certain microbes and also exclude colonization by others. For instance, some microbes have features to facilitate colonization of more rigid mucus such as flagella, pili and fimbriae.

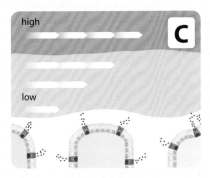

Fluid Shear Gradients

Panel C illustrates another gradient effect, fluid shear, across the lumen, outer mucus layer and the inner mucus layers. Fluid shear stress is highest in the lumen, and decreases so that the lowest shear stress is experienced by the microbes associated with the enterocytes in the inner mucus layer.

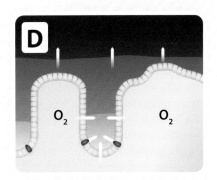

Oxygen Gradients

An oxygen gradient is also present within the colonic microbiota. Oxygen leaks from epithelial cells and consequently dilutes into the mucus layer. Some anaerobic bacteria have been shown to tolerate low concentrations of oxygen such as *F. prausnitzii* and *Bacteroides spp* within the mucus layers due to this oxygen gradient.

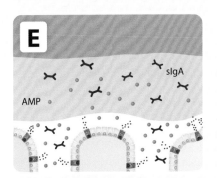

Host Defense Molecules

Host defense molecules are another factor shaping the micro-niche environment of the colonic microbiome. Such host defense molecules include antimicrobial peptides (AMPs) and secretory IgA (sIgA), by the colonic epithelial cells; compared to the small intestine, the colon secretes much lower amounts of AMPs and sIgA. Nonetheless, these antimicrobial components in the mucus layer impact the colonization ability of several microorganisms. Interestingly, the mucosal microbes are not only affected by the secretion of these host defense molecules, but also are capable of regulating host secretion of these molecules, and thereby are capable of modulating the mucosal micro-niche community. Colon mucosal biofilm formation is shaped by the build-up of host defense molecules in the thick mucus layer, with antimicrobial activities comparable to, or even greater than, those in the small intestine.

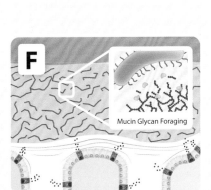

Mucosal Nutrient Platform

Another factor impacting the various micro-niche communities within the colon is the diverse nutrient availability within the lumen, outer mucus layer and the inner layer. According to De Weirdt and Van de Wiele (2015), "the colonic mucosal nutrient platform is enriched with asaccharolytic microbes that primarily metabolize peptones and amino acids, which are probably derived from proteinaceous substrates from mucus and shedded epithelium."

An example of a mucin degrading microbe is *A. muciniphila* which uses mucin as a sole carbon and nitrogen source. Mucin degradation requires a diverse enzyme set, and mucin degraders may interact with other microbes to stimulate their growth.

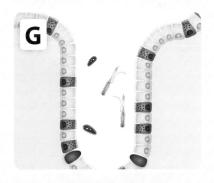

Crypt Niche

Further niche specialization may occur in certain unique environments within the colonic microbiota – such an example is the colonic crypt. Crypts are vulnerable areas of the gut epithelium as they contain stem cells and are the site of epithelial proliferation and restitution. Although the crypt niche is difficult to study in humans due to sampling limitations, the crypt micro-environment is proposed to be characterized by low mucus viscosity, a high partial oxygen pressure that, in mice, selects for aerobic species and the presence of specific types and concentrations of host glycans mediating saturable crypt occupancy by *Bacteroides spp*.

Microbiome Development: From Birth to Biosenescence

As we develop and mature from birth to old age, our various microbiome(s) develop in a predictable succession of species and function, much like other complex ecosystems.[42] Certain organisms that play a vital role in an earlier phase of microbiome development may be undetectable as a person matures, though their influence may last much longer than our ability to detect their presence. Therefore, disturbing the developing microbiome at critical stages of its development may create permanent vulnerabilities for which the host may need to compensate in order to prevent GI or other dysfunctions later in life.

While it may no longer be correct to assume the human GI tract is sterile at birth, owing to some evidence of a placental microbiome, it is still safe to assume whatever microbial ecosystem is present, appears to have limited function.[43,44] However, immediately after birth, the gut microbial community begins being seeded by microbes from the outside environment and is greatly affected by the type of delivery and initial food sources selected by the mother.[45]

It is clear that cesarean birth (C-section) alters the initial inoculation of the infant gut microbiome compared to vaginal delivery. Infants born by C-section have delayed colonization of *Bifidobacterium* and *Bacteroides* and have an initial microbiome that is often heavily influenced by the mother's skin microbiota.[46,47,48] This initial development within the microbiome is considered to be a key contributor to alterations in immune system regulation that increase the risk for certain allergic, inflammatory and metabolic disorders in individuals born by C-section (part of the hygiene hypothesis).[49,50,51] The practice of vaginal microbial transfer or "vaginal seeding," whereby a swab of vaginal fluid is transferred to the infant after C-section birth, is becoming a common practice, though there is currently little known as to its efficacy for long-term health outcomes. Nonetheless, the procedure does appear to allow a cesarean-born infant's microbiota to closely mirror that of a vaginally-born infant, though some have raised the potential for safety concerns related to transferring vaginal pathogens.[52,53]

The gut microbiota is also influenced greatly by whether, and for how long, the infant consumes breast milk or formula. The microbiota within the breast milk secretions along with the specific types of milk oligosaccharides, help establish a foundational gut microbiome in the infant.[54,55] Introduction of solid food is considered the beginning of the transition to an "adult" microbiome, though many factors influence this as well. The most studied influential factors are dietary patterns, hygiene factors, age and antibiotic use, though many other factors, such as host genetics, stress, circadian dysrhythmia, and a host of GI disorders, have been implicated (see Figure 20). We will discuss several of these factors in detail below.

How Stable Is An Adult's Microbiome Over Time?

Before discussing the many factors that can alter the gut microbiome, it is important to establish the relative stability of a person's microbiota. This is especially important for the clinician using fecal samples to analyze a person's microbiota, and whether this analysis represents only a transient snapshot or are semi-permanent features of the patient's core microbiome. Recently, several studies have attempted to answer this question by analyzing the microbiome (via fecal samples) of the same individuals over time, often tracking dietary or other changes along the way. In general, they have discovered that a fairly large core microbiome (~40 species of bacteria) remains stable in an individual over at least one year.[56] In fact, a landmark study published in *Science* (2013) using fecal samples from 37 individuals showed that a person's "core" gut microbiota is remarkably stable for greater than five years (they speculate for decades).[57] They also showed that the core species of family members is very similar, and that species within the Bacteroidetes and Actinobacteria phyla are more stable than those in other phyla (e.g., Firmicutes).

One of the most comprehensive analyses of the core microbiome of adults was published recently by Falony et al. called the Flemish Gut Flora Project (FGFP). The study was originally designed to investigate the global core microbiome and to study the impact of host and environmental factors on microbiota variation within an average, healthy Western European population in Flanders, Belgium.[58] In addition, they combined the FGFP with other large metagenomics data sets from recent adult cohorts in the Netherlands, United Kingdom and United States, characterizing the fecal microbiome of 4,000 individuals. Their overall dataset estimated a core Western microbiota (i.e., the genera shared by 95% of samples) of 17 genera and a total genus richness of 664 genera. This value still underestimates the total Western

INFANT

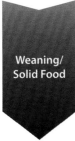

Weaning/
Solid Food

Rapidly Changing Microbiota

Colonization and development dependent on many factors-changes rapidly

Early Life Experiences Critical to the Establishment of the Gut Microbiota:

- **Birth Mode**
  Cesarean birth delays colonization by *Bifidobacterium* and *Bacteroides*, initial gut community resembles mother's skin and oral microbiota and environmental bacteria *(Staphylococcus, Propionibacterium and Corynebacterium)*; Vaginally born infant gut microbiota resembles maternal vaginal and gut microbiota *(Lactobacillus, Prevotella and Sneathia)*

- **Length of gestation**
  Preterm associated with ↑ bacterial translocation, ↑ inflammation, oxidative stress, ↑ necrotizing enterocolitis (NEC) compared to infants born at term

- **Mode of feeding**
  Breastmilk associated with ↑ *Bifidobacterium* and ↓ *Enterobacteriaceae*

- **Environment (NICU)**

- **Medications**
  Antibiotics and proton pump inhibitors

- **Vaccination**

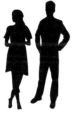

ADULT

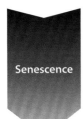

Senescence

Relatively Stable Microbiota

Firmicutes > Bacteroidetes >Proteobacteria > Actinobacteria

Core species fairly stable over time

Core Adult Factors That Affect Gut Microbiota:

- **Hygiene factors**
- **Circadian dysrhythmia**
- **Stress**
- **Inflammation**
- **GI Disorders**
- **Sex-hormone effects**
- **Diet**
  - ➤ Mediterranean diet linked to more diverse and healthy gut microbiome compared to standard Western dietary pattern
  - ➤ Microbiota quickly adapts to dietary shifts
  - ➤ Vegetarians: ↑ Bacteroidetes, ↓ Clostridia
  - ➤ See page 104 for dietary recommendations

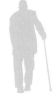

AGING

Vulnerable/Deteriorating Microbiota

↑ Bacteroidetes, ↓ *Bifidobacteria*

Microbiota more vulnerable to change due to alterations in diet, activity, bowel transit and immunosenescence

Factors Affecting all Stages of Development:

Host Genetics

Probiotics

Inulin
(FOS)

Prebiotics

**Medication/
Antibiotics**

Malnutrition
In children:
↑ Proteobacteria,
↓ Bacteroidetes

Geography

Figure 20: The Microbiome from Birth to Aging. This figure illustrates the many factors that influence the health and diversity of an individual's gut microbiota. See text for more details.

genus richness, which has been estimated to be 784 ± 40 genera. In order to obtain an estimated global core microbiota, the group added 308 more samples from Papua New Guinea, Peru and Tanzania and estimated the global core human microbiota was reduced to 14 genera.

Perhaps more applicable for the clinician are their findings related to host and environmental factors on the gut microbiota community composition, linked by exhaustive phenotyping via online questionnaires, standardized medical histories and health assessment by general practitioners. Of the 503 metadata variables that emerged, 69 factors were shown to correlate significantly with overall microbiome community variation. The association between BMI and microbiome composition was found to be small but significant. Of all the covariates detected, 63% were driven by medication (mostly the use of antibiotics and laxatives), making the use of any medication the largest predefined explanatory variable tested in this study. However, when breaking down the covariates into smaller categories, stool consistency as measured by the Bristol Stool Scale (BSS) emerged as the top single non-redundant microbiome covariate in the FGFP metadata. BSS score reflects transit time, water availability, and potential niche differentiation within the colon ecosystem. For 12 of the 20 FGFP core genera, core abundance was shown to increase with looser stools. The authors note medication use and BSS scores have been largely ignored in microbiome studies, and should be considered in future studies based on the strong findings in the FGFP cohort. (For more about the BSS, see page 52).

This connection between stool consistency and microbiota abundance/diversity has been further analyzed in a subgroup of this same cohort. Vandeputte et al. (2016) found stool consistency (as measured by BSS) was strongly associated with fecal microbial richness.[59] Species richness was shown to significantly decline as stool firmness declined (p=0.0007), reaching its minimum in those with diarrhea. The group also found enterotypes were distributed over BSS scores, the Prevotella enterotype was more abundant in looser stools (p=0.019) and the Ruminococcaceae-Bacteroides (RB) enterotype completely dominated firmer samples (p=0.019) perhaps suggesting that enterotypes may be a surrogate marker for bowel transit time since transit time may "select" for bacteria with certain traits. For instance, individuals with a short transit time may have greater amounts of fast-growing bacterial species, while those with slow transit times may instead be favorable for bacteria with greater adherence to host tissue.

What these and other data seem to reveal is that while a core microbiome (structure and species) is part of a person's development, and is formed as part of an individual's early inoculation and environmental exposure, subtle and important changes in the variable commensal microbiome can occur without fundamentally altering the long-term stability of the core species (at least as determined by analysis of fecal microbiota). This means differences in fecal microbiota (beyond the core species enumeration and ratio) may reflect adaptations to environmental or pathophysiological changes that can be meaningfully followed in clinical research or in clinical application. Lastly, there is also a significant

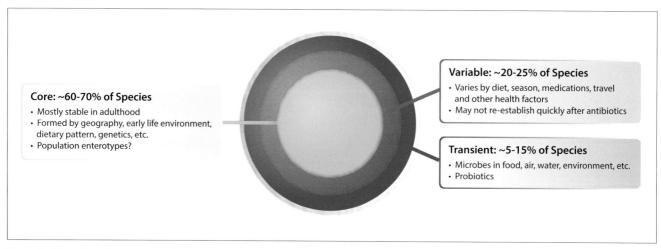

Figure 21: Three Microbiomes in One. This figure illustrates the relative abundance of bacterial species within the core, variable and transient microbiomes in adults. This allows for a balance between metabolic stability and adaptability.

portion of the microbiota that is transient; coming from our food (including probiotics), water, air, and environment. These microorganisms rarely persist beyond a week or two, but they can be important modulators of both the core and variable microbiome, and greatly influence host physiology (see Figure 21). Therefore, sampling and analyzing a person's fecal microbiota as a routine part of a yearly physical exam may be a way to note subtle (or radical) changes in the microbiome consistent with noted changes in a patient's overall health (see fecal metagenomics analysis on page 94). We predict microbiome testing will soon be a routine practice for annual exams, like standard blood tests, and will be part of the health assessment of most subjects.

Is There An Ideal Microbiome?

This is a very tricky question. If the question implies a basic set of microbial species that is ideal for any human subject living anywhere, then the answer is "no." However, we believe there is likely a *suitable* microbiome for each person, one that is properly adapted to their particular geography, genetics, diet and environment. In fact, if we are correct in understanding the microbiome as the ultimate adaptable organ system, the microbiota within the GI tract (and therefore in the fecal sample) should change with age, with seasonal dietary changes and with health status. Comparing the microbiome of Western subjects consuming monotonous and poor diets to the microbiome of hunter-gatherers eating seasonally shows dramatic differences. While some would describe the microbiota of these hunter-gatherers as ideal, it probably would be poorly sustained and ill-suited to benefit the Western subject eating a standard Western diet.

As we shall see, general changes in the fecal microbiota are indicative of certain gastrointestinal disorders (when compared to "healthy" individuals). Some of these alterations reflect wholesale changes at the phylum-level, while others are subtle changes in one or two species. Most of the time, however, the clinician's first analysis of a patient's microbiome is performed after a dysfunctional change has already occurred (often the first encounter with the patient) and therefore clinicians don't usually have access to a patient's former ("baseline") core microbiome for comparison. Nonetheless, analyzing a patient's gut microbiota (via fecal microbiota testing) is often helpful in both diagnosing a complex GI-related issue as well as for confirming therapeutic impact (via follow-up testing).

Dysbiosis: Imbalance within the Microbiome

Most integrative and functional medicine clinicians are familiar with the term dysbiosis. Essentially, it describes any significant imbalance in the gut microbial ecosystem, especially one that leads to a negative host response. This includes either an abundance or depletion of a particular commensal species, family or phylum of bacteria, or a geographic dislocation of one or more species (i.e., colon bacteria colonizing the small

Genetic Dysbiosis: When Immune Cells Misinterpret the Microbiota

When an imbalance in the number and types of commensal microbes develops in the gut, the immune system is activated to respond in a variety of ways. New research now suggests that in some patients, the immune system can misinterpret a "normal" microbiome as "dysbiotic" due to genetic polymorphisms in a variety of immune receptors tasked with interpreting the gut microbial environment.[60] Pattern recognition receptors are an important component of both the innate and adaptive immune response, and are an important mechanism for helping the host immune system interface with the gut microbiome. However, similar to an overreaction to a benign food protein that causes an immune response in some individuals (based on genetics), certain commensal organisms may trigger an inappropriate response when the host immune system misinterprets their molecular pattern as "pathogenic" (e.g., inflammation, auto-immune cross-reactivity, etc.).

Likewise, inappropriate receptor expression caused by changes in genetics (gene/protein sequence) or genomics (altered expression pattern of one or more receptors) can result in dysfunctional immune regulation of the commensal organisms within the gut (e.g., reduced levels of sIgA to target pathobionts). This lowers the precision of the immune surveillance within the GI tract, allowing for an imbalance in the commensal organisms; creating a host-derived genetics-induced dysbiosis.[61] Clinicians attempting to help correct a patient's gut dysbiosis must understand that host factors, including genetics, may profoundly affect how they respond to therapies intended to re-balance the gut microbiome (via diet, probiotics, prebiotics, etc.). Therefore, some recommendations or products may work better or quicker (or not at all) in some patients compared to others.

intestines). While an infection by a pathogenic microbe such as *Salmonella* is not usually called "dysbiosis," the opportunistic overgrowth of bacteria like *Clostridium difficile* or a yeast like *Candida albicans* is often directly related to an infection or an antibiotic-induced alteration in the gut microbiota (i.e., dysbiosis-induced). Ironically, with the advanced technologies now available to help the clinician analyze specific changes in the gut microbiota,

this term has almost become too generic for the research setting, and clinicians should be aware that more specific terms might be used to define specific microbiome-host dysfunctions. Still, the notion that a disturbance in the gut microbial ecosystem—dysbiosis— may be a major trigger in a wide range of gastrointestinal and systemic disorders is an important factor often missed by clinicians uninformed by these recent discoveries.

Re-establishing A Healthy Microbiome

One of the main goals for any clinician is to help all patients, especially those with GI-related dysfunction, maintain a healthy microbiome. Within the 4R model, this has been defined as "re-inoculate," though we think the goal to "re-establish" a healthy microbiome is a more correct way to understand this idea. Certainly, adding microorganisms (i.e., inoculation) in the form of probiotics or fecal transplantation can be a major therapeutic strategy to help maintain a healthy microbiome, but there are many fundamental strategies that do not involve adding live organisms.

Diet and the Microbiome
A person's diet (historical and current) is likely the single greatest influence on their gut microbiome since it serves as both a source of inoculation of microbes and provides the nutrients upon which the resident commensal organisms feed. Research looking at diverse dietary patterns has revealed significant differences in the gut microbiota from vegetarians compared to meat-eaters, Western urban children vs. rural African children, and a range of elderly subjects consuming different dietary patterns over time.[12,62,63] Not surprisingly, healthy dietary patterns like the Mediterranean diet have been shown to be associated with a more diverse and healthy gut microbiota, compared to standard unhealthy Western dietary patterns.[64]

To investigate the adaptability of the microbiota to changes in dietary patterns, researchers at Harvard University analyzed the fecal microbiota of individuals when shifted between an exclusively plant-based diet to an exclusively animal-based diet.[65] They found that the microbiota pattern was noticeably shifted shortly after changing diets in a similar and predictable manner in multiple subjects

(n=11). This suggests the microbiota within the gut appear to adapt to changing nutrient availability, and can do so quite rapidly (within days). Clinicians should be aware of this adaptability when they are using dietary analysis and stool microbiota analysis to understand a patient's health. Since some patients delay taking their stool test for weeks after receiving the sample kit, they may have changed (or improved) their diet based on the advice of their clinician long enough to alter the microbiota prior to sampling. Therefore, the analysis may not accurately reflect the "baseline" microbiota.

Basic Dietary Principles to Benefit the Microbiome

It is not surprising that the basic dietary principles that promote overall health and reduce the risk for most chronic diseases are also those which promote a healthy gut microbial community.

- Diversity is key; the diet should contain a wide range of foods, especially those derived from plants with different phytochemicals.

- Dietary fiber and complex carbohydrates should be emphasized.

- Eat food as fresh and unprocessed as possible (safely).

- Eating in seasonal rotation (using local foods) may help diversify gut microbiota

- Individuals should avoid foods they suspect will trigger GI discomfort, allergic reactions or cause noticeable changes in bowel transit time.

- Limit access to foods (meats) that contain antibiotics.

Artificial Sweeteners and the Microbiome

Artificial sweeteners such as aspartame (NutraSweet®, Equal®), sucralose (Splenda®), and saccharin (Sweet'N Low®) are ubiquitous in processed foods and beverages; and are regularly consumed by 1/3 of all Americans in a variety of "diet" products.[1] While designed to be low calorie alternatives to sugar, research has repeatedly shown that consumption of these artificial sweeteners is still linked to metabolic derangements such as weight gain, impaired glucose tolerance and increased incidence of type 2 diabetes.[2,3] Now, research has discovered that while most of these synthetic sweeteners are excreted unchanged in either the urine or feces, they affect metabolism through alterations of the gut microbiota.

In an animal model, Suez et al. showed aspartame, sucralose and saccharin induced glucose intolerance over eight and eleven weeks; further study of saccharin demonstrated the effects were mediated through compositional and functional changes to the gut microbiota, with more than 40 operational taxonomic units altered in the saccharin-fed group.[4] Interestingly, *Akkermansia muciniphila* was underrepresented in the mice fed saccharin. Using antibiotics and transplanting fecal microbiota samples into germ-free mice, the group linked the impaired glucose tolerance to an altered microbiome.

The group then studied the effects of artificial sweeteners in a small-scale human intervention study. Seven subjects (who did not normally consume artificial sweeteners) consumed a regular diet supplemented with the upper limit of daily saccharin dose (5 mg/kg/day) for one week. Four of the seven volunteers showed an elevated glycemic response (responders), and the other three individuals showed no response. The researchers transplanted the four responders' microbiota into germ-free mice and replicated the impaired glucose response, again linking the metabolic effects to the altered microbiota. The responder/non-responder effect suggests that not all individuals are affected equally by artificial sweetener consumption, and the response may depend on an individual's baseline microbiota.[5] Although this is one of the few human intervention trials available to show the effect of artificial sweeteners on the microbiome, other animal studies using these ingredients (at relevant dietary doses) suggest that this phenomena is an important link between artificial sweeteners and metabolic dysregulation.[6,7]

Ironically, many "light" yogurt products include these artificial sweeteners as a key ingredient in the effort to retain palatability while reducing total sugars and calories.[3] Consuming yogurt products in an effort to favorably modify the microbiome while consuming these "light" or "reduced calorie" additives may detrimentally undermine any beneficial changes to the microbiome the consumer anticipates.

References

1. Sylvetsky AC, Welsh JA, Brown RJ, Vos MB. Low-calorie sweetener consumption is increasing in the United States. *Am J Clin Nutr*. 2012 Sep;96(3):640-6.
2. Suez J, Korem T, Zilberman-Schapira G, et al. Non-caloric artificial sweeteners and the microbiome: findings and challenges. *Gut Microbes*. 2015;6(2):149-55.
3. Spencer M, Gupta A, Dam LV, et al. Artificial Sweeteners: A Systematic Review and Primer for Gastroenterologists. *J Neurogastroenterol Motil*. 2016 Apr 30;22(2):168-80.
4. Suez J, Korem T, Zeevi D, et al. Artificial sweeteners induce glucose intolerance by altering the gut microbiota. *Nature*. 2014 Oct 9;514(7521):181-6.
5. Nettleton JE, Reimer RA, Shearer J. Reshaping the gut microbiota: Impact of low calorie sweeteners and the link to insulin resistance? *Physiol Behav*. 2016 Apr 15. pii: S0031-9384(16)30164-0.
6. Palmnäs MS, Cowan TE, Bomhof MR, et al. Low-dose aspartame consumption differentially affects gut microbiota-host metabolic interactions in the diet-induced obese rat. *PLoS One*. 2014 Oct 14;9(10):e109841.
7. Abou-Donia MB, El-Masry EM, Abdel-Rahman AA, et al. Splenda alters gut microflora and increases intestinal p-glycoprotein and cytochrome p-450 in male rats. *J Toxicol Environ Health A*. 2008;71(21):1415-29.

There are several components of the diet that appear to have the greatest influence on the species diversity and abundance of the gut microbiota (at least as measured by fecal metagenomics).[66] Most of the population research has focused on macronutrient content (especially the diversity and complexity of the carbohydrate components), and phytonutrient diversity, though individuals consuming foods that radically alter bowel transit time or that cause a major inflammatory response will also experience an altered gut microbiota.

Carbohydrates

Overall, carbohydrates are the principal energy source for a majority of the gut microbiota. Individuals who consume a more diverse diet including high amounts of dietary fiber and complex carbohydrates will typically have a more diverse (and healthy) gut microbiota. In fact, fermentation of complex carbohydrates by specific species of bacteria in the colon produces several important short-chain fatty acids (SCFA) such as acetate, propionate and butyrate. These, as well as other organic acids produced by fermentation (e.g., lactate, succinate, etc.) influence colonic pH, inhibiting the growth of pathogenic bacteria. While it is well-known that butyrate serves as the principal source of metabolic energy for the colonocytes, the SCFAs produced through fermentation are important signaling molecules for critical metabolic functions throughout the body.[67,68] For more details on complex carbohydrate intake and the use of prebiotics for improving microbial/GI health, see the prebiotic section on page 108.

Proteins

Dietary protein is also very important with respect to the gut microbiota, as it provides the major source of nitrogen for these organisms. However, while fermentation of amino acids is also an important by-product of colonic bacterial metabolism (e.g., isobutyrate and isovalerate), the availability of certain undigested peptides and amino acids can result in by-products known as putrefactive short-chain fatty acids that are thought to play a role in inflammatory bowel diseases and colorectal cancer.[69,70] This has spurred the debate around the role of diets that are skewed toward animal protein and the risk for colorectal cancer, mediated by changes in the microbiota and their metabolites.[71] While there is still much we do not know about these relationships, it appears that the potential negative effects happen when excessive fermentation of amino acids occurs as a result of a depletion of available fermentable carbohydrates (e.g., resistant starches), suggesting that eating excessive animal protein in the context of low dietary fiber may actually be the underlying culprit (fecal putrefactive SCFA may also be a sign of poor protein digestion; see page 46).[72]

Fats

The effect of dietary fat intake (amount and type) on changes in the microbiota have been studied, mostly in the context of high-fat Western (or experimental) diets. Generally, these diets show a similar shift in the microbiota as other studies of Western diets (characterized as low in both food diversity and dietary fiber, and high in saturated fat and animal protein). Curiously, high-fat intake is associated with increased circulating levels of bacteria-derived lipopolysaccharides (LPS), presumably from an alteration in gut permeability to LPS.[73] While more research is needed, there is some evidence to suggest this phenomenon is higher for saturated and omega-6 fatty acid intake, while omega-3 fatty acid intake may limit these negative outcomes.[74]

Another way fat intake can modify the gut microbiota is via bile acid availability. When fat intake is increased, so is the amount of bile that avoids enterohepatic recycling and enters the colon where these bile acids can be metabolized into secondary bile acids by colonic bacteria.[75] The implications of this mechanism may be far-reaching, as recent research has shown that secondary bile acids are absorbed from the colon and have a number of metabolic-signaling effects that impact health and disease in a range of tissues.[76,77] Changes in the gut microbiota are now known to influence the types and amounts of these secondary bile acids leading to some of the negative consequences related to dysbiosis.

Phytonutrients

A healthy diet should include a wide range of fresh fruits, vegetables, herbs and spices. Not only will this provide a large amount of dietary fiber to benefit a healthy gut microbiota, it will also provide a diverse array of bioactive plant compounds generally referred to as phytonutrients. These include, for example, carotenoids, glucosinolates, and a large family of compounds called polyphenols, many of which have been studied for their health-related benefits when part of the diet (or via supplementation). Since many of these compounds are known to have poor gastrointestinal absorption, their higher concentrations throughout the GI tract allow for microbial metabolism and signaling.

Ironically, much of the early studies on polyphenolic compounds (e.g., flavonoids, catechins, anthocyanins, isoflavones, lignans, stilbenoids, curcuminoids, tannins, etc.) were related to their potential antimicrobial activities.[78] In fact, while many are still commonly used as antimicrobial agents, today researchers are realizing that many of these dietary plant compounds have a diverse range of specific influences on the microbiome that can help explain their health-promoting outcomes. In addition to these findings, it is now appreciated that many of these polyphenolic compounds would be of little health benefit to the host without first being metabolized by the gut microbiota, either to produce the "active" compound or to alter the compound to improve its bioavailability. Therefore, the relative efficacy of certain plant phytonutrients (either from dietary intervention or supplementation) may greatly depend upon the metabolic activities expressed by an individual's gut microbiota.[79]

There are numerous well-studied examples of microbial metabolism altering the biological effect of dietary phytonutrients. One of the most well studied is the conversion of the soy isoflavone compounds daidzin and genistin into the more absorbable daidzein and genistein, along with the deconjugation of their liver metabolites and the creation of secondary metabolites with specific estrogen-like effects (e.g., equol; see Figure 22).[80] Therefore, the ability for these compounds to generate a biological effect in those consuming soy is partly (perhaps mainly) influenced by the availability of certain bacterial species, which are themselves influenced by the diet and genetics of the host.[81,82] This may explain many of the differences between certain epidemiological disease risk in populations that regularly consume soy from early life and intervention trials using concentrated soy isoflavones in populations with little history of soy consumption.

Another example of this back and forth relationship between the microbiota and a well-known phytonutrient is with the alkaloid berberine, known to possess "antimicrobial" activity and used in a variety of

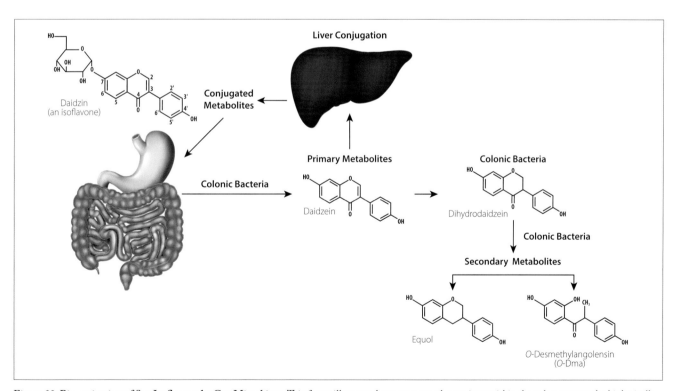

Figure 22: Bio-activation of Soy Isoflavone by Gut Microbiota. This figure illustrates how commensal organisms within the colon convert the biologically inactive soy isoflavone daidzin by converting it to the aglycone daidzein and then further metabolizing that compound to biologically active secondary metabolites, like equol. Conjugated isoflavone metabolites from the liver are also modified by the gut microbiota into bioactive compounds.

Prebiotics and the Gut Microbiome

The term "prebiotic," like many terms used by scientists, marketers, clinicians and regulators, has yet to reach a consensus. The original definition proposed by Gibson and Roberfroid in 1995 was, *"Non-digestible food ingredients that beneficially affects the host by selectively stimulating the growth and/or activity of one or a limited number of bacteria in the colon, and thus improves host health."*[1] The last 20 years have seen numerous challenges, disputes, refinements and a host of new proposed definitions for the term. These have been posited mostly in the attempt to include other sites beyond the colon (small bowel, oral, vaginal, skin bacteria, etc.), to broaden (or remove) the term "selectively," and in nuanced ways to define what specific changes in the microbiota are deemed beneficial to the host. While these definitions may seem trivial for some, the definition radically alters the list of fibers that meet these definitions (from as few as two to as many as a dozen or more). For those interested, there are several recent publications outlining these changes in prebiotic nomenclature.[2,3,4]

For the most part, the list of proposed prebiotics includes mostly complex carbohydrates defined as oligosaccharides, though several resistant starches and a few disaccharides are also proposed by some. Figure A shows the various structures of many of these proposed compounds. For clinicians attempting to understand the functional role of prebiotics, they are essentially complex carbohydrates (from the diet or from specifically designed functional foods or supplements) for which humans lack the enzymes to hydrolyze, allowing commensal organisms the opportunity to metabolize (ferment) them, resulting in some tangible benefit for the consumer.[5] For many years, clinicians were told that prebiotics exclusively promoted *Bifidobacteria*, though more advanced metagenomic analysis of fecal samples after the consumption of consensus prebiotics (e.g., FOS, inulin) shows that other genera increase as well.[6,7]

Since we generally encourage the consumption of a diverse diet containing a wide array of fruits and vegetables (with an emphasis on increasing dietary fiber), we do not generally provide a separate recommendation for dietary prebiotic consumption. However, when patients are specifically targeting both increased dietary fiber and prebiotic fibers, they will want to increase consumption of the foods listed in Table 5. Clinical trials using various prebiotic fibers range in dose from around 5 grams to over 25 grams per day. We will discuss some of these trials in the therapeutic sections where some of these prebiotics are known to benefit GI-related outcomes (most studies of prebiotics are now focused on metabolic-related outcomes).[8,9] Clinicians should be aware that high levels of prebiotic fibers are not tolerated by every patient, and most will need to allow their gut microbiota to adjust to increasing levels. Gas, bloating and related GI discomfort often accompanies the increased intake of fermentable fiber and can be modulated by reducing the dose or the addition of probiotics. Also, patients who have been prescribed certain carbohydrate restrictions, such as the low FODMAP diet, should refrain from consuming most prebiotic fibers (see FODMAP diet on page 236).

Supplementing Prebiotics (and Synbiotics)

There are numerous products designed to deliver one or more prebiotic available to consumers worldwide. These products usually deliver several grams of prebiotic fiber in ready-to-drink beverages, powders, bars or other functional foods (capsules or tablets are also available, though it is often difficult to deliver adequate doses). Products combining prebiotic fibers with probiotic organisms are called "synbiotics." Since the probiotic must remain inert prior to ingestion, there is no particular benefit to delivering both a prebiotic and a probiotic in the same product, with the exception of convenience. Manufacturers not careful to ensure fibers mixed with probiotics have been specially prepared to maintain a low water activity may inadvertently reduce the viability/shelf life of a probiotic by introducing moisture during the manufacturing process.

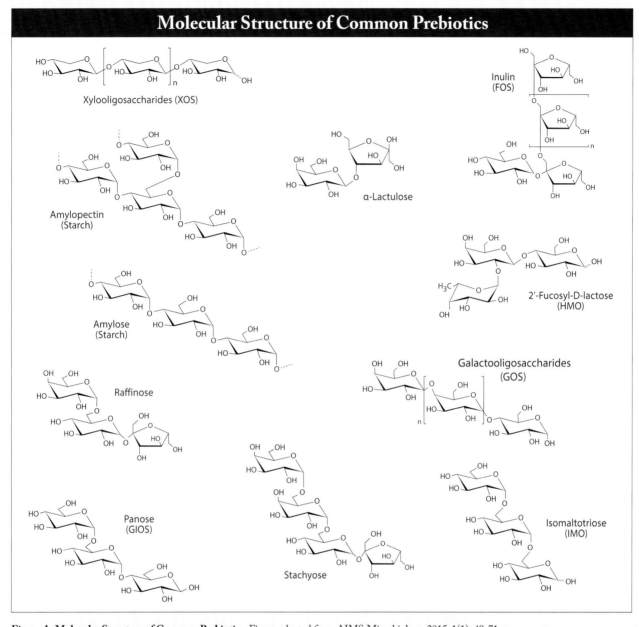

Figure A: Molecular Structure of Common Prebiotics. Figure adapted from AIMS Microbiology, 2015, 1(1): 48-71.

References

1. Gibson GR, Roberfroid MB. Dietary modulation of the human colonic microbiota: introducing the concept of prebiotics. *J Nutr*. 1995 Jun;125(6):1401-12.
2. Hutkins RW, Krumbeck JA, Bindels LB, et al. Prebiotics: why definitions matter. *Curr Opin Biotechnol*. 2016 Feb;37:1-7.
3. Bindels LB, Delzenne NM, Cani PD, Walter J. Towards a more comprehensive concept for prebiotics. *Nat Rev Gastroenterol Hepatol*. 2015 May;12(5):303-10.
4. Valcheva R, Dieleman LA. Prebiotics: Definition and protective mechanisms. *Best Pract Res Clin Gastroenterol*. 2016 Feb;30(1):27-37.
5. Verspreet J, Damen B, Broekaert WF, et al. A Critical Look at Prebiotics Within the Dietary Fiber Concept. *Annu Rev Food Sci Technol*. 2016;7:167-90.
6. Kato T, Fukuda S, Fujiwara A, et al. Multiple omics uncovers host-gut microbial mutualism during prebiotic fructooligosaccharide supplementation. *DNA Res*. 2014 Oct;21(5):469-80.
7. Dewulf EM, Cani PD, Claus SP, et al. Insight into the prebiotic concept: lessons from an exploratory, double blind intervention study with inulin-type fructans in obese women. *Gut*. 2013 Aug;62(8):1112-21.
8. Rastall RA, Gibson GR. Recent developments in prebiotics to selectively impact beneficial microbes and promote intestinal health. *Curr Opin Biotechnol*. 2015 Apr;32:42-6.
9. Beserra BT, Fernandes R, do Rosario VA, et al. A systematic review and meta-analysis of the prebiotics and synbiotics effects on glycaemia, insulin concentrations and lipid parameters in adult patients with overweight or obesity. *Clin Nutr*. 2015 Oct;34(5):845-58.

ancient medicinal traditions. More recently, berberine has demonstrated profound metabolic benefits, especially in subjects with metabolic syndrome, type 2 diabetes, hypertension and certain dyslipidemias.[83] Along with its well-described cellular signaling effects, berberine has been shown to alter the microbiota to a metabolically-favorable profile; perhaps accounting for some of its clinical efficacy.[84,85] Furthermore, it has now been shown that the efficacy of berberine is itself altered by microbial metabolism, through the gastrointestinal conversion of ingested berberine (which is poorly absorbable) to dihydroberberine (which has high bioavailability).[86] Therefore, the microbiota may be the target of and the facilitator for the metabolic effects of this alkaloid.

These are merely two examples of perhaps thousands of different phytonutrients that modify, or are modified by, the microbiota. We should caution, then, that while poor bioavailability of certain phytonutrients is often considered to be a detrimental factor leading many drug and supplement companies to modify these compounds to improve their bioavailability (e.g., liposomal technologies), these changes may inadvertently avoid the necessary microbial interaction that activates these compounds, while delivering higher levels of an inactive precursor. If, as is becoming clearer, the microbiome is one of the most active metabolic "organs" in the body, we may need to readjust our understanding of the biological potential of compounds with limited human bioavailability and consider a plant compound's microbial accessibility as equally important.[87]

Fecal Microbiota Transplantation (FMT)

The transfer of microbiota from one person (or animal) to another through fecal transplantation is being explored as a therapeutic strategy to re-establish a healthy microbiome. In humans, this technique primarily involves diluting donor feces in a manner to be infused into the recipient either through a retention enema, colonoscope, or nasogastric/nasoduodenal tube.[88] While FMT has been investigated for a range of microbiome-related conditions, the treatment of *Clostridium difficile* infection is by far the most studied and successful indication (see page 166 for FMT use in *C. difficile* infections). Other indications being explored for FMT include inflammatory bowel diseases, functional bowel disorders like IBS, and obesity/type 2 diabetes; though many others have been proposed.[89,90]

The use of FMT may prove to be an extremely helpful remedy for a number of important conditions for which dysbiosis is a major contributing factor. We encourage clinicians to investigate the most up-to-date methods, guidelines and regulations in order to ensure the use of this therapy maximizes the benefits to their patients.

The Effects of Antibiotics on the Gut Microbiome

The discovery and use of antibiotics is considered one of the great watershed moments in medical history, helping to turn the tide on a host of microbial pathogens that ravaged the world for centuries. Today, however, we are acutely aware of the immense collateral impact the sustained use of antibiotics has had on the host-microbe relationship. Two of those impacts are the rise of antibiotic-resistant strains of pathogenic organisms and the alteration of the human microbiome, both individually and globally.[91,92]

Broad-spectrum antibiotics have been prescribed for decades in the attempt to protect patients from pathogenic organisms. Commonly, these include ampicillin, ciprofloxacin, tetracyclines, clarithromycin, clindomycin and metronidazole. Since they kill a broad spectrum of potentially pathogenic bacteria, these antibiotics also kill a wide range of commensal organisms in the gut and elsewhere on or in the patient. How destabilizing a particular antibiotic is for an individual subject is still debated.

Some studies suggested the "core" species of an adult commensal microbiota are somewhat resilient to antibiotic therapy, or at least would recover to pre-antibiotic levels once therapy is discontinued.[93] However, when the microbiota in healthy subjects is analyzed after treatment with a broad-spectrum antibiotic (via fecal sampling or biopsy) there is an immediate reduction in species diversity, which often does not fully mirror the pre-antibiotic sample for up to 12 months after ceasing the antibiotic.[94,95,96,97] Perhaps even more important than the alterations in species diversity caused by antibiotic therapy is the altered function of the microbiome. Using multi-metagenomic analysis (transcripts, proteins and metabolites from gut microbes), research now shows that the metabolic

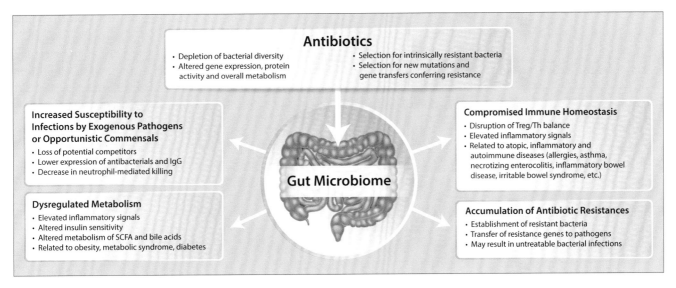

Figure 23: The Devastating Effects of Antibiotics on the Gut Microbiome. This figure shows the basic changes (upper box) in the gut microbiome that occur with the use of broad-spectrum antibiotics; along with the physiological and global ramifications of these changes.

functions can be quickly and significantly altered in the gut microbes that survive the antibiotic therapy and are altered in ways that can detrimentally affect the host.[98]

This destabilization of the gut microbiota (antibiotic-induced dysbiosis) has both immediate and long-term consequences. The immediate consequences can be seen in the dramatic increase in antibiotic associated diarrhea (AAD), often attributed to an increased proliferation of *Clostridium difficile*.[99,100] According to the Centers for Disease Control, *C. diff* infections (CDI) were estimated to cause almost half a million infections in the United States in 2011, and 29,000 deaths within 30 days of the initial diagnosis; this is mostly attributable to the use of antibiotics.[101] The relationship between antibiotic use and CDI is two-fold: the increased selection of antibiotic-resistant strains of *C.diff* within the human population, coupled with an antibiotic-induced depletion of the commensal organisms that normally prevent *C.diff* from colonizing the gut.[102] The phenomenal success of fecal microbiota transplants in the treatment of CDI confirms the important role of commensal organism protection (see page 165 for discussion of CDI therapeutic options).[103]

The long-term alterations of the gut microbiome related to antibiotic use may not be as immediate, but likely affect more individuals in subtler ways. These impacts are now being seen in the increased risk of metabolic (obesity, type 2 diabetes, etc.) and immune-related disorders (inflammatory disorders, atopic disease, autoimmunity, etc.) related to frequent and early use of antibiotics.[104,105,106,107,108] This should come as little surprise now that we understand the intricate relationship between the metabolic activity of our gut microbiota and most human metabolism and cell signaling. In fact, we predict that most chronic disease conditions will eventually be shown to have a link to an imbalance in the gut microbiota and/or the frequent and early use of antibiotics. We agree with those that call for a judicious use of antibiotics, especially in children or for prophylactic use, encouraging the use of targeted antimicrobials where available. In most cases, the concomitant use of probiotics will diminish some of the dysbiotic consequences of antibiotic use (see page 134).

References

1. Marchesi JR, Adams DH, Fava F, et al. The gut microbiota and host health: a new clinical frontier. *Gut.* 2016 Feb;65(2):330-9.
2. Power SE, O'Toole PW, Stanton C, Ross RP, Fitzgerald GF. Intestinal microbiota, diet and health. *Br J Nutr.* 2014 Feb;111(3):387-402.
3. Goulet O. Potential role of the intestinal microbiota in programming health and disease. *Nutr Rev.* 2015 Aug;73 Suppl 1:32-40.
4. Updates can be found at the NIH Human Microbiome Project Website: http://hmpdacc.org/
5. Sankar SA, Lagier JC, Pontarotti P, Raoult D, Fournier PE. The human gut microbiome, a taxonomic conundrum. *Syst Appl Microbiol.* 2015 Jun;38(4):276-86.
6. Dugas LR, Fuller M, Gilbert J, Layden BT. The obese gut microbiome across the epidemiologic transition. *Emerg Themes Epidemiol.* 2016 Jan 11;13:2.
7. Rosenbaum M, Knight R, Leibel RL. The gut microbiota in human energy homeostasis and obesity. *Trends Endocrinol Metab.* 2015 Sep;26(9):493-501.

8.   Bauer PV, Hamr SC, Duca FA. Regulation of energy balance by a gut-brain axis and involvement of the gut microbiota. *Cell Mol Life Sci*. 2016 Feb;73(4):737-55.
9.   Arumugam M, Raes J, Pelletier E, et al. Enterotypes of the human gut microbiome. *Nature*. 2011 May 12;473(7346):174-80.
10.   Jeffery IB, Claesson MJ, O'Toole PW, Shanahan F. Categorization of the gut microbiota: enterotypes or gradients? *Nat Rev Microbiol*. 2012 Sep;10(9):591-2.
11.   Knights D, Ward TL, McKinlay CE, et al. Rethinking "enterotypes." *Cell Host Microbe*. 2014 Oct 8;16(4):433-7.
12.   Claesson MJ, Jeffery IB, Conde S, et al. Gut microbiota composition correlates with diet and health in the elderly. *Nature*. 2012 Aug 9;488(7410):178-84.
13.   Donaldson GP, Lee SM, Mazmanian SK. Gut biogeography of the bacterial microbiota. *Nat Rev Microbiol*. 2016 Jan;14(1):20-32.
14.   Hong PY, Croix JA, Greenberg E, Gaskins HR, Mackie RI. Pyrosequencing-based analysis of the mucosal microbiota in healthy individuals reveals ubiquitous bacterial groups and micro-heterogeneity. *PLoS One*. 2011;6(9):e25042.
15.   hang Z, Geng J, Tang X, et al. Spatial heterogeneity and co-occurrence patterns of human mucosal-associated intestinal microbiota. *ISME J*. 2014 Apr;8(4):881-93.
16.   Jamal M, Tasneem U, Hussain T, Andleeb S. Bacterial Biofilm: Its composition, formation and role in human infections. Research and Review: *J. Microb. and Biotech*. P-ISSN: 2347 - 2286.
17.   Chandra J, Mukherjee PK. Candida Biofilms: Development, Architecture, and Resistance. *Microbiol Spectr*. 2015 Aug;3(4).
18.   Pais-Correia AM, Sachse M, Guadagnini S, et al. Biofilm-like extracellular viral assemblies mediate HTLV-1 cell-to-cell transmission at virological synapses. *Nat Med*. 2010 Jan;16(1):83-9.
19.   Fux CA, Costerton JW, Stewart PS, Stoodley P. Survival strategies of infectious biofilms. *Trends Microbiol*. 2005 Jan;13(1):34-40.
20.   J.W. Costerton, et al. Bacterial biofilms: a common cause of persistent infections. *Science*, 284 (1999), pp. 1318–1322.
21.   Olsen I. Biofilm-specific antibiotic tolerance and resistance. *Eur J Clin Microbiol Infect Dis*. 2015 May;34(5):877-86.
22.   Antunes LC, Ferreira RB, Buckner MM, Finlay BB. Quorum sensing in bacterial virulence. *Microbiology*. 2010 Aug;156(Pt 8):2271-82.
23.   Abraham WR. Going beyond the Control of Quorum-Sensing to Combat Biofilm Infections. *Antibiotics (Basel)*. 2016 Jan 9;5(1).
24.   Zhou L, Zheng H, Tang Y, Yu W, Gong Q. Eugenol inhibits quorum sensing at sub-inhibitory concentrations. *Biotechnol Lett*. 2013 Apr;35(4):631-7.
25.   Packiavathy IA, Priya S, Pandian SK, Ravi AV. Inhibition of biofilm development of uropathogens by curcumin - an anti-quorum sensing agent from Curcuma longa. *Food Chem*. 2014 Apr 1;148:453-60.
26.   Jakobsen T, van Gennip M, Phipps RK, et al. Ajoene, a sulfur-rich molecule from garlic, inhibits genes controlled by quorum sensing. *Antimicrob Agents Chemother*. 2012 May;56(5):2314-25.
27.   Kalia M, Yadav VK, Singh PK, et al. Effect of Cinnamon Oil on Quorum Sensing-Controlled Virulence Factors and Biofilm Formation in Pseudomonas aeruginosa. *PLoS One*. 2015 Aug 11;10(8):e0135495.
28.   Qin N, Tan X, Jiao Y, et al. RNA-Seq-based transcriptome analysis of methicillin-resistant Staphylococcus aureus biofilm inhibition by ursolic acid and resveratrol. *Sci Rep*. 2014 Jun 27;4:5467.
29.   Cho HS, Lee JH, Cho MH, Lee J. et al. Red wines and flavonoids diminish Staphylococcus aureus virulence with anti-biofilm and anti-hemolytic activities. *Biofouling*. 2015;31(1):1-11.
30.   Vasavi HS, Arun AB, Rekha PD. Anti-quorum sensing activity of flavonoid-rich fraction from Centella asiatica L. against Pseudomonas aeruginosa PAO1. *J Microbiol Immunol Infect*. 2016 Feb;49(1):8-15.
31.   Fletcher MH, Jennings MC, Wuest WM. Draining the moat: Disrupting bacterial biofilms with natural products. *Tetrahedron*. 2014 July; 70(37):6373.
32.   Chan BK, Abedon ST. Bacteriophages and their enzymes in biofilm control. *Curr Pharm Des*. 2015;21(1):85-99.
33.   von Rosenvinge EC, O'May GA, Macfarlane S, Macfarlane GT, Shirtliff ME. Microbial biofilms and gastrointestinal diseases. *Pathog Dis*. 2013 Feb;67(1):25-38.
34.   De Weirdt R, Van de Wiele T. Micromanagement in the gut: microenvironmental factors govern colon mucosal biofilm structure and functionality. *npj Biofilms and Microbiomes* (2015) 1, 15026.
35.   Macfarlane S, Bahrami B, Macfarlane GT. Mucosal biofilm communities in the human intestinal tract. *Adv Appl Microbiol*. 2011;75:111-43.
36.   Zoetendal EG, von Wright A, Vilpponen-Salmela T et al. Mucosa-associated bacteria in the human gastrointestinal tract are uniformly distributed along the colon and differ from the community recovered from feces. *Appl Environ Microbiol*. 2002 Jul;68(7):3401-7.
37.   Hidalgo-Cantabrana C, Sánchez B, Milani C, et al. Genomic overview and biological functions of exopolysaccharide biosynthesis in Bifidobacterium spp. *Appl Environ Microbiol*. 2014 Jan;80(1):9-18.
38.   Nikolic M, López P, Strahinic I, Suárez A, et al. Characterisation of the exopolysaccharide (EPS)-producing Lactobacillus paraplantarum BGCG11 and its non-EPS producing derivative strains as potential probiotics. *Int J Food Microbiol*. 2012 Aug 17;158(2):155-62.
39.   Salazar N, Prieto A, Leal JA, Mayo B, et al. Production of exopolysaccharides by Lactobacillus and Bifidobacterium strains of human origin, and metabolic activity of the producing bacteria in milk. *J Dairy Sci*. 2009 Sep;92(9):4158-68.
40.   Beloin C, Renard S, Ghigo JM, Lebeaux D. Novel approaches to combat bacterial biofilms. *Curr Opin Pharmacol*. 2014 Oct;18:61-8.
41.   Simonetti O, Cirioni O, Mocchegiani F, et al. The efficacy of the quorum sensing inhibitor FS8 and tigecycline in preventing prosthesis biofilm in an animal model of staphylococcal infection. *Int J Mol Sci*. 2013 Aug 7;14(8):16321-32.
42.   Rodríguez JM, Murphy K, Stanton C, et al. The composition of the gut microbiota throughout life, with an emphasis on early life. *Microb Ecol Health Dis*. 2015 Feb 2;26:26050.
43.   Collado MC, Rautava S, Aakko J, Isolauri E, Salminen S. Human gut colonisation may be initiated in utero by distinct microbial communities in the placenta and amniotic fluid. *Sci Rep*. 2016 Mar 22;6:23129.
44.   Koleva PT, Kim JS, Scott JA, Kozyrskyj AL. Microbial programming of health and disease starts during fetal life. *Birth Defects Res C Embryo Today*. 2015 Dec;105(4):265-77.
45.   Munyaka PM, Khafipour E, Ghia JE. External influence of early childhood establishment of gut microbiota and subsequent health implications. *Front Pediatr*. 2014 Oct 9;2:109.
46.   Huurre A, Kalliomäki M, Rautava S, et al. Mode of delivery - effects on gut microbiota and humoral immunity. *Neonatology*. 2008;93(4):236-40.
47.   Dominguez-Bello MG, Costello EK, Contreras M, Magris M, Hidalgo G, Fierer N, Knight R. Delivery mode shapes the acquisition and structure of the initial microbiota across multiple body habitats in newborns. *Proc Natl Acad Sci U S A*. 2010 Jun 29;107(26):11971-5.
48.   Jakobsson HE, Abrahamsson TR, Jenmalm MC, et al. Decreased gut microbiota diversity, delayed Bacteroidetes colonisation and reduced Th1 responses in infants delivered by caesarean section. *Gut*. 2014 Apr;63(4):559-66.
49.   Blustein J, Attina T, Liu M, et al. Association of caesarean delivery with child adiposity from age 6 weeks to 15 years. *Int J Obes* (Lond). 2013 Jul;37(7):900-6.
50.   Puff R, D'Orlando O, Heninger AK, et al. Compromised immune response in infants at risk for type 1 diabetes born by Caesarean Section. *Clin Immunol*. 2015 Oct;160(2):282-5.
51.   Mulder IE, Schmidt B, Lewis M, et al. Restricting microbial exposure in early life negates the immune benefits associated with gut colonization in environments of high microbial diversity. *PLoS One*. 2011;6(12):e28279.
52.   Dominguez-Bello MG, De Jesus-Laboy KM, Shen N, et al. Partial restoration of the microbiota of cesarean-born infants via vaginal microbial transfer. *Nat Med*. 2016 Mar;22(3):250-3.
53.   Banda C. Offering women safer options than "vaginal seeding" for infants born by caesarean section. *BMJ*. 2016 Mar 31;352:i1734.
54.   Jost T, Lacroix C, Braegger C, Chassard C. Impact of human milk bacteria and oligosaccharides on neonatal gut microbiota establishment and gut health. *Nutr Rev*. 2015 Jul;73(7):426-37.
55.   Pacheco AR, Barile D, Underwood MA, Mills DA. The impact of the milk glycobiome on the neonate gut microbiota. *Annu Rev Anim Biosci*. 2015;3:419-45.
56.   Martínez I, Muller CE, Walter J. Long-term temporal analysis of the human fecal microbiota revealed a stable core of dominant bacterial species. *PLoS One*. 2013 Jul 16;8(7):e69621.
57.   Faith JJ, Guruge JL, Charbonneau M, et al. The long-term stability of the human gut microbiota. *Science*. 2013 Jul 5;341(6141):1237439.
58.   Falony G, Joossens M, Vieira-Silva S, et al. Population-level analysis of gut microbiome variation. *Science*. 2016 Apr 29;352(6285):560-4.

59. Vandeputte D, Falony G, Vieira-Silva S, et al. Stool consistency is strongly associated with gut microbiota richness and composition, enterotypes and bacterial growth rates. *Gut*. 2016 Jan;65(1):57-62.
60. Nibali L, Henderson B, Sadiq ST, Donos N. Genetic dysbiosis: the role of microbial insults in chronic inflammatory diseases. *J Oral Microbiol*. 2014 Feb 25;6.
61. Frosali S, Pagliari D, Gambassi G, et al. How the Intricate Interaction among Toll-Like Receptors, Microbiota, and Intestinal Immunity Can Influence Gastrointestinal Pathology. *J Immunol Res*. 2015;2015:489821.
62. Glick-Bauer M, Yeh MC. The health advantage of a vegan diet: exploring the gut microbiota connection. *Nutrients*. 2014 Oct 31;6(11):4822-38.
63. De Filippo C, Cavalieri D, Di Paola M, et al. Impact of diet in shaping gut microbiota revealed by a comparative study in children from Europe and rural Africa. *Proc Natl Acad Sci U S A*. 2010 Aug 17;107(33):14691-6.
64. De Filippis F, Pellegrini N, Vannini L, et al. High-level adherence to a Mediterranean diet beneficially impacts the gut microbiota and associated metabolome. *Gut*. 2015 Sep 28. pii: gutjnl-2015-309957.
65. David LA, Maurice CF, Carmody RN, et al. Diet rapidly and reproducibly alters the human gut microbiome. *Nature*. 2014 Jan 23;505(7484):559-63.
66. Conlon MA, Bird AR. The impact of diet and lifestyle on gut microbiota and human health. *Nutrients*. 2014 Dec 24;7(1):17-44.
67. Leonel AJ, Alvarez-Leite JI. Butyrate: implications for intestinal function. *Curr Opin Clin Nutr Metab Care*. 2012 Sep;15(5):474-9.
68. Ríos-Covián D, Ruas-Madiedo P, et al. Intestinal Short Chain Fatty Acids and their Link with Diet and Human Health. *Front Microbiol*. 2016 Feb 17;7:185.
69. Windey K, De Preter V, Verbeke K. Relevance of protein fermentation to gut health. *Mol Nutr Food Res*. 2012 Jan;56(1):184-96.
70. Macfarlane GT, Macfarlane S. Bacteria, colonic fermentation, and gastrointestinal health. *J AOAC Int*. 2012 Jan-Feb;95(1):50-60.
71. Kim E, Coelho D, Blachier F. Review of the association between meat consumption and risk of colorectal cancer. *Nutr Res*. 2013 Dec;33(12):983-94.
72. Conlon MA, Kerr CA, McSweeney CS, et al. Resistant starches protect against colonic DNA damage and alter microbiota and gene expression in rats fed a Western diet. *J Nutr*. 2012 May;142(5):832-40.
73. Moreira AP, Texeira TF, Ferreira AB, Peluzio Mdo C, Alfenas Rde C. Influence of a high-fat diet on gut microbiota, intestinal permeability and metabolic endotoxaemia. *Br J Nutr*. 2012 Sep;108(5):801-9.
74. Kaliannan K, Wang B, Li XY, Kim KJ, Kang JX. A host-microbiome interaction mediates the opposing effects of omega-6 and omega-3 fatty acids on metabolic endotoxemia. *Sci Rep*. 2015 Jun 11;5:11276.
75. Ridlon JM, Kang DJ, Hylemon PB, Bajaj JS. Bile acids and the gut microbiome. *Curr Opin Gastroenterol*. 2014 May;30(3):332-8.
76. Li T, Chiang JY. Bile acids as metabolic regulators. *Curr Opin Gastroenterol*. 2015 Mar;31(2):159-65.
77. Tsuei J, Chau T, Mills D, Wan YJ. Bile acid dysregulation, gut dysbiosis, and gastrointestinal cancer. *Exp Biol Med (Maywood)*. 2014 Nov;239(11):1489-504.
78. Etxeberria U, Fernández-Quintela A, Milagro FI, et al. Impact of polyphenols and polyphenol-rich dietary sources on gut microbiota composition. *J Agric Food Chem*. 2013 Oct 9;61(40):9517-33.
79. Bolca S, Van de Wiele T, Possemiers S. Gut metabotypes govern health effects of dietary polyphenols. *Curr Opin Biotechnol*. 2013 Apr;24(2):220-5.
80. Rafii F. The role of colonic bacteria in the metabolism of the natural isoflavone daidzin to equol. *Metabolites*. 2015 Jan 14;5(1):56-73.
81. Brown, N.M.; Galandi, S.L.; Summer, S.S.; Zhao, X.; Heubi, J.E.; King, E.C.; Setchell, K.D. S-(-)-Equol production is developmentally regulated and related to early diet composition. *Nutr. Res*. 2014, 34, 401–409.
82. Setchell KD, Brown NM, Summer S, et al. Dietary factors influence production of the soy isoflavone metabolite s-(-)equol in healthy adults. *J Nutr*. 2013 Dec;143(12):1950-8.
83. Pirillo A, Catapano AL. Berberine, a plant alkaloid with lipid- and glucose-lowering properties: From in vitro evidence to clinical studies. *Atherosclerosis*. 2015 Dec;243(2):449-61.
84. Han J, Lin H, Huang W. Modulating gut microbiota as an anti-diabetic mechanism of berberine. *Med Sci Monit*. 2011 Jul;17(7):RA164-7.
85. Zhang X, Zhao Y, Xu J, et al. Modulation of gut microbiota by berberine and metformin during the treatment of high-fat diet-induced obesity in rats. *Sci Rep*. 2015 Sep 23;5:14405.
86. Feng R, Shou JW, Zhao ZX, He CY, et al. Transforming berberine into its intestine-absorbable form by the gut microbiota. *Sci Rep*. 2015 Jul 15;5:12155.
87. Chen F, Wen Q, Jiang J, et al. Could the gut microbiota reconcile the oral bioavailability conundrum of traditional herbs? *J Ethnopharmacol*. 2016 Feb 17;179:253-64.
88. Bakken JS, Borody T, Brandt LJ, et al. Treating Clostridium difficile Infection with Fecal Microbiota Transplantation. *Clin Gastroenterol Hepatol*. 2011 Dec; 9(12): 1044–1049.
89. Gupta S, Allen-Vercoe E, Petrof EO. Fecal microbiota transplantation: in perspective. *Therap Adv Gastroenterol*. 2016 Mar;9(2):229-39.
90. Choi HH, Cho YS. Fecal Microbiota Transplantation: Current Applications, Effectiveness, and Future Perspectives. *Clin Endosc*. 2016 Mar 9. doi: 10.5946/ce.2015.117.
91. Macfarlane S. Antibiotic treatments and microbes in the gut. *Environ Microbiol*. 2014 Apr;16(4):919-24.
92. Langdon A, Crook N, Dantas G. The effects of antibiotics on the microbiome throughout development and alternative approaches for therapeutic modulation. *Genome Med*. 2016 Apr 13;8(1):39.
93. De La Cochetière MF, Durand T, Lepage P, et al. Resilience of the dominant human fecal microbiota upon short-course antibiotic challenge. *J Clin Microbiol*. 2005 Nov;43(11):5588-92.
94. Mangin I, Lévêque C, Magne F, Suau A, Pochart P. Long-term changes in human colonic Bifidobacterium populations induced by a 5-day oral amoxicillin-clavulanic acid treatment. *PLoS One*. 2012;7(11):e50257.
95. Heinsen FA, Knecht H, Neulinger SC, et al. Dynamic changes of the luminal and mucosa-associated gut microbiota during and after antibiotic therapy with paromomycin. *Gut Microbes*. 2015 Jul 4;6(4):243-54.
96. Rashid MU, Zaura E, Buijs MJ, et al. Determining the Long-term Effect of Antibiotic Administration on the Human Normal Intestinal Microbiota Using Culture and Pyrosequencing Methods. *Clin Infect Dis*. 2015 May 15;60 Suppl 2:S77-84.
97. Dethlefsen L, Huse S, Sogin ML, Relman DA. The pervasive effects of an antibiotic on the human gut microbiota, as revealed by deep 16S rRNA sequencing. *PLoS Biol*. 2008 Nov 18;6(11):e280.
98. Pérez-Cobas AE, Gosalbes MJ, Friedrichs A, et al. Gut microbiota disturbance during antibiotic therapy: a multi-omic approach. *Gut*. 2013 Nov;62(11):1591-601.
99. Johanesen PA, Mackin KE, Hutton ML, et al. Disruption of the Gut Microbiome: Clostridium difficile Infection and the Threat of Antibiotic Resistance. *Genes (Basel)*. 2015 Dec 21;6(4):1347-60.
100. Seekatz AM, Young VB. Clostridium difficile and the microbiota. *J Clin Invest*. 2014 Oct;124(10):4182-9.
101. http://www.cdc.gov/HAI/organisms/cdiff/Cdiff_infect.html
102. Vincent C, Manges AR. Antimicrobial Use, Human Gut Microbiota and Clostridium difficile Colonization and Infection. *Antibiotics (Basel)*. 2015 Jul 3;4(3):230-53.
103. Britton RA, Young VB. Role of the intestinal microbiota in resistance to colonization by Clostridium difficile. *Gastroenterology*. 2014 May;146(6):1547-53.
104. Francino MP. Antibiotics and the Human Gut Microbiome: Dysbiosis and Accumulation of Resistances. *Front Microbiol*. 2016 Jan 12;6:1543.
105. Janssen AW, Kersten S. The role of the gut microbiota in metabolic health. *FASEB J*. 2015 Aug;29(8):3111-23.
106. Principi N, Esposito S. Antibiotic administration and the development of obesity in children. *Int J Antimicrob Agents*. 2016 Mar;47(3):171-7.
107. Cox LM, Blaser MJ. Antibiotics in early life and obesity. *Nat Rev Endocrinol*. 2015 Mar;11(3):182-90.
108. Tsakok T, McKeever TM, Yeo L, Flohr C. Does early life exposure to antibiotics increase the risk of eczema? A systematic review. *Br J Dermatol*. 2013 Nov;169(5):983-91.

Probiotics: Therapeutic Agents for Dysbiosis and Beyond

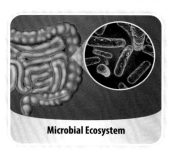

Microbial Ecosystem

The use of probiotics to help re-establish a healthy gut microbiome is now a well-accepted practice across the globe. Research into various types, combinations and doses of probiotics for nearly every potential outcome is expanding at a rapid pace, making it difficult for clinicians to assess the validity of the products that are available for their use or recommendation. In this section, we will outline critical information clinicians should know about using probiotics within the clinical setting, focusing on those factors that may help distinguish one particular product from another. Here, we will also discuss the use of probiotics for basic therapies such as dysbiosis and microbiota maintenance; however, specific recommendations for probiotic therapies will be left to their respective sections.

Probiotics: Definitions and Distinctions

Within the context of this discussion, probiotics describe microorganisms that are intentionally consumed for an intended health benefit, usually to help re-establish a healthy gut microbiome. We specifically distinguish the term "probiotics" from both foodborne microbes (e.g., from soil on vegetables) and microbes used in the production of foods (for fermentation, etc.).[1] While both of the latter can be important influences on a person's gut microbiota over time, the overwhelming majority of research on probiotics in human health is based on commercially-prepared products derived from concentrated bacterial strains. In some cases, these probiotics are added to fermented foods in order to deliver added benefits to the consumer (e.g., yogurt, kefir).

It is also import to establish that commercial probiotics should not be confused with commensal (or indigenous) organisms and, therefore, the therapeutic use of probiotics should not be strictly viewed as "re-inoculating" or "re-colonizing" the gut (see 4R model on page 22). Instead, probiotics should be viewed as highly domesticated varieties of a very limited subset of the "wild" population of microbes living in the human gut. Depending on the strain, probiotics retain some of their "wild-type" characteristics, allowing them to confer benefit alongside the commensal organisms, though they usually lack other characteristics that would permit them to become permanent residents within the host (discussed further below). Probiotics, then, can benefit the host by direct (but transient)

effects, and/or by modifying various gut micro-environments that benefit commensal organisms (limiting pathogenic or pathobiont organisms, altering pH, signaling immune cell function, etc.).

From a regulatory standpoint, probiotics are controlled based on the type of products in which they are contained (food, dietary supplement, investigational drug, etc.), based on the types of claims made for those products. In the United States, probiotics are sold mainly as dietary supplements or foods, though the definition of a dietary supplement in the Dietary Supplement Health and Education Act (DSHEA) does not specifically include probiotics. Probiotic research in the United States is often complicated by these definitions since the FDA (or institutional review boards) can require an Investigational New Drug (IND) application prior to conducting research involving certain disease-related endpoints or patient types.[2] This can stall important research or cause researchers and probiotic marketers to go outside the United States to perform their clinical trials.

The definition of a probiotic assumes two other features: they are "live" organisms and they have a defined health benefit. While both of these are prominently part of the agreed-upon definition of a probiotic *"live microorganism that, when administered in adequate amounts, confer a health benefit on the host,"* they are not as easily defined, and even more difficult to regulate.[3] As we shall discuss further in this section, "live" is a relative term when it comes to probiotics, since most strains are prepared in a manner as to suspend their biological activity (i.e., freeze-drying), many do not survive the transit to the intestines, and some are in the form of spores. Also, there is evidence that some limited benefits can be realized with "dead" probiotics.[4] We will use the term "viability" when discussing both the ability of a probiotic to survive and become "live" in the intestines after consumption and also as a measure of product stability and shelf life (measured in the laboratory).

Finally, the level of evidence required before a particular strain can be deemed to "*confer health benefit on the host*" is highly variable and unregulated. There are many probiotic strains with dozens of randomized clinical trials, and others with no published data that are still marketed as "probiotics." For instance, many so-called soil-based probiotics claim to contain many different strains of bacteria (usually of unknown quantities), most of which have never been shown to have demonstrable health benefits when administered to humans.

As Figure 26 shows, there are several types of mechanisms (and outcomes) that can be demonstrated for probiotics, partly dependent on how they are studied. Most probiotic strains share common benefits, while some trials have demonstrated species-specific and even strain-specific benefits. We will review, where available, the evidence for specific strains, strain combinations, and doses of probiotics for a wide range of gastrointestinal conditions.

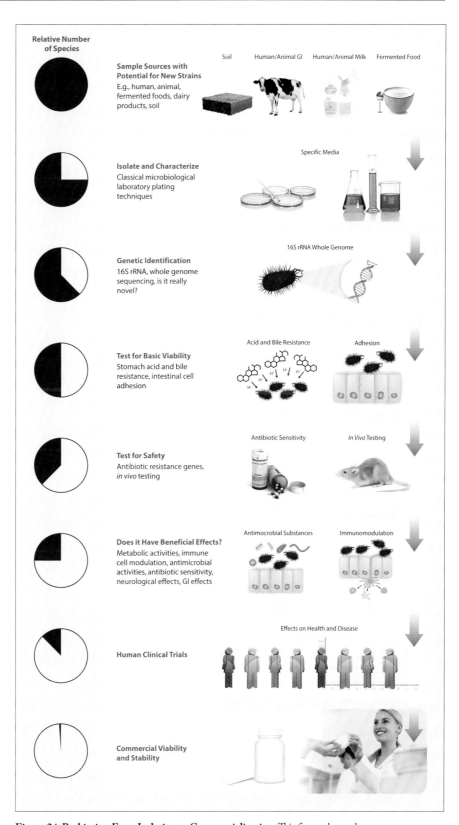

Figure 24: Probiotics: From Isolation to Commercialization. This figure shows the many steps involved in taking an organism from its original isolation to its commercial use as a beneficial therapeutic product. The left side shows that relatively few species of bacteria make it into commercialization. See text for specifics.

Probiotics: From Isolation to Utilization

While there may be over 1, 300 different commensal species of microorganisms identified within the human gut microbiome (globally), only a small handful of species are currently used as probiotics. This is because most of these gut bacteria cannot be effectively isolated and grown outside the human GI tract, and therefore cannot be delivered in sufficient amounts as therapeutic agents. Therefore, the majority of the research on probiotics has focused on those strains which are commercially-viable and readily available (mostly *Lactobacilli* and *Bifidobacterium*), even if they are found as minor contributors to the overall species abundance in the human gut microbiota.

Sources of Probiotics

It is often assumed that probiotic strains must be isolated (originally) from the human gut to be beneficial probiotics. This is not true. In fact, effective probiotic strains have been isolated from a number of sources including animals, soil, fermented foods, breast milk, as well as the human gut. However, in order for a particular microorganism to be considered an effective probiotic (regardless of where it was sourced), it must be able to pass a series of important hurdles (see Figure 24). Essentially, these hurdles involve the strain's ability to show effective benefit in humans while also having the capability of production on a commercial scale (or even viable growth outside the human GI tract).

- **Strain Isolation:** As we have already mentioned, the vast majority of microbes identified within the human GI tract have yet to be properly isolated and grown outside the GI tract. While their genetic material has been routinely identified in fecal samples or intestinal biopsies, many strains have never been grown in the laboratory and characterized in classical microbiological techniques.

- **Genetic Identity:** In classic microbiology, single organisms can be plated on media that allow them to divide and form a colony of genetically identical cells. This colony of cells can then be characterized chemically, metabolically and genetically. Thousands of such microorganisms have been identified, catalogued and stored for future research based on their strain identity.

Most of the common probiotic species used today are represented by a variety of strains, many of which differ only by small genetic differences (often with unknown functional differences). These strain identities may be listed on the label after the species (i.e., *Lactobacillus rhamnosus*- Lr32).

- **Oral Delivery to Intestines:** Strains that can be isolated and genetically identified must be grown in sufficient amounts to be used in further research studies. Initial studies for bile and stomach resistance are followed by cell culture studies of intestinal cell adhesion and animal studies regarding safety. Strains need not be completely resistant to stomach acid, enzymes and bile to be considered transit-viable, nor is intestinal cell adhesion mandatory for use as a probiotic, as many commensals have limited or no attachment to intestinal cells.

- **Biological Effects:** Strains that are considered to be safe and "transit-viable" can be explored for a variety of beneficial effects, such as metabolic activities, immune cell modulation, antimicrobial activities, antibiotic sensitivity, etc. This might include studies done *in vitro*, in cell culture, or using laboratory animals.

- **Human Clinical Trials:** Strains that are safe and have the potential for positive health outcomes might then be used in a clinical trial with a variety of clinical endpoints. Most often, these clinical trials are done on strains that have become commercially available, though some may be performed on strains made available through small laboratory scale preparation.

- **Commercial Viability:** Strains that pass each of the steps above are unlikely to be used in clinical practice unless they are also commercially viable. This means that they have the capacity to be grown in large quantities using relatively economical means, can be prepared for long-term storage (usually through freeze-drying), and maintain their beneficial activities through the process of manufacturing (capsules, tablets, powder) and oral consumption.

Commercial Preparation of Probiotics

Regardless of where a particular strain may have been originally isolated, all probiotics used for food or therapeutic potential are prepared commercially in large monocultures using special nutrient media for optimal growth and viability. Probiotic strains, regardless of their therapeutic potential, can be rendered inert if manufacturers fail to use proper growth conditions, preparation or storage techniques. These processes allow for the production of highly-concentrated organisms that, when dried, can yield powders exceeding 500 billion cells/gram (measured as colony forming units[CFU], see below) for use in foods and dietary supplements.

First, we should note that the many steps involved in making these commercial probiotics change them in a way that is best described as "domestication." Unlike commensal GI organisms that must vie for nutrients in a competitive ecosystem, these probiotics develop and divide in growth medium that is strain-optimized for maximal growth with no competition from other strains or need to adhere to cells or biofilm. Research has shown that in such a domesticated ecosystem, these organisms often fail to express important genes and proteins that prepare them for life "in the wild" of the human GI tract and may even contribute to genetic and/or epigenetic changes over time.[5] Therefore, sub-lethal stressors during the fermentation process (e.g., heat or altered pH) are sometimes used to increase the fitness, robustness and stability of the probiotic bacteria during manufacturing, storage or GI transit.[6] Nonetheless, these probiotics still have a slightly altered phenotype than their wild-type counterparts, even if they are genetically indistinguishable.

Mass Fermentation of Single Strains: Years of research and development has been invested in taking large quantities of multiplying probiotic organisms living in enormous stainless steel vessels of broth and producing a dosage form such as a capsule or tablet. First, well-characterized stock cultures are inoculated into a small vessel containing a broth designed to promote optimal growth for the selected strain.

This culture is allowed to grow at the appropriate temperature until it has reached a sufficient concentration and can then be used to inoculate a larger vessel. This process is repeated several times until one or more large fermentation vessels have reached the desired level of growth (this is often monitored by pH or other measures of bacterial/yeast growth). The fermentation process is stopped by cooling the vessel and adjusting the pH.

Drying to Concentrated Powders: The organisms must then be preserved through one of several different drying techniques or they would quickly die. Freeze-drying is the most common technique, though spray-drying, fluid-bed drying and vacuum-drying techniques are employed for many commercially-available strains of probiotics.[7] Depending on the drying technique employed, various protective agents may be added to help maintain the integrity of the microbe through the drying process. For instance, various carbohydrate-based cryoprotectants are used to stabilize the bacterial cell wall during the process of freeze-drying, cold storage and subsequent thawing and rehydration.

The goal for each of these drying processes is to reduce the moisture content (water activity), one of the most important factors for long-term viability prior to ingestion. These dried powders of concentrated probiotics are then milled for powder consistency (if necessary) and stored frozen for later preparation into dosage forms.

Preparation of Dosage Forms: Frozen drums of probiotics must be thawed (tempered) prior to manufacturing the dosage forms in a prescribed manner to ensure maximum viability. Depending on the final formula, single-strain powders can be mixed to produce multi-strain formulas, diluted with appropriate low-moisture excipients to provide the correct concentration of each strain and then placed in pouches, stick packs, capsules or tablets. Extreme caution should be taken by the manufacturer to ensure the process does not introduce moisture or heat to the probiotic at any stage of manufacturing. Packaging materials should be selected to help protect the probiotic from heat, light, oxygen and, especially, moisture. Therefore, bottles should include desiccants or have a desiccant liner to maintain low moisture throughout the shelf life of the product.

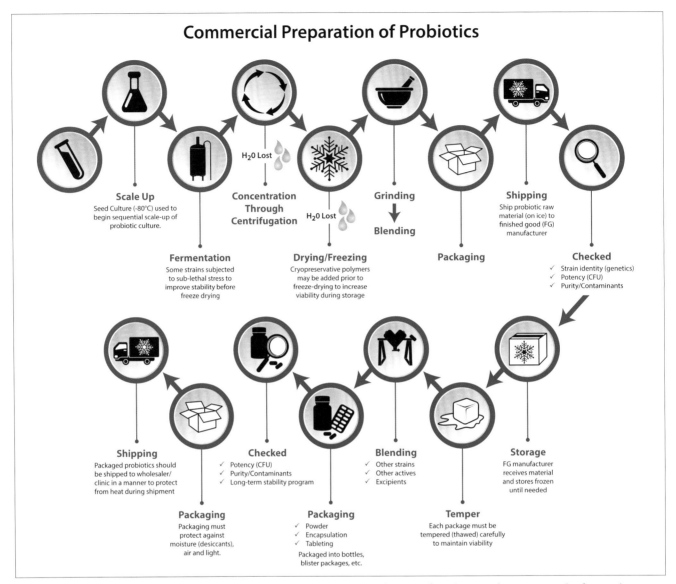

Figure 25: This figure depicts the general flow chart that allows for the commercial manufacturing of a probiotic product; starting with a frozen culture, through fermentation, and the various processes that eventually creates the final finished dosage form. Each of these steps is critical for ensuring the potency, stability, and identity of the product. See text for further details.

Shelf Life of Probiotic Products—*Do Products Need Refrigeration?*

Probiotic organisms within foods or supplements are prone to easy degradation and must be manufactured with great care. We advise clinicians only to recommend probiotics that have a listed shelf-life/expiration date printed on the bottle from reputable companies known to have strict manufacturing procedures, robust quality control procedures and an ongoing product stability program.[†] Procedures must be put in place to limit exposure to heat, oxygen and moisture throughout the manufacturing, storage and shipping process. Even when all these factors are considered, companies must still add a significant overage at the time of manufacturing to maintain their stated potency at the *time of expiration* (do not recommend products which claim potency only at "time of manufacturing").

[†] Technically, dietary supplements in the US are not currently required to have a printed expiration date and some manufacturers use no date, or a "manufactured on" date instead. While the FDA interprets this to mean the product will always meet its label claim, this often means the manufacturer has no stability data. These products should be avoided.

While it is generally true that all probiotics will have a longer shelf life when kept refrigerated, a significant amount of innovation has been developed to allow manufacturers to make products that have significant shelf life at room temperature. This is done to allow the consumer months of shelf life without the need for refrigeration. Companies are required to have real-time data to show that products still meet their label claim potency at the time of expiration, which is usually 9-18 months after the original manufacturing date. Still, when receiving product from companies with room temperature shelf-life dates, they should be shipped to retail or clinical settings in insulated containers with cold packs (or similar packaging) to prevent temperatures from reaching very high levels during the shipping process.

Once a probiotic product is opened and exposed to oxygen and moisture, the shelf life greatly diminishes. Product packages should be small enough that a patient will use up the product within a month or two. Once products are opened, refrigeration may actually contribute additional moisture through condensation, and should not be relied upon as a way to extend shelf life. As a general rule of thumb, once products have been opened, they should be consumed fairly quickly.

Common Probiotic Genera

| *Lactobacillus spp.* | Phylum: Firmicutes | Family: Lactobacillaceae |

Lactobacilli are Gram-positive bacilli (rod-shape) that are non-spore forming, non-motile, facultative anaerobes commonly found in the normal microbiome of the mouth, gastrointestinal tract and female genitourinary tract.[1] Within the GI tract, most *Lactobacilli* are found in the stomach and small intestine where they are metabolically active and have a more unfettered interaction with the immune system. *Lactobacilli* are prototypical lactic acid bacteria (LAB), because lactic acid is their major metabolite of fermentation.[11] Other minor metabolites include acetic acid and succinic acids.

There are well over 100 different species of *Lactobacilli* that have been isolated and identified from a variety of human, animal, soil, or dairy (hence, lacto) sources. Many of these are used in food preparation/ fermentation and as probiotic organisms. *L. acidophilus* is likely the most used probiotic species (historically), though many other species and subspecies of this genera have now surpassed *L. acidophilus* in the number of clinical studies performed and biological mechanisms proposed.

| *Bifidobacterium spp.* | Phylum: Actinobacteria | Family: Bifidobacteriaceae |

Bifidobacterium are non-motile, non-spore-forming, Gram-positive, Y-shaped ("bifid"), anaerobic bacteria resident to the gastrointestinal and female genitourinary tract. Within the GI tract, most *Bifidobacteria* are localized in the colon and terminal ileum. *Bifidobacteria* represent up to 25% of the cultivatable fecal bacteria in adults and 80% in infants (Henry Tissier originally isolated *Bifidobacteria* from the feces of breast-fed infants).[2] *Bifidobacterium* are known to ferment a variety of oligosaccharides usually referred to as "prebiotics" and produce a number of short-chain fatty acids, such as butyrate.

Several dozen species of this genera have been isolated and identified, many of which have confirmed probiotic characteristics. Along with *Lactobacilli*, *Bifidobacterium* species are some of the most widely used commercial probiotic strains.

| *Streptococcus spp.* | Phylum: Firmicutes | Family: Streptococcaceae |

Streptococci are spherical, non-motile, Gram-positive bacteria. The term "*Streptococci*" means "twisted berry" and describes the bacteria's characteristic growth pattern in chains or pairs. Like *Lactobacilli*, many members of the genus *Streptococcus* are facultative anaerobes, reside in the upper part of the GI tract, and produce lactic acid as a major metabolic end product (as such, they are termed LAB). Many members of the *Streptococci* genus are pathogenic; however, *Streptococcus salivarius subsp. thermophilus* (often called *S. thermophilus*) is generally recognized as safe by the FDA and is an important dairy starter culture.[3] It is also recognized to have probiotic characteristics and is sometimes added to probiotic formulas.

Enterococcus spp.	**Phylum:** Firmicutes	**Family:** Enterococcaceae

Bacteria belonging to the genera *Enterococcus* are Gram-positive, facultative anaerobic, non-spore forming cocci that occur as single cells, diplococci (pairs), or short chains.[4] *Enterococci* morphology and phenotypic characteristics are similar to *Streptococci*, and until DNA hybridization studies and 16S rRNA sequencing technology became available in the 1980s, *Enterococci* were originally classified as *Streptococci*. Despite their inability to form spores, *Enterococci* are able to survive in diverse environmental conditions, such as extreme temperature ranges, high sodium chloride concentrations and wide pH ranges, a feature not shared among *Streptococci*. *Enterococci* belong to the clade *Lactobacillales* and as such are lactic-acid-producing bacteria.

As of 2011, approximately 37 species of *Enterococci* had been described; however, two are important medically and from a food microbiological perspective: *E. faecalis* and *E. faecium*.[5] The two species are commensal to the GI tract and involved in food fermentation and food spoilage, but also implicated as opportunistic pathogens in many human infections, including urinary tract infections, bacteremia, bacterial endocarditis, diverticulitis, and meningitis. Many *Enterococci* strains have a high level of intrinsic antibiotic resistance and virulence factors, contributing to their pathogenic nature.[6]

Both *E. faecium* and *E. faecalis* are used as probiotics in humans and animals. According to Franz et al., the strains used commonly as probiotics, *E. faecium* SF68 (NCIMB10415) and *E. faecalis* Symbioflor 1, have been used for more than 20 years without any reported safety concerns. Still, the safety of currently used *Enterococci* probiotic strains and potential probiotic strains should be carefully monitored for safety based on the possibility of genetic transfer from virulent traits.[5] In humans, these probiotics have been studied to treat diarrhea, antibiotic-associated diarrhea, and irritable bowel syndrome; lower cholesterol; and to improve host immunity.

Saccharomyces boulardii	**Phylum:** Ascomycota (Fungi)	**Family:** Saccharomycetaceae

Originally isolated from the litchi fruit (*Litchi chinensis*) in 1923 by Henri Boulard, *Saccharomyces boulardii* differs from other probiotics in that it is a non-pathogenic yeast, not a bacterium.[7] *S. boulardii* is phylogenetically related to, but distinct genetically and metabolically from the baker's yeast used in bread and beer making (*S. cerevisiae*). Although yeast represent less than 0.1% of the resident microbes within the microbiome, yeast cells are about 10 times larger than bacterial cells—a proposed beneficial property of *S. boulardii*, as it may contribute steric hindrance against pathogens within the GI microbiome.[8]

According to Czerucka et al., yeast cells typically reside within the stomach and colon.[8] Additionally, *S. boulardii* is particularly hardy and able to withstand many local stresses within the GI tract, including pH variability, bile salts, enzymes, antibacterial antibiotics, and organic acids. Therefore, *S. boulardii* has shown great probiotic potential for the treatment and prevention of numerous GI-related conditions such as *Clostridium difficile* infection and antibiotic associated diarrhea.[9,10]

Bacillus spp.	**Phylum:** Firmicutes	**Family:** Bacillaceae

Bacilli are Gram-negative, motile, sporulating, facultative anaerobic, rod-shaped bacteria.[11] The ability of vegetative cells to form spores in response to environmental stress (e.g., reduced nutrient availability) sets *Bacilli* apart from many other microbes.[12] The spore coat, rich in peptidoglycan and protein, forms under stressful conditions to protect the dehydrated endospore from UV radiation, extreme heat, solvent exposure, freezing, radiation, hydrogen peroxide and enzymes – a characteristic that greatly increases shelf live and stability of *Bacillus* spore products. Once exposed to the appropriate nutrients, the endospore will transition to a vegetative cell once again. *Bacillus* species are almost entirely isolated from the soil, water, dust and air.[13]

Bacillus species are ubiquitous in nature and have a wide-range of characteristics and enzymatic activities. Notable *Bacillus* species include *B. clausii*, *B. coagulans* (often mislabeled as *Lactobacillus sporogenes*), *B. substilis*, *B. cereus* (a known human food borne pathogen, though not all strains are virulent) and *B. anthracis* (a human pathogen).[12,13,14] *B. subtilis* strain natto is used in the fermentation of soybeans to make the Japanese food natto. Vegetative cells of this strain produce a serine protease, nattokinase, which is used as a dietary supplement.[12] In 2008, *B. coagulans* strain GanedenBC[30] was the first *Bacillus* strain to be given self-affirmed GRAS approval in the United States.[12] While other *Bacillus* species have been added to dietary supplements sold to consumers as probiotics (or beneficial soil-based organisms), most of these strains have not been characterized as having probiotic features or function within the human gut microbiome.

Spore-forming organisms are marketed primarily for their shelf-stability, as they are more resistant to manufacturing and shipping factors that harm the viability of most other probiotic strains. However, as technology has improved the viability of most other strains of probiotics, and conscientious manufacturers with sophisticated product stability programs have learned ways to ensure probiotic viability, spore-forming probiotics are less desirable options, especially since most of the data pointing to clinical efficacy have been with other types of probiotics. Also, since spores are small, light and difficult to destroy, many manufacturers find them difficult to work with, as they persist within the manufacturing environment and require special handling to prevent cross-contamination.

References

1. Slover CM & Danziger L. Lactobacillus: a Review. *Clinical Microbiology Newsletter*. 2008 Feb 15;30(4) 23-27.
2. Picard C, Fioramonti J, Francois A, et al. Review article: bifidobacteria as probiotic agents -- physiological effects and clinical benefits. *Aliment Pharmacol Ther*. 2005 Sep 15;22(6):495-512.
3. Sharma R, Bhaskar B, Sanodiya, BS, et al. Probiotic Efficacy and Potential of Streptococcus thermophilus modulating human health: A synoptic review. *IOSR Journal of Pharmacy and Biological Sciences*. 2014;9(3) 52-58.
4. Arias CA, Murray BE. Enterococcal Infections. In: Kasper D, Fauci A, Hauser S, Longo D, Jameson J, Loscalzo J. eds. Harrison's Principles of Internal Medicine, 19e. New York, NY: McGraw-Hill; 2015.
5. Franz CM, Huch M, Abriouel H, et al. Enterococci as probiotics and their implications in food safety. *Int J Food Microbiol*. 2011 Dec 2;151(2):125-40.
6. Hollenbeck BL, Rice LB. Intrinsic and acquired resistance mechanisms in enterococcus. *Virulence*. 2012 Aug 15;3(5):421-33.
7. Saccharomyces boulardii in Gastrointestinal Related Disorders. 2008. (Point Institute)
8. Czerucka D, Piche T, & Rampal P. Review article: yeast as probiotics –Saccharomyces boulardii. *Alimentary Pharmacology & Therapeutics*. 2007 Sep;26(6) 767-778.
9. Szajewska H, Kołodziej M. Systematic review with meta-analysis: Saccharomyces boulardii in the prevention of antibiotic-associated diarrhoea. *Aliment Pharmacol Ther*. 2015 Oct;42(7):793-801.
10. McFarland LV. Probiotics for the Primary and Secondary Prevention of C. difficile Infections: A Meta-analysis and Systematic Review. *Antibiotics (Basel)*. 2015 Apr 13;4(2):160-78.
11. Juturu V, Wu JC. Microbial production of lactic acid: the latest development. *Crit Rev Biotechnol*. 2015 Aug 17:1-11.
12. Cutting SM. Bacillus probiotics. *Food Microbiology*. 2011;28 214-220.
13. Sanders ME, Morelli L, & Tompkins TA. Sporeformers as human probiotics: Bacillus, Sporolactobacillus, and Brevibacillus. *Comprehensive Reviews in Food Science and Food Safety*. 2003;2 101-110.
14. Jurenka JS. Bacillus coagulans: Monograph. *Altern Med Rev*. 2012 Mar;17(1):76-81.

How Cell Viability is Measured

Probiotics are usually measured (enumerated) by colony forming units (CFU or c.f.u.). This method requires that the bacteria (or yeast), which is usually in a freeze-dried state, be prepared in a manner as to allow them to slowly revive prior to dilution and plating on an appropriate medium. When sufficiently diluted, single cells then produce visible colonies after several days of growth in an incubator. The number of colonies formed, multiplied by the dilution used, allows for a calculation of the starting material in CFU/gram. The FDA does not mandate that probiotics be labeled using this, or any, specific enumeration; though most products list the number of CFU per dose (for each strain, or for the total) in the supplement facts panel. Because the number of cells is so large, the probiotic dose is often expressed in the literature (and some product labels) using scientific notation (powers of 10) where $3x10^6$ would represent 3 million CFU, while $3.5x10^{10}$ would represent 35 billion CFU and so on.

The CFU method of enumeration is currently the industry standard, though it is quite unsophisticated and often, problematic. Besides the well-known method variability associated with this enumeration technique, it is not uniformly consistent between different strains of bacteria and is difficult to use after several strains of similar species are blended together.[8] Furthermore, research suggests that some strains of probiotics can enter a "viable but non-culturable" state that allows them to become viable when placed in the appropriate (i.e., GI) environment, but lose their ability to form a colony on an agar plate.[9] New methods (e.g., flow cytometry) may soon be readily available to allow more accurate and timely ways to determine the functional viability of probiotic strains prior to manufacturing and finished probiotic products after manufacturing and storage.

The Efficacy of Dead Probiotics
Does Viability Matter?

As we have alluded to on several occasions, the official definition of a probiotic includes the provision that it is "alive." We have already discussed two technical challenges to this definition, in that most probiotics are inert when consumed (freeze-dried, spores, etc.) with the potential to become alive or viable if they reach a

suitable environment; and the laboratory challenge of defining cell viability, since some stored products show viability (using flow-cytometry), but cannot be cultured using traditional plating techniques. Beyond these technicalities, there is a growing list of published research documenting beneficial biological outcomes when using heat-killed or dead probiotic strains.[10]

First, we should mention that the majority of these studies are in cell-culture experiments, though animal and human studies (mostly in Japan and China) have confirmed some of these outcomes.[11,12,13] Secondly, while these effects are not limited to a single species or strain of bacteria (though virtually all have been *Lactobacilli spp.*), most of the documented effects are related to immune system modulation, presumably because dead cells still contain membranes with lipopolysaccharides for toll-like receptor interactions (see page 151 for microbe-immune system interactions).[14,15] Therefore, while intentionally-killed probiotic cells appear to mimic some of the immune-modulating effects of "live" probiotics (those deemed viable by traditional CFU/plate counting prior to ingestion), they have not been documented to have any of the other direct antimicrobial, microbiome-altering, or metabolic functions attributed to probiotic species.

The notion of using intentionally killed probiotics is an intriguing development in the area of immune-modulation, there is not enough evidence to recommend this as a method for replacing traditionally prepared probiotics (nor are we aware of such products available to the clinician in the US). While these data might also suggest that some probiotics may still have some immune-modulating benefits after their viable (culturable) shelf life has passed, we do not recommend clinicians or patients rely upon the efficacy of expired products.

Which Strains are Best?

One question that always comes up when discussing probiotics is, "What strain, or strain combination, is the best?" Of course, this begs the follow-up question: "For what purpose?" The use of a probiotic as a preventative measure against potential dysbiosis (as one would use a multivitamin), is quite different than using a probiotic to treat a subject with antibiotic-associated diarrhea or inflammatory bowel disease. Therefore, this question must be answered in a step-wise fashion, owing to the unique nature in which probiotic research has been done over the years.

First, while there are many different strains of probiotic organisms currently available, the majority of these are very similar to each other, especially when compared to the overall diversity within the gut commensal community. Most have never been compared head-to-head in human clinical trial settings. Therefore, while some studies may suggest one strain is preferable to another for a particular outcome, this is often simply because that particular strain was used to perform one or more (positive) clinical trial, a trial which simply was not done with, or compared to, other similar strains. Therefore, choosing the strain(s) used in positive clinical trials may be "evidence-based," but large gaps in study design and the lack of strain-to-strain comparison often limit definitive strain-specific recommendations.

A good way to illustrate the clinical data for different probiotic strains is shown in Figure 26. The vast majority of probiotic species share common activities that are expected to benefit most individuals, related mostly to a minimal dose or intake frequency. Beyond these common benefits, we know that certain species provide particular activities not found in other species;

in some cases, these have been reinforced by positive clinical trials. Finally, research has uncovered certain activities that may even be strain-specific, allowing for the potential of targeted probiotic therapies for discrete clinical outcomes. Again, we must emphasize that few head-to-head studies are performed, as this type of research is difficult and expensive to conduct, and therefore these differences are likely exaggerated by the design of the clinical study.

We believe it is safe to say that there is not one strain or strain combination of probiotics that is ideally suited for each individual or clinical outcome. For the most part, increasing commensal diversity is likely to benefit most individuals, something that is likely to occur when consuming a product containing a diverse mix of probiotic species or strains; what we call a multi-species or multi-strain approach. Choosing a specific strain or strain combination (or a higher dose) may be warranted when that dose or strain(s) has shown consistent clinical evidence for the specific goal of the therapy. Healthcare providers should stay abreast of the published literature in this area as new studies (and some new probiotic strains) are likely to influence clinical decision-making for recommending probiotics to patients.

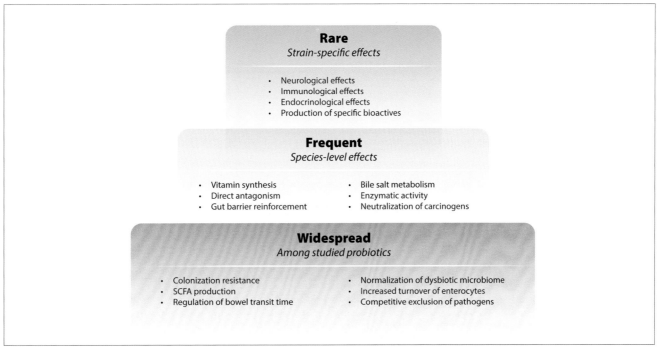

Figure 26: Hierarchy of Strain-Specificity. This figure shows that the majority of probiotic functions are shared by most proven strains of probiotics; while certain functions are shared only by certain families or species of bacteria; and finally, some features may only be recognized with one or a few sub-species of strains. Systematic head-to-head research limits the reliability of many strain-specific claims.

Health Benefits of Fermented Foods

The natural or intentional application of microbes to various foods, resulting in a fermented end-product ready for consumption, has been used for thousands of years in many cultures throughout the world. Fermentation has been used for enhancing taste, for slowing spoilage, and in some cases to aid in the digestion of some dietary components (e.g., lactose in milk, in the case of yogurt).[1] The most commonly used bacteria for food fermentation are lactic acid bacteria (LAB) which includes a broad category of bacterial genera including: *Lactobacillus, Bifidobacterium, Streptococcus, Enterococcus, Lactococcus,* etc. Various species of yeast (esp. *Saccharomyces cerevisiae*) are also widely used in the brewing, baking, and cheese-making industries; characteristically producing ethanol and carbon dioxide in the fermentation of sugars.

While some fermented foods are made by spontaneous fermentation using no "starter culture" (e.g., sauerkraut), most others are made by using a common starter culture which is usually a small portion of a previously prepared fermented culture

(e.g., sourdough bread and kombucha). Today, most commercially prepared fermented foods are produced in large-scale batches that are designed for efficiency and reliable reproduction of culture conditions (to meet rigorous regulatory, quality control, taste, texture and shelf life standards). This process, as well as the selection of microbial strains that function best in commercial-scale operations, has led to the "domestication" of many wild-type microbial strains. This domestication has resulted in documented genetic changes in these strains, compared to their wild-type counterparts, to better adapt to the food production environment (similar to what we have described for commercially prepared probiotics).[2] Therefore, some have claimed certain commercially prepared fermented foods differ in their health benefits compared to traditionally prepared or small-batch home preparations. While such differences may exist, we are not aware of any evaluation comparing the microbes, fermented by-products or health outcomes between different methods of fermenting the same foods.

Should Fermented Foods be Considered Probiotics?

There is no doubt certain fermented foods account for a portion of the ingested microbes in many diets and therefore are capable of being part of the transient gut microbiota. In fact, the analysis of three standard dietary plans revealed that the presence of yogurt and cottage cheese as recommended foods greatly enhanced the amount of microbes present in the diet.[3] However, in most cases, these microbes do not meet the definition of a probiotic.[4] First, many of the strains used to ferment various food substrates prior to ingestion have not been shown to have independent health benefits for the host, an important requirement for the definition of a probiotic. Also many commercially prepared fermented products are processed in ways that limit or kill the microorganisms prior to packaging (e.g., pasteurization, food additives) in order to stop the fermentation process, sanitize or increase the shelf life of these products. Therefore, most fermented foods do not typically report a CFU count on their label (or the types of microbes present), limiting the consumer's ability to know if, and how much of, any potential viable probiotic organisms are present.

The National Yogurt Association (NYA) offers a "live and active cultures" seal to yogurt manufacturers and/or distributers. To qualify for the seal, companies must submit an application fee of $2,500 and document, via third-party laboratory testing, that each refrigerated yogurt product contains at least 10^8 CFU/gram of live starter culture (*Lactobacillus delbrueckii* subsp. *bulgaricus* and *Streptococcus thermophilus*) at the time of manufacture.[5] Frozen yogurt must contain 10^7 CFU/gram of live starter culture at the time of manufacture. In 2011, a scientific, global authority committee upheld a health claim for the live yogurt starter cultures, *Lactobacillus delbrueckii subsp. bulgaricus* and *Streptococcus salvarius subsp. thermophilus*.[6] The claim reads, "Live yogurt cultures in yogurt improve digestion of lactose in yogurt in individuals with lactose maldigestion." The group used randomized clinical trials and *in vitro* studies as scientific substantiation. Yogurt manufacturers may elect to add probiotic strains to the yogurt in addition to the starter cultures (after pasteurization), allowing some yogurts to fit the definition of a "probiotics" or functional food.[7]

Foods/Beverages	Organisms
TRADITIONAL FERMENTED FOODS	
Kimchi (cabbage)	Leuconostoc mesenteroides and other LAB
Cortido (cabbage, onions, carrots)	Not specified
Sourdough	L. reuteri, S. cerevisiae
Kvass (beverage from black or rye bread)	Lactobacillus spp.
Kombucha tea (black, green, white, pekoe, oolong or darjeeling, water, sugar)	Gluconacetobacter and Zygosaccharomyces
Pulque (beverage from agave plant sap)	Zymomonas mobilis
Kaffir beer (beverage from Kaffir maize)	Lactobacillus spp.
Ogi (cereal)	Lactobacillus spp., Saccharomyces spp., Candida spp.
Igunaq (fermented walrus)	Not specified
Miso (soybeans)	Aspergillus oryzae, Zygosaccharomyces, Pediococcus spp.
Tepa (Stinkhead fermented fish)	Not specified
Dosa (fermented rice batter and lentils)	L. plantarum
Surströmming (fermented herring, brine)	Haloanaerobium praevalens, Haloanaerobium alcaliphilum
Crème fraîche (soured dessert cream)	L. cremoris, L. lactis
Fermented sausage	Lactobacillus, Pediococcus, or Micrococcus
Traditional preparation of cod liver oil	Not specified
Hákarl (fermented shark meat, dried)	Not specified
Kefir	Kefir grains (combination of LAB and yeasts)
Garum (fish sauce, ancient Roman condiment)	Fish intestine microbiota
Natto	Bacillus subtilis var. natto
COMMERCIAL/NON-TRADITIONAL FERMENTED FOODS	
Yogurt	L. delbrueckii ssp. bulgaricus, S. thermophilus (starter cultures), adjunct cultures of Bifidobacterium spp., Lactobacillus spp., etc. may be added
Kefir	Commercially produced kefir may use kefir grains at large scale, or pure cultures isolated from kefir grains or commercial cultures to keep flavor consistent; adjunct cultures Bifidobacteria spp., Lactobacillus spp., Lactococcus spp., Streptococcus spp., Saccharomyces spp., etc. may be added
Cheese	LAB starter cultures; adjunct cultures (for flavor/textures) Lactobacillus spp., Propionibacterium spp. (eye formation in Swiss cheese), Penicillium spp., etc.
Pickled Vegetables	LAB (Streptococci spp., Leuconostoc spp., Pediococcus spp., Lactobacillus spp.)
Sauerkraut (cabbage)	LAB (Lactobacillus spp., Leuconostoc spp., Pediococcus spp.)
Soy sauce	Aspergillus oryzae or Aspergillus sojae molds, other related microbes (S. cerevisiae, Bacillus spp., Lactobacillus spp.); can be made by fermentation or by acid hydrolysis
Tempeh	Rhizopus spp.
Olives	LAB (Lactobacillus spp., Pediococcus spp.)
Beer	Saccharomyces cerevisiae, Saccharomyces uvarum, Dekkera spp., Brettanomyces spp.
Wine	Various yeast organisms particularly Saccharomyces cerevisiae; LAB added in a second step to make red wine

Benefits of Fermented Foods, Beyond Their Microbes

Even though most fermented foods do not meet the definition of a probiotic and should not be considered a therapeutic alternative to probiotics, but this does not mean that they are devoid of potential health benefits. Fermented foods often contain substrates upon which commensal microbes can thrive (and ferment), as well as many bioactive compounds derived from the fermentation process, both of which can benefit the host or their gut microbiota.[8]

In many cases, foods containing beneficial nutrients are easier to consume or are more bioavailable after fermentation.[9,10] Unfortunately, most traditionally fermented foods with a history of health-promoting attributes have not been rigorously tested using modern scientific research and, therefore, specific recommendations as to the type, dose or means of fermentation cannot yet be given.[11] Some fermented foods have been documented to have beneficial outcomes, but with the exception of particular yogurt and kefir preparations, these benefits should not generally be considered "probiotic" in nature (though this term is still often used of fermented food microbes).[12,13,14,15,16,17] Though we do not believe clinicians should consider fermented foods as therapeutically equivalent to proven probiotic strains, we do recommend their consumption as part of a diverse, GI-enriching diet.

References

1.   Chilton SN, Burton JP, Reid G. Inclusion of fermented foods in food guides around the world. *Nutrients*. 2015 Jan 8;7(1):390-404.
2.   Gibbons JG, Rinker DC. The genomics of microbial domestication in the fermented food environment. *Curr Opin Genet Dev*. 2015 Dec;35:1-8.
3.   Lang JM, Eisen JA, Zivkovic AM. The microbes we eat: abundance and taxonomy of microbes consumed in a day's worth of meals for three diet types. *PeerJ*. 2014 Dec 9;2:e659.
4.   Hill C, Guarner F, Reid G, et al. Expert consensus document. The International Scientific Association for Probiotics and Prebiotics consensus statement on the scope and appropriate use of the term probiotic. *Nat Rev Gastroenterol Hepatol*. 2014 Aug;11(8):506-14.
5.   National Yogurt Association. Live and Active Culture Yogurt Seal Program: Procedures and Guidelines. Updated December 2013. Retrieved from: http://aboutyogurt.com/AboutYogurt08/files/ccLibraryFiles/Filename/000000000046/12%2013%2013_LAC%20Seal%20Guidelines%20with%20Appendices.pdf
6.   EFSA Panel on Dietetic Products, Nutrition and Allergies. Scientific Opinion on the substantiation of health claims related to live yoghurt cultures and improved lactose digestion (ID 1143, 2976) pursuant to Article 13(1) of Regulation (EC) No 1924/2006. EFSA Journal 8, 1763 (2010).
7.   Glanville JM, Brown S, Shamir R, et al. The scale of the evidence base on the health effects of conventional yogurt consumption: findings of a scoping review. *Front Pharmacol*. 2015 Oct 30;6:246.
8.   Budak NH, Aykin E, Seydim AC, Greene AK, Guzel-Seydim ZB. Functional properties of vinegar. *J Food Sci*. 2014 May;79(5):R757-64.
9.   Scheers N, Rossander-Hulthen L, Torsdottir I, Sandberg AS. Increased iron bioavailability from lactic-fermented vegetables is likely an effect of promoting the formation of ferric iron (Fe(3+)). *Eur J Nutr*. 2016 Feb;55(1):373-82.
10. Humer E, Schedle K. Fermentation of food and feed: A technology for efficient utilization of macro and trace elements in monogastrics. *J Trace Elem Med Biol*. 2016 Mar 15. pii: S0946-672X(16)30028-1.
11. Chilton SN, Burton JP, Reid G. Inclusion of fermented foods in food guides around the world. *Nutrients*. 2015 Jan 8;7(1):390-404.
12. Tamang JP, Shin DH, Jung SJ, Chae SW. Functional Properties of Microorganisms in Fermented Foods. *Front Microbiol*. 2016 Apr 26;7:578.
13. Leroy F, De Vuyst L. Fermented food in the context of a healthy diet: how to produce novel functional foods? *Curr Opin Clin Nutr Metab Care*. 2014 Nov;17(6):574-81.
14. Vīna I, Semjonovs P, Linde R, Deniņa I. Current evidence on physiological activity and expected health effects of kombucha fermented beverage. *J Med Food*. 2014 Feb;17(2):179-88.
15. Park KY, Jeong JK, Lee YE, Daily JW 3rd. Health benefits of kimchi (Korean fermented vegetables) as a probiotic food. *J Med Food*. 2014 Jan;17(1):6-20.
16. Shiby VK, Mishra HN. Fermented milks and milk products as functional foods--a review. *Crit Rev Food Sci Nutr*. 2013;53(5):482-96.
17. Borresen EC, Henderson AJ, Kumar A, Weir TL, Ryan EP. Fermented foods: patented approaches and formulations for nutritional supplementation and health promotion. *Recent Pat Food Nutr Agric*. 2012 Aug;4(2):134-40.

Multi-Strain vs. Single-Strain vs. Rotating Strains

Since there are many purposes for which a probiotic may be recommended, and the published literature includes a wide range of probiotic formulas, strains and doses, many different theories of proper probiotic recommendations have emerged. Two, in particular, are the multi-strain and rotation of single-strain approaches. We advocate for using a multi-strain approach for the vast majority of applications within the clinical setting. First, since a diverse blend of commensal species appears to be one of the most important factors in maintaining a healthy gut microbiome, using a range of different strains has the best chance of promoting a wider array of commensal organisms. In addition, because of individual differences in strain survival, compatibility and metabolic potential, a multi-strain approach allows for a more diverse benefit in a wider range of individuals. Finally, recall that probiotics represent a part of the transient microbiome (see page 102), which is normally encountered as a range of organisms ingested in the diet, and through contact with the soil and air. A multi-strain approach is therefore more consistent with this natural encounter with ingested microorganisms.

There are several ways to define a multi-strain approach. In general, we define this as a product with five or more proven probiotic strains containing at least two Lactobacilli and two Bifidobacterium strains. One way to enhance the potential for diversity using this multi-strain approach is to choose products that contain species (or sub-species) with a range of genetic variability (see phylogenetic relationship of common probiotic strains in Figure 27). By combining strains that are more genetically diverse, rather than clustering the diversity with closely related sub-species, a greater potential for diversity may be achieved. Inclusion of *Streptococci*, *Saccharomyces boulardii*, or other non-LAB strains will expand this diversity even further.

The other popular means of attempting to achieve diversity is to rotate single-strain probiotics, consuming a different strain for a few months and then switching to a different strain and so on. The difficulty in recommending this approach is that there is virtually no information available to evaluate this strategy and, in comparison to the multi-strain approach above, does not mimic the way we encounter transient microbes from our food or environment. Also, since many probiotics require several weeks or months of continuous use to achieve noticeable benefit, the subject might be planning to rotate to a new strain just as tangible benefits may be realized from the current product, and switching may not be in the best interest of the patient. While switching from one product to another may be necessary to find a product more suited for an individual or a therapeutic purpose, rotating single-strain products in an attempt to increase overall microbiota diversity is likely a hold-over from the days when only single-strain products were available and is accomplished more efficiently by the use of multi-strain products. As a final note, rotating different multi-strain products is not discouraged, provided they are equally diverse, though research investigating this approach is also lacking.

Changes in Commensal Population from Probiotic Intake

Compared to the changes detected in commensal populations that occur after radical dietary changes, bariatric surgery or antibiotic use (or fecal microbiota transplants), detectible changes in the commensal microbiota after probiotic consumption are much more limited.[16,17] This should come as little surprise since the strains used as probiotics are generally limited to just a few genera, are almost exclusively transient in nature (because of their species and/or commercial domestication), and are usually given in doses that are difficult to detect in fecal samples (by culture or genetic methods). However, there are several important points that need to be considered before determining such subtle changes are unimportant.

First, as we shall show in subsequent sections, even when no major changes are detectible in commensal microbiota after ingestion of certain probiotics, there is often still a demonstrable improvement in GI or other health outcomes. This suggests that subtle changes in commensal species abundance or function, along with the direct metabolic contributions of the transient probiotic species, can have profound and important health benefits for the host. Second, the dose of most probiotics is likely to alter the immediate microbial balance within the small intestine where there are fewer numbers and species of microorganisms, though this population is poorly represented in fecal microbial analysis. This means that probiotics, especially *Lactobacilli* strains, may profoundly alter the balance of microbial species in the small intestine and subsequently benefit the host, without demonstrably altering the total gut microbiota when measured via fecal analysis.[18,19,20]

In some cases, resident commensal microbiota may be more or less permissive to an incoming probiotic strain. A recent animal study published in February 2016 evaluated whether the host's resident gut microbiota may influence niche permissivity (i.e., colonization resistance) for transient probiotic bacteria administered in a fermented milk product containing five strains.[21] Zhang et al. used a GI transit marker to evaluate whether the administered probiotic appeared in the feces at the same rate. Two phenotypes emerged based on probiotic transit: one termed "resistant," where the administered probiotic appeared in the feces at the same rate as the GI transit marker, and the other termed "permissive," where the group shed *L. lactis* CNCM I-1631 over an additional 24-48 hours. Therefore, the resistant rats were less susceptible to transient probiotic colonization from the fermented milk drink compared to the permissive group.

Further gut microbiome analysis of the two phenotypes showed differences in their relative abundance of Lachnospiraceae. The authors conclude: "evaluation of gut microbiota directed therapies involving administration of allochthonous microbes [i.e., probiotics] should consider the endogenous gut microbiota as a stratifying factor." Further, "our results suggest that the composition of the autochthonous [i.e., commensal] gut microbial community might account for the amplitude and persistence of effects of supplements containing allochthonous microbes."

Finally, it is not generally agreed that radical microbiome alterations would be a desirable outcome of probiotic use, since the potential for monoculture or core microbiome disruption could be more harmful than other "natural" forms of dysbiosis. Recall that probiotic therapy should not be considered a re-inoculation of commensal strains as much as providing a commensal-friendly transient population. Oral doses of commensal organisms in the form of encapsulated frozen feces may have the effect of "re-inoculation" and have been studied for use in subjects with recurring *C. difficile* infections with some success, though these products are not technically "probiotics" and their regulatory status is currently unknown (see FMT on

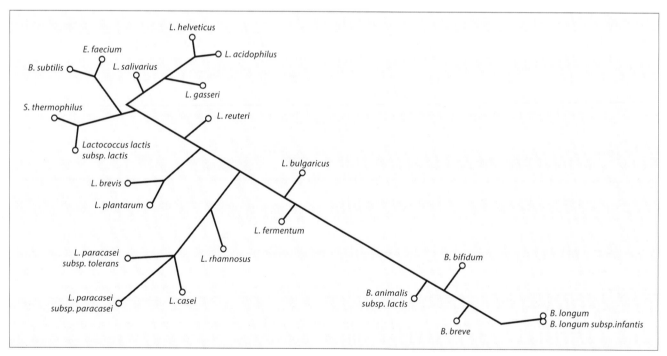

Figure 27: Phylogenetic relationship between common probiotic strains based on unrooted maximum parsimony clustering of partial 16S rRNA gene sequences (courtesy of Danisco/Dupont).

page 110).[22] Therefore, it is currently more reliable to use patient signs and symptoms (or other biomarkers of disease progression, if they exist), rather than changes in fecal microbiota, to judge the efficacy of probiotic therapies.

Probiotics: Part of the Transient Microbiome

We have already emphasized the idea that the strains of commercially-prepared probiotics currently available should be considered temporary, rather than permanent, members of the gut microbiome. While many view the temporary status of probiotics as a negative feature, this is likely due to the lack of appreciation for the importance of the transient microbiome (see Figure 21, page 102).

Perhaps one of the key reasons that probiotic strains are generally safe and applicable for most individuals is related to the fact that they are transient. This feature allows them to function primarily to promote an environment that is friendly for the variable and core species of the microbiome, which is different in each individual. In addition, while their residence may be temporary, certain effects (immune modulation, pathogen diminution, etc.) may persist long after their presence in the gut has ceased.

Generally, probiotics that survive the initial transit are considered to persist in the GI tract for one to two weeks after ingestion, though this is strain, dose and host dependent.[23] Most of these studies define persistence as the detection (usually metagenomics) of the consumed strain using fecal samples, though biopsies and simulated gastrointestinal environments have also been used with similar results.[24,25]

While the relative persistence of every strain has not been confirmed in human subjects, similar persistence has been seen in most strains tested, including Lactobacilli, Bifidobacterium, Saccharomyces boulardii and spore-forming Bacilli.[26,27] Obviously, probiotics consumed on a regular basis will continually replenish this transient portion of the microbiome and, depending on dose, can significantly alter the patient's health during that time.

What is the Right Dose?

The use of probiotics is now commonplace in the United States and around much of the world. These probiotics can be delivered in relatively low-dose functional foods (primarily yogurts) providing up to a few billion colony forming units (CFU); or in modest doses, in the form of dietary supplements of 5-25 billion CFU. However, over the past several years, a trend has emerged in which much higher doses of probiotics are being used in both clinical practice and research. Since most strains or strain combinations have not been clinically researched using dose-response relationships as a primary analytical goal, we review below the limited available evidence on dose-to-dose outcomes and also the types of studies where high-dose probiotic therapies (defined here as >100 billion CFU/day[†]) have been successful.

Dose Comparison Studies

Few dose-response or dose-comparison clinical trials (high vs. low) using probiotics have been performed in human subjects. Two studies, using very different definitions of "high-dose" therapy, have evaluated the dose-effects of probiotics in subjects using antibiotics and their subsequent risk for antibiotic-associated diarrhea (AAD) or C. difficile associated diarrhea (CDAD). In both cases, the higher dose reduced the incidence of AAD and/or CDAD in a statistically and clinically significant way, compared to the lower dose (see details on page 167).

Also, a few dose-response studies looked at bowel transit and stool consistency. One study assessed two different doses of Bifidobacterium lactis on whole gut transit time (WGTT, assessed by abdominal X-ray) and GI symptoms in subjects with an average of one to three bowel movements per week.[28] Subjects were given capsules containing placebo, 1.8 billion CFU (low-dose), or 17.2 billion CFU (high-dose) at breakfast for two weeks (capsules opened and eaten with yogurt). After 14 days, both doses of B. lactis improved transit time and functional GI symptoms, though the high-dose therapy was slightly better (and more statistically different compared to placebo) than the low-dose therapy. Another study investigated the effect of supplementing

---

†   This definition of "high-dose" is somewhat arbitrary based on the recent trend of available products. Some would argue that therapies delivering >20 billion CFU should be deemed "high," while others may suggest that "high-dose" therapy is not reached until >450 billion CFU has been exceeded.

healthy young adults with a combination of *Lactobacillus paracasei* and *Bifidobacterium lactis* at doses ranging from 100 million CFU/day to 100 billion CFU/day in tenfold increments.[29] They reported a significant dose-dependent improvement in fecal consistency (looser stools) as the dose increased.

While these data suggest that the dose of certain probiotics may influence certain outcomes in certain patients, it is difficult to generalize beyond these particular strains and the limited outcomes reviewed here. Since the vast majority of clinical trials using probiotics use only one dose (comparing to placebo), often with no explanation as to the reason the particular dose (or strain[s]) was chosen, clinicians should consider altering the suggested dose before concluding that a patient can receive no benefit from the particular probiotic product chosen.

High-dose Therapies

Over the past decade, there has been an emerging increase in probiotic dosing seen in both clinical research and clinical practice. Not surprisingly, the initial focus of the clinical research on high-dose probiotics has been on GI disorders such as inflammatory bowel disease (IBD), irritable bowel syndrome (IBS), and antibiotic-associated diarrhea (AAD). These conditions represent extreme examples of dysbiosis or dysfunction within the mucosal immune system of the gut, a system which is integrally associated with the gut microbiota (see page 164). Although supplemental probiotics are only transient members of the intestinal microbiota, the introduction of large quantities of probiotics may sufficiently alter this environment allowing the probiotic to act as potent bio-therapeutic agents in a manner that lower doses may not.

The majority of these high-dose clinical trials have been performed using various doses of one particular combination of probiotic strains (VSL#3: containing three strains of *Bifidobacteria*, four strains of *Lactobacilli*, and one strain of *Streptococcus salivarius* ssp.). Figure 28 shows these doses have ranged from 450 billion CFU/day to as high as 3.6 trillion CFU/day, and from as short as four weeks of supplementation to as long as 12 months. Positive benefits (most statistically significant compared to placebo) were noted in patients with ulcerative colitis, pouchitis, and antibiotic-associated diarrhea (details for each will be covered in their respective section). However,

as mentioned earlier, only one very high dose was used in each clinical trial (compared to placebo), and it is therefore difficult to determine if lower doses would have accomplished similar results in similar subjects. As we will outline in other sections, lower doses and different strain combinations have been shown to have clinically meaningful and statistically significant benefits in similar patients, suggesting that high-dose therapies may not always be necessary to achieve meaningful clinical results.

Proposed Mechanisms of High-dose Probiotic Therapy

Numerous mechanisms are attributed to a wide dose range of probiotic therapies which mirror the mechanisms of beneficial commensal organisms (see Figure 16, earlier). As mentioned earlier, adding significantly more metabolically active cells into the GI microbiome can have significant implications for the balance of commensal organisms, resulting in more pathogen/pathobiont exclusion, nutrient fixation, bacteriocin production, etc. These transient intraluminal effects may account for much of the benefits seen in AAD and CDAD studies when higher doses are used.

Another major focus of this research is the interaction between bacterial organisms in the gut and specific cells within the gut associated lymphoid tissue (GALT), especially the dendritic cells which act as specialized antigen-presenting cells within the gastric mucosa. These dendritic cells are critical for both the maturation and tolerance of the immune system. A recent study showed that by increasing the number of probiotic organisms interacting with dendritic cells *in vitro* (this study used *Lactobacillus rhamnosus*), a much different genomic response was elicited.[30] When researchers increased the multiplicity of infection (MOI), or the number of *L. rhamnosus* plated with immature human dendritic cells by hundredfold, they induced a sharp change in gene expression of over 1,700 different genes compared to dendritic cells in the presence of fewer bacteria. Most of the changes in gene expression were for genes that control immune and inflammatory signaling or dendritic cell maturation. In fact, these data showed a progressive dose-response increase in specific dendritic cell surface markers at five different probiotic:dendritic cell ratios. This genomic effect is an exciting new line of research that is likely to lead to a greater understanding

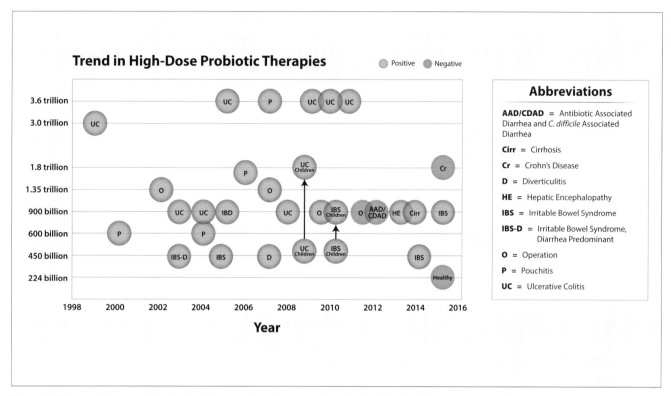

Figure 28: This graph shows the GI-related publications for studies using the high-dose formula VSL#3 by year, type of patients studied and dose (Y axis not to scale).

of how commensal and probiotic organisms help regulate immune function and attenuate numerous conditions related to the gut. In this case, progressively higher bacterial concentration triggered a much different response in immune system regulation than a lower concentration, suggesting one broad mechanism by which high-dose probiotic therapies may differ from similar strains at lower doses.

Since this study has not been repeated with other strains or other species (or directly in humans), it is unknown how applicable these findings would be to other probiotic strains, though similar modulations of immune cell functions are likely with many other strains of probiotics. In fact, a study comparing two different doses of *Lactobacillus plantarum* ("low-dose" 500 million CFU and "high-dose" 5 billion) in institutionalized elderly subjects showed significant differences in immune cell activation that differed based on dose.[31] Since many clinicians would consider both of these doses "low," it should be noted that high doses are not necessarily needed to achieve meaningful benefits in some subjects, only that high (or very high) doses may achieve different (or additional) benefits.

Final Thoughts on High-dose Therapy

While the available clinical research on high-dose probiotic therapy is relatively recent, a trend is emerging in clinical practice to begin increasing probiotic doses, primarily for GI-related dysfunctions. More data are needed in order to discern whether specific GI disorders would be better supported using specific probiotic strains or combinations of strains (at different doses). Until such a time, doses of between 200 billion and several trillion CFU/day of products consisting of mixed probiotic strains should be considered safe for adjunct therapies for patients with IBD, IBS and AAD. This approach should be considered short term (four to eight weeks for functional bowel disorders or until symptoms cease for AAD), although cost may limit the accessibility of this therapy for many patients.

When to Take Probiotics

As with many other therapeutic products taken orally, questions about when to take them, especially in relation to a meal, is often asked by patients and clinicians alike. Knowing that most probiotics are negatively affected by stomach acid, bile and pancreatic secretions makes this question all the more relevant. Although many clinical opinions exist, this question is relatively un-researched. In fact, many clinical studies using probiotics do not even describe (or control for) the probiotic dose respective to the timing of meals.

That said, attempting to answer this question in the research setting is not easy. As mentioned previously, identifying consumed probiotic strains using fecal sampling is not a reliable method, and is certainly not able to act as a quantitative measure of viability. And unlike animal studies, biopsies of the stomach, small intestines and colon for such an enumeration study are also not feasible. Therefore, the limited research investigating this question so far has come from the use of simulated gastric or intestinal environments with varying degrees of sophistication.

One study has attempted to answer this question directly using an *in vitro* digestive system model, designed to simulate both the gastric and duodenal environment. They used a four-strain, non-enteric coated capsule containing *Lactobacillus helveticus*, *Lactobacillus rhamnosus*, *Bifidobacterium longum* and *Saccharomyces boulardii*.[32] Two capsules were added to the system 30 minutes before, during, or 30 minutes after the addition of a "meal" consisting of oatmeal and 1% milk. Capsules added before the oatmeal had 250 ml of spring water added. Additionally, they tested the differential effect of apple juice, 1% milk or water on the probiotic survival.

In this model system, probiotic survival was slightly better when added to the system before or during the oatmeal and slightly lower when added 30 minutes after the oatmeal. In most cases, these differences were not statistically significant nor, in our opinion, clinically significant. A more noticeable difference was seen when using water or apple juice, both of which significantly decrease *Lactobacillus* and *Bifidobacterium* strain survival compared to the oatmeal or 1% milk alone. The authors believe this was due either to a protective effect of the 1% fat content, a longer buffering of stomach acid by the milk and oatmeal, or a quicker gastric emptying

rate (especially water). It should be noted that in each case, the *Bifidobacterim longum* was more vulnerable to these changes than the *Lactobacillus* strains, while the *Saccharomyces boulardii* had a universally high survival that was unaffected by beverage selection or meal timing. The delivery of probiotic strains in milk-based or other food-derived vehicles has been suggested to improve viability in other *in vitro* gastric-simulated test environments, though the lack of uniformity in measures of viability, testing environments, delivery vehicles and probiotic strains used in these studies make it very difficult to generalize these conclusions to most other commercially available products.[33,34,35,36]

Still, many other host factors that could not be replicated in these artificial GI environments affect probiotic survival and efficacy and may be patient-specific. Therefore, with the limited data available to answer this question, we suggest that patients consume probiotics when it is most convenient for them, as the differences noted in these studies are likely to be insignificant (clinically), compared to the cumulative benefits of daily supplementation, or conversely, non-compliance. Since only water, apple juice and 1% milk were compared, it may be suggested that when probiotics are consumed away from a meal that 1% milk may benefit survival over water or apple juice. Whether milk substitutes with fat (almond, soy or rice) or other fruit juices will behave in the same manner is unknown.

Safety and Tolerability of Probiotic Therapy

Overall, oral administration of even high-dose probiotic formulas is well tolerated and proven to be safe in hundreds of human clinical trials. Extremely rare cases of local or systemic infections have occurred with probiotic therapy, mainly in immune-compromised individuals.[37,38,39] In particular, septicemia and endocarditis were found to occur in immune-compromised patients with aplasia,[40] HIV,[41] and organ transplantation[42] who had been administered *Lactobacilli* species. Further investigation revealed that in most of these cases, the source of the infection was a commensal *Lactobacillus*. It is safe to assume that most *Bifidobacteria* and *Lactobacilli* used in the food industry, as well as those reported in clinical trials, are safe for the general adult and pediatric populations.[43]

Available products range from as little as 1 billion CFU/dose to as high as 450 billion CFU/dose. For the purposes of non-disease-specific balancing of the GI microflora, daily doses of 20 to 40 billion CFU in adults and 1 to 5 billion in children are usually sufficient. Much higher doses (some well over 1 trillion CFU/day) have been reported in the literature to benefit patients with specific clinical conditions (like IBD), but are rarely needed to help most patients without specific dysbiotic abnormalities.

D-Lactate-Producing Probiotics:
Do they need to be avoided in some patients?

Lactic acid-producing commensal and probiotic organisms can convert simple sugars into either or both racemic isomers of lactic acid/lactate (D or L). Since humans produce high levels of L-lactate (primarily skeletal muscles), the body has adequate capacity to metabolize this isomer, while most individuals lack the capacity to metabolize high amounts of D-lactate (produced mostly by the gut microbiota; see exception below). Therefore, elevated levels of D-lactate in the blood (also measured in urine or feces) can lead to D-lactic acidosis with detrimental neurological consequences, defined primarily in subjects with short bowel syndrome (SBS).[44]

In most individuals (without SBS), other bacteria within the GI tract are capable of metabolizing the D-lactate produced, rendering this isomer inert to the host. Subjects with increased intestinal permeability have elevated serum and urine levels of D-lactate since the molecule can absorb before being metabolized in the gut. However, some have argued that based on a few published case-studies over the past three decades that changes in urinary D-lactate may also suggest microbial-induced acidosis occurs in subjects with jejuno-ileostomy, pancreatic insufficiency, or appendicitis,[45] though others document that such phenomena is exceedingly rare.[46] However, one potential confounder to linking elevated serum or urine D-lactate levels with changes in gut microbial metabolism is the fact that hyperglycemia can trigger the production of D-lactate from methylglyoxal (MG) metabolism through the glyoxalase pathway.[47] Accordingly, the serum (and urine) D-lactate levels in type 2 diabetic patients are significantly elevated compared to normoglycemic controls.[48]

The reason this issue is considered here is that some lab interpretative guides suggest that when patient urine D-lactate is high (above reference range), clinicians should advise against the use of D-lactate-producing probiotics, or avoid probiotics altogether until D-lactate-producing organisms are eliminated (usually through the judicious use of antibiotics). Though this recommendation is sometimes given by clinicians, and widely circulated on the Internet, limited data are available linking the use of D-lactate-producing probiotics to elevated D-lactate in subjects *without* SBS.[49] Nonetheless, if clinicians choose to avoid D-lactate-producing probiotics for this, or other reasons, they can select from products containing strains such as *L. casei, L. paracasei, L. salivarius, L. rhamnosus*, any *Bifidobacterium spp.*, and *Saccharomyces boulardii*.

Probiotics and Histamine Sensitivity

In discussions with clinicians, there have been two primary assertions related to the intake of probiotics and histamine sensitivity, though they are polar opposite in nature. The first is the concern that consuming particular species or strains of probiotics will trigger the production of histamine leading to an unwanted reaction in subjects with food-histamine sensitivities. We believe this concern has stemmed from a misapplication of articles published on the histamine and tyramine production capabilities of certain bacteria used in the processing of food (e.g., fermentation of cheese) that are also potential probiotic strains.[50] We are not aware of any reported relationship between the consumption of any probiotic and a resulting negative histamine-related reaction (though there are mechanistic reports that some probiotics benefit IBD patients, ironically, by stimulating histamine receptors).[51]

At the same time, there are those who suggest that certain strains of probiotics will help those with histamine-sensitivity due to their expression of enzymes that metabolize histamine (e.g., diamine oxidase).[52] Again, we are not aware of clinical studies attempting to confirm the benefits of any particular strain in human subjects with reported histamine sensitivity. We advise clinicians to monitor the use of probiotics in subjects with histamine sensitivity, noting whether one product or strain either exacerbates or relieves histamine-associated symptoms; however, there are limited data upon which to make definitive suggestions as to specific strains to avoid or include for such subjects.

Probiotic Supplementation During Antibiotic Use

A common question among clinicians is whether probiotic use is appropriate, effective or contraindicated during antibiotic therapy. These questions stem from the fact that antibiotic use has a well-known detrimental effect on commensal bacterial species, causing an antibiotic-associated dysbiosis that often leads to bowel symptoms, especially diarrhea. We will address three basic questions related to probiotic use during antibiotic therapy.

- **Does antibiotic therapy render probiotic therapy inert?** While some strains of probiotics are susceptible to certain antibiotics, most strains are resistant or partially resistant to many common antibiotics used today. Broad spectrum antibiotics, such as amoxicillin, ampicillin and penicillin G, are particularly harsh on most commercially produced probiotic strains. The yeast probiotic *Saccharomyces boulardii* is resistant to all antibiotics. Using a multi-strain probiotic that includes *S. boulardii* is recommended during antibiotic therapy to offset potentially

harmful dysbiosis caused by the use of broad spectrum antibiotics. Taking probiotics at least 2 hours after an antibiotic dose is a generally recognized way to limit probiotic susceptibility to antibiotics.

- **Do probiotics make antibiotics less effective?** There is no evidence to suggest probiotics change the effectiveness of any particular antibiotic. Since a dose of even 100 billion CFU (if all survived to the gut) would still only represent about 0.1% of the total bacterial organisms in the gut, even susceptible strains would offer a small percentage of likely "targets" for any antibiotic, leaving the antibiotic dose undiminished to target other organisms. Again, consuming probiotics at least 2 hours after an antibiotic dose will limit the interaction between these therapies.

- **Are probiotics effective for preventing or treating antibiotic-associated GI side effects?** Yes, though not all strains or doses are equally effective. A large number of studies have attempted to answer this question, mainly focused on antibiotic-associated diarrhea (AAD), often connected with preferential overgrowth of *Clostridium difficile* (CDAD). Unfortunately, these studies have included a wide range of doses, strains, strain combinations, antibiotics and patient-types, leading to a wide range of reported efficacy. See page 164 for our discussion of treatment strategies, including the use of probiotics, for AAD and CDAD.

References for Probiotic Section on page 139.

Probiotic Supplementation in Infants and Children

With the growing acknowledgment of the importance of the GI microbiome for proper metabolic and immune system development, along with the safe use of probiotics in adult populations, there has been an accumulating body of research on the use of probiotics in infants and children. Here, we will briefly summarize data on the use of probiotics for GI-related conditions in infants and children, along with the safety of using probiotics in these populations. There are several recent comprehensive reviews covering more details, including many non-GI indications.[1,2,3,4]

Safety

In the general pediatric population (aged zero to 18 years), probiotics have been well-tolerated and are generally regarded as safe with few adverse events; however, extra precautions should be taken in at-risk pediatric populations when supplementing with probiotics.[5] Such at-risk patient populations are immune-compromised children; premature infants; those with critical illness, structural heart disease, or a central venous catheter; and in those with potential for translocation of probiotics from the gut lumen to the bloodstream.

A meta-analysis of 57 clinical trials (and eight follow-up studies) including 10,056 infants under the age of two years found supplementation with probiotics and synbiotics to be safe; furthermore, no serious adverse events or safety concerns were found to be associated with the probiotics and prebiotics studied.[6] Rarely probiotics may cause bacteremia, fungemia and sepsis in immune-compromised, critically ill children.[7] We should note the number of species (and strains) used in the pediatric population is limited, and therefore the number of strains demonstrated to be safe (compared to adult populations) is also limited. However, based on what is known about the isolation of probiotic strains and their overall record of safety in foods and supplements worldwide, we believe that most currently available strains are likely to be safe in the pediatric population (with the noted exceptions listed above).

Probiotic Use in Selected Childhood Conditions

Acute Gastroenteritis

The probiotic strains most studied for treatment of acute gastroenteritis (AGE) in pediatric populations include: *L. rhamnosus* GG[8,9] *S. boulardii*,[10, 11, 12] and *L. retueri* DSM 17938.[13,14] In fact, a working group from the European Society for Pediatric Gastroenterology, Hepatology and Nutrition (ESPGHAN) strongly recommends the use of *L. rhamnosus* GG ($\geq$10 billion CFU/day) and *S. boulardii* (250-750 mg/day) for AGE in children, along with a "weak" recommendation for *L. reuteri* DSM 17938 (10^8 to 4×10^8 CFU/day) for the same indication.[15] Most of these probiotics are recommended to be taken for five to seven days. The only probiotic with a negative recommendation based on this report by ESPGHAN was for *Enterococcus faecium* (SF68 strain); the group strongly recommends avoiding this strain due to safety concerns (specifically related to a possible recipient of vancomycin-resistant genes).

Antibiotic-Associated Diarrhea

A 2015 Cochrane Review by Goldenberg et al. included 23 RCTs studying 3,938 children (two weeks to 17 years old) found significantly reduced incidence of AAD in the probiotic groups (*Lactobacilli spp.*, *Bifidobacterium spp.*, *Streptococcus spp.*, or *Saccharomyces*

---

† The limited number of strains used in the pediatric population (perhaps due to their selection by researchers or IRB reviewers based on previous safety data) severely limits the strength of strain-specific recommendations. That is, since most strains (or strain combinations) have never been tested for particular outcomes in children, any strain-specific recommendation is made by default; simply using those limited strains with positive clinical evidence.

‡ Historically, *S. boulardii* has been dosed in mg rather than CFU, though the products used have generally been thought to contain 20 billion CFU/gram of material (i.e., 5 billion CFU/250 mg). Since most of the materials and method sections for these clinical trials do not specify further, it is difficult to confirm the exact dosing used in these trials.

boulardii alone or in combination) compared to the control groups (RR: 0.46; 95% CI: 0.35 to 0.61).[16] The authors concluded, "L. rhamnosus and S. boulardii at 5 to 40 billion CFU/day may be appropriate for preventing AAD in children receiving antibiotics;" however, no other recommendations were made about other strains.

Many RCTs and meta-analyses recommend probiotics for the prevention of AAD. Strains with the most evidence include L. rhamnosus GG (five RCTs, n= 445, RR: 0.48; 95% CI: 0.26 to 0.89)[17] and S. boulardii (six RCTs, n=1653, RR: 0.43, 95% CI 0.3 to 0.6)[18]; both of which are recommended by the ESPGHAN working group guidelines (2016).[19] Mcfarland (2015) notes in a mini-review on deciphering meta-analytic results that the best evidence for a probiotic in pediatric AAD is for S. boulardii because the favorable pooled effect for L. rhamnosus GG is skewed by one large positive trial.[20] As we mentioned previously, the lack of clinical trials (positive or negative) for other strains is not evidence of their lack of efficacy, and the use of other strains or strain combination in adult AAD suggest other strains are likely beneficial for this outcome. (see page 164 for discussion of AAD in adults).

Clostridium difficile Infection (CDI)
Compared to the literature surrounding probiotics for C. difficile infections in adults, information concerning the use of probiotics in children is limited. A 2013 Cochrane review by Goldenberg et al. considered probiotics for prevention of CDI in both adults and children.[21] After pooling 23 trials including 4,213 participants, use of probiotics was found to decrease the risk of CDI by 64% (RR: 0.36; CI: 0.26-0.51) (see page 165 for C. difficile-related therapies in adults).

Helicobacter Pylori Infection
A meta-analysis completed in 2014 that pooled seven studies (508 pediatric patients) found that probiotic supplementation (different strains and doses), when combined with triple antibiotic therapy for H. pylori, was able to increase eradication rate (OR: 1.96, 95% CI: 1.28-3.02) and was associated with reduced risk of therapy-related side effects (five RCTs, RR: 0.32).[22] Since there was significant heterogeneity

between these trials, it was unclear which probiotic strains or doses might be more effective.

A 2015 meta-analysis by Szajewska et al. pooling nine RCTs that included 1,708 participants (330 children) found supplementation with S. boulardii was significantly associated with increased H. pylori eradication rate compared to standard triple therapy; though the treatment was still below the desired eradication rate.[23] Nonetheless, S. boulardii therapy did reduce the overall risk of H. pylori therapy-related side effects (RR: 0.44, 95% CI 0.31-0.64). The evidence for both associations was rated as moderate, and the authors call for further research—especially in pediatric populations, as only two studies in this systematic review considered children. In these two studies, which included 330 children, the H. pylori eradication rate was improved in the S. boulardii group compared with the control group (RR: 1.13, 95% CI 1.03-1.25).

Necrotizing Enterocolitis (NEC)
Numerous reviews have recently been published on the promising benefits of using probiotics in infants with NEC.[24,25,26] According to Szajewska (2016), preventing NEC is possibly the most promising indication for the use of probiotics in preterm infants. An updated Cochrane review studied 24 RCTs and compared to the control group, preterm neonates in the probiotics group had reduced risks of NEC stage ≥2 (20 RCTs, RR: 0.43) and all-cause mortality (17 RCTs, RR: 0.65), but there was no difference between groups in the risk of nosocomial sepsis (19 RCTs, RR: 0.91).[27]

According to those who have studied this in depth, despite the potential benefit of probiotics in NEC, many questions remain unanswered, including the optimal probiotic formulation and the safety and efficacy of using probiotics in very low-birthweight (birthweight < 1, 500 g) and extremely low-birthweight infants (birthweight <1, 000 g)".[1]

Infantile Colic
In reviewing data related to the use of probiotics and infantile colic, it was unusual to find nearly all were performed with a single strain of L. reuteri. Four independent RCTs showed L. reuteri DSM 17938 (generally dosed 100 million CFU/day)

reduced crying times in breastfed infants with infantile colic.[28,29,30,31,32] However, another study involving both breast-fed and formula-fed infants did not confirm this benefit, perhaps because it enrolled children predominantly from the emergency department and included children on proton pump inhibitors.[33] Interestingly, the formula-fed infants after one month of supplementation with *L. reuteri* DSM 17938 showed significantly more fussing time with treatment compared to placebo (p = 0.005).

Systematic reviews and meta-analyses have shown benefit for *L. reuteri* in breast-fed infants for infantile colic.[34,35] A 2016 systematic review found supplementation with *L. reuteri* in breast-fed infants associated with a 2.3-fold greater chance of having a 50% or greater decrease in crying/fussing time compared to controls (p=0.01).[36]

In the investigation of the *prevention* of infantile colic, a 2014 trial by Indrio et al. enrolled 589 Italian neonates in the first week of life and compared the incidence of developing a functional GI disorder (FGIDs) in babies receiving *L. reuteri* compared with those receiving placebo.[37] FGIDs were defined as "inconsolable crying time, regurgitation, and modification of bowel movements." The study showed a significant difference in crying time from 70.9 min/day in the placebo group to 37.7 min/day in the probiotic group; approximately 1.5 less regurgitations/day in treatment group (4.6/day in control and 2.9 in treatment); and increased stool frequency (3.6/day vs. 4.2 stools/day treatment).

While these studies appear quite promising, it is difficult to know whether these effects are strain or even species-specific. Since probiotic therapy is safe in most infants, the clinician should consider recommending a probiotic designed for children, perhaps selecting one with this or similar strains of *L. reuteri*.

Other GI-Related Outcomes

Probiotics have been investigated as a therapeutic intervention for a number of other GI-related conditions in infants and children. For the most part, there is simply not enough evidence to make specific recommendations, as clinical trials have had a range of positive and negative outcomes. There is

limited evidence to recommend selected probiotics for ulcerative colitis. The European Crohn's and Colitis organization (ECCO) and ESPGHAN consider VSL#3 and *E. Coli* Nissle 1917 as effective treatment for maintenance in patients with UC, but this recommendation is based on limited evidence.[38,39,40,41] According to ECCO/ESPGHAN guidelines, there is not enough evidence to suggest probiotics are beneficial for the maintenance or remission of Crohn's disease in children.[42]

For abdominal-pain-related functional gastrointestinal disorders (FGID), Korerink et al. performed a systematic review of all available RCTs in children with FGID and concluded that *L. rhamnosus* GG, *L. reuteri* DSM 17938 and VSL#3 strains are possibly effective in decreasing pain-related FGID with a pooled risk ratio of 1.5.[43] The studies, however, were relatively heterogeneous and therefore prevented firm conclusions on efficacy.[1] There is also limited evidence to make specific recommendations for either functional constipation or irritable bowel syndrome, though probiotics are likely to be safe in such populations and some small clinical trials have shown benefit.[44,45,46,47]

Probiotics for Non-GI Conditions

There are many possible therapeutic benefits related to probiotic therapy in children for non-GI-related conditions such as atopic/allergic treatment and prevention, immune-related outcomes, upper respiratory infections, mood-related outcomes and even metabolic-related outcomes. While these topics are outside the scope of this handbook, clinicians should be aware of the broader potential for non-GI-related outcomes for the use of probiotics in children (and adults).

References

1. Szajewska H. What are the indications for using probiotics in children? *Arch Dis Child*. 2016 Apr;101(4):398-403.
2. Barnes D, Yeh AM. Bugs and Guts: Practical Applications of Probiotics for Gastrointestinal Disorders in Children. *Nutr Clin Pract*. 2015 Dec;30(6):747-59.
3. Singhi SC, Kumar S. Probiotics in critically ill children. *F1000Res*. 2016 Mar 29;5.
4. Hashemi A, Villa CR, Comelli EM. Probiotics in early life: a preventative and treatment approach. *Food Funct*. 2016 Apr 20;7(4):1752-68.
5. van den Nieuwboer M, Brummer RJ, Guarner F, et al. Safety of probiotics and synbiotics in children under 18 years of age. *Benef Microbes*. 2015;6(5):615-30.

6.   van den Nieuwboer M, Claassen E, Morelli L, et al. Probiotic and synbiotic safety in infants under two years of age. *Benef Microbes*. 2014 Mar;5(1):45-60.
7.   Singhi SC, Kumar S. Probiotics in critically ill children. *F1000Res*. 2016 Mar 29;5.
8.   Szajewska H, Skórka A, Ruszczyński M, Gieruszczak-Białek D. Metaanalysis: Lactobacillus GG for treating acute gastroenteritis in children— updated analysis of randomised controlled trials. *Aliment Pharmacol Ther*. 2013;38(5):467-476.
9.   Sindhu KNC, Sowmyanarayanan TV, Paul A, et al. Immune response and intestinal permeability in children with acute gastroenteritis treated with Lactobacillus rhamnosus GG: a randomized, double-blind, placebo-controlledtrial. *Clin Infect Dis*. 2014;58(8):1107-1115.
10.   Szajewska H, Skórka A. Saccharomyces boulardii for treating acute gastroenteritis in children: updated meta-analysis of randomized controlled trials. *Aliment Pharmacol Ther*. 2009;30(9):960-961.
11.   Feizizadeh S, Salehi-Abargouei A, Akbari V. Efficacy and safety of Saccharomyces boulardii for acute diarrhea. *Pediatrics*. 2014;134(1):e176-e191.
12.   Dinleyici EC, Eren M, Ozen M, et al. Effectiveness and safety of Saccharomyces boulardii for acute infectious diarrhea. Expert *Opin Biol Ther*. 2012;12:395–410.
13.   Szajewska H, Urban´ska M, Chmielewska A, et al. Meta-analysis: Lactobacillus reuteri strain DSM 17938 (and the original strain ATCC 55730) for treating acute gastroenteritis in children. *Benef Microbes*. 2014;Jan 24:1–9.
14.   Dinleyici EC, Dalgic N, Guven S, et al. Lactobacillus reuteri DSM 17938 shortens acute infectious diarrhea in a pediatric outpatient setting. *J Pediatr (Rio J)*. 2015 Jul-Aug;91(4):392-6.
15.   Szajewska H, Guarino A, Hojsak I, et al. European Society for Pediatric Gastroenterology, Hepatology, and Nutrition. Use of probiotics for management of acute gastroenteritis: a position paper by the ESPGHAN Working Group for Probiotics and Prebiotics. *J Pediatr Gastroenterol Nutr*. 2014;58:531–9.
16.   Goldenberg JZ, Lytvyn L, Steurich J, et al. Probiotics for the prevention of pediatric antibiotic associated diarrhea. *Cochrane Database Syst Rev Online*. 2015 Dec 22;(12):CD004827.
17.   Szajewska H, Kołodziej M. Systematic review with meta-analysis: Lactobacillus rhamnosus GG in the prevention of antibiotic-associated diarrhoea in children and adults. *Aliment Pharmacol Ther*. 2015 Nov;42(10):1149-57.
18.   Szajewska H, Kołodziej M: Systematic review with meta-analysis: Saccharomyces boulardii in the prevention of antibiotic-associated diarrhoea. *Aliment Pharmacol Ther*. 2015; 42(7): 793–801.
19.   Szajewska H, Canani RB, Guarino A, et al. Probiotics for the Prevention of Antibiotic-Associated Diarrhea in Children. *J Pediatr Gastroenterol Nutr*. 2016 Mar;62(3):495-506.
20.   McFarland LV. Deciphering meta-analytic results: a mini-review of probiotics for the prevention of paediatric antibiotic-associated diarrhoea and Clostridium difficile infections. *Benef Microbes*. 2015;6(2):189-94.
21.   Goldenberg JZ, Ma SS, Saxton JD, et al. Probiotics for the prevention of Clostridium difficile-associated diarrhea in adults and children. *Cochrane Database Syst Rev*. 2013 May 31;(5):CD006095.
22.   Li S, Huang XL, Sui JZ, et al. Meta-analysis of randomized controlled trials on the efficacy of probiotics in Helicobacter pylori eradication therapy in children. *Eur J Pediatr* 2014;173:153–61.
23.   Szajewska H, Horvath A, Kołodziej M. Systematic review with meta-analysis: Saccharomyces boulardii supplementation and eradication of Helicobacter pylori infection. *Aliment Pharmacol Ther* 2015;41:1237–45.
24.   Warner BB, Tarr PI. Necrotizing enterocolitis and preterm infant gut bacteria. *Semin Fetal Neonatal Med*. 2016 Jun 22. pii: S1744-165X(16)30027-0.
25.   Aceti A, Gori D, Barone G, et al. Probiotics for prevention of necrotizing enterocolitis in preterm infants: systematic review and meta-analysis. *Ital J Pediatr*. 2015 Nov 14;41:89.
26.   Fleming P, Hall NJ, Eaton S. Probiotics and necrotizing enterocolitis. *Pediatr Surg Int*. 2015 Dec;31(12):1111-8.
27.   AlFaleh K, Anabrees J. Probiotics for prevention of necrotizing enterocolitis in preterm infants. *Cochrane Database Syst Rev* 2014;4:CD005496.
28.   Szajewska H, Gyrczuk E, Horvath A. Lactobacillus reuteri DSM 17938 for the management of infantile colic in breastfed infants: a randomized, double-blind, placebo-controlled trial. *J Pediatr* 2013;162:257–62.
29.   Savino F, Cordisco L, Tarasco V, et al. Lactobacillus reuteri DSM 17938 in infantile colic: a randomized, double-blind, placebo-controlled trial. *Pediatrics* 2010;126: e526–33.
30.   Savino F, Pelle E, Palumeri E, Oggero R, Miniero R. Lactobacillus reuteri (American Type Culture Collection Strain 55730) versus simethicone in the treatment of infantile colic: a prospective randomized study. *Pediatrics*. 2007;119(1):e124-e130.
31.   Chau K, Lau E, Greenberg S, et al. Probiotics for infantile colic: a randomized, double-blind, placebo-controlled trial investigating Lactobacillus reuteri DSM 17938. *J Pediatr* 2015;166:74–8.
32.   Mi GL, Zhao L, Qiao DD, et al. Effectiveness of Lactobacillus reuteri in infantile colic and colicky induced maternal depression: a prospective single blind randomized trial. *Antonie Van Leeuwenhoek* 2015;107:1547–53.
33.   Sung V, Hiscock H, Tang ML, et al. Treating infant colic with the probiotic Lactobacillus reuteri: double blind, placebo controlled randomised trial. *BMJ* 2014;348:g2107.
34.   Harb T, Matsuyama M, David M, et al. Infant Colic-What works: A Systematic Review of Interventions for Breast-fed Infants. *J Pediatr Gastroenterol Nutr*. 2016 May;62(5):668-86.
35.   Urbańska M, Szajewska H. The efficacy of Lactobacillus reuteri DSM 17938 in infants and children: a review of the current evidence. *Eur J Pediatr* 2014;173:1327–37.
36.   Schreck Bird A, Gregory PJ, Jalloh MA, et al. Probiotics for the Treatment of Infantile Colic: A Systematic Review. *J Pharm Pract*. 2016 Mar 2. pii: 0897190016634516.
37.   Indrio F, Di Mauro A, Riezzo G, et al. Prophylactic use of a probiotic in the prevention of colic, regurgitation, and functional constipation: a randomized clinical trial. *JAMA Pediatr*. 2014;168(3):228-233.
38.   Turner D, Levine A, Escher JC, et al. European Crohn's and Colitis Organization; European Society for Paediatric Gastroenterology, Hepatology, and Nutrition. Management of pediatric ulcerative colitis: joint ECCO and ESPGHAN evidence-based consensus guidelines. *J Pediatr Gastroenterol Nutr* 2012;55:340–61.
39.   Henker J, Muller S, Laass MW, et al. Probiotic Escherichia coli Nissle 1917 (EcN) for successful remission maintenance of ulcerative colitis in children and adolescents: an open-label pilot study. *Z Gastroenterol* 2008;46:874–5.
40.   Huynh HQ, deBruyn J, Guan L, et al. Probiotic preparation VSL#3 induces remission in children with mild to moderate acute ulcerative colitis: a pilot study. *Inflamm Bowel Dis* 2009;15:760–8.
41.   Miele E, Pascarella F, Giannetti E, et al. Effect of a probiotic preparation (VSL#3) on induction and maintenance of remission in children with ulcerative colitis. *Am J Gastroenterol* 2009;104:437–43.
42.   Ruemmele FM, Veres G, Kolho KL, et al. ECCO/ESPGHAN. Consensus guidelines of ECCO/ESPGHAN on the medical management of pediatric Crohn's disease. *J Crohns Colitis* 2014;8:1179–207.
43.   Korterink JJ, Ockeloen L, Benninga MA, Tabbers MM, Hilbink M, Deckers-Kocken JM. Probiotics for childhood functional gastrointestinal disorders: a systematic review and meta-analysis. *Acta Paediatr*. 2014;103(4):365-372.
44.   Tabbers MM, DiLorenzo C, Berger MY, et al. European Society for Pediatric Gastroenterology, Hepatology, and Nutrition; North American Society for Pediatric Gastroenterology. Evaluation and treatment of functional constipation in infants and children: evidence-based recommendations from ESPGHAN and NASPGHAN. *J Pediatr Gastroenterol Nutr* 2014;58:258–74.
45.   Bu L-N, Chang M-H, Ni Y-H, et al. Lactobacillus casei rhamnosus Lcr35 in children with chronic constipation. *Pediatrics International* 2007;49:485–90.
46.   Guerra PV, Lima LN, Souza TC, et al. Pediatric functional constipation treatment with Bifidobacterium-containing yogurt: a crossover, double-blind, controlled trial. *World J Gastroenterol* 2011;17:3916–21.
47.   Guandalini S, Magazzù G, Chiaro A, et al. VSL#3 improves symptoms in children with irritable bowel syndrome: a multicenter, randomized, placebo-controlled, double-blind, crossover study. *J Pediatr Gastroenterol Nutr*. 2010;51(1):24-30.

References

1. Sanders ME. Probiotics: definition, sources, selection, and uses. *Clin Infect Dis*. 2008 Feb 1;46 Suppl 2:S58-61; discussion S144-51.
2. Sanders ME, Shane AL, Merenstein DJ. Advancing probiotic research in humans in the United States: Challenges and strategies. *Gut Microbes*. 2016 Mar 3;7(2):97-100.
3. Hill C, Guarner F, Reid G, et al. Expert consensus document. The International Scientific Association for Probiotics and Prebiotics consensus statement on the scope and appropriate use of the term probiotic. *Nat Rev Gastroenterol Hepatol*. 2014 Aug;11(8):506-14.
4. Adams CA. The probiotic paradox: live and dead cells are biological response modifiers. *Nutr Res Rev*. 2010 Jun;23(1):37-46.
5. Bull MJ, Jolley KA, Bray JE, et al. The domestication of the probiotic bacterium Lactobacillus acidophilus. *Sci Rep*. 2014 Nov 26;4:7202.
6. Lacroix C, Yildirim S. Fermentation technologies for the production of probiotics with high viability and functionality. *Curr Opin Biotechnol*. 2007 Apr;18(2):176-83.
7. Broeckx G, Vandenheuvel D, Claes IJ, et al. Drying techniques of probiotic bacteria as an important step towards the development of novel pharmabiotics. *Int J Pharm*. 2016 May 30;505(1-2):303-18.
8. Sutton, S. The limitations of CFU: Compliance to CGMP requires good science. *Journal of GXP Compliance*. 2012; 16(1): 74-80.
9. Davis C. Enumeration of probiotic strains: Review of culture-dependent and alternative techniques to quantify viable bacteria. *J Microbiol Methods*. 2014 Aug;103:9-17.
10. Kataria J, Li N, Wynn JL, Neu J. Probiotic microbes: do they need to be alive to be beneficial? *Nutr Rev*. 2009 Sep;67(9):546-50.
11. Ting WJ, Kuo WW, Hsieh DJ, et al. Heat Killed Lactobacillus reuteri GMNL-263 Reduces Fibrosis Effects on the Liver and Heart in High Fat Diet-Hamsters via TGF-β Suppression. *Int J Mol Sci*. 2015 Oct 28;16(10):25881-96.
12. Miyazawa K, Kawase M, Kubota A, et al. Heat-killed Lactobacillus gasseri can enhance immunity in the elderly in a double-blind, placebo-controlled clinical study. *Benef Microbes*. 2015;6(4):441-9.
13. Inoue Y, Kambara T, Murata N, et al. Effects of oral administration of Lactobacillus acidophilus L-92 on the symptoms and serum cytokines of atopic dermatitis in Japanese adults: a double-blind, randomized, clinical trial. *Int Arch Allergy Immunol*. 2014;165(4):247-54.
14. Thakur BK, Saha P, Banik G, et al. Live and heat-killed probiotic Lactobacillus casei Lbs2 protects from experimental colitis through Toll-like receptor 2-dependent induction of T-regulatory response. *Int Immunopharmacol*. 2016 Jul;36:39-50.
15. Adams CA. The probiotic paradox: live and dead cells are biological response modifiers. *Nutr Res Rev*. 2010 Jun;23(1):37-46.
16. Derrien M, van Hylckama Vlieg JE. Fate, activity, and impact of ingested bacteria within the human gut microbiota. *Trends Microbiol*. 2015 Jun;23(6):354-66.
17. Plaza-Díaz J, Fernández-Caballero JÁ, Chueca N, et al. Pyrosequencing analysis reveals changes in intestinal microbiota of healthy adults who received a daily dose of immunomodulatory probiotic strains. *Nutrients*. 2015 May 26;7(6):3999-4015.
18. El Aidy S, van den Bogert B, Kleerebezem M. The small intestine microbiota, nutritional modulation and relevance for health. *Curr Opin Biotechnol*. 2015 Apr;32:14-20.
19. Wang M, Ahrné S, Jeppsson B, Molin G, et al. Comparison of bacterial diversity along the human intestinal tract by direct cloning and sequencing of 16S rRNA genes. *FEMS Microbiol Ecol*. 2005 Oct 1;54(2):219-31.
20. Quartieri A, Simone M, Gozzoli C, et al. Comparison of culture-dependent and independent approaches to characterize fecal bifidobacteria and lactobacilli. *Anaerobe*. 2016 Apr;38:130-7.
21. Zhang C, Derrien M, Levenez F, et al. Ecological robustness of the gut microbiota in response to ingestion of transient food-borne microbes. *ISME J*. 2016 Mar 8. doi: 10.1038/ismej.2016.13.
22. Youngster I, Russell GH, Pindar C, et al. Oral, capsulized, frozen fecal microbiota transplantation for relapsing Clostridium difficile infection. *JAMA*. 2014 Nov 5;312(17):1772-8.
23. Hütt P, Kõll P, Stsepetova J, Alvarez B, et al. Safety and persistence of orally administered human Lactobacillus sp. strains in healthy adults. *Benef Microbes*. 2011 Mar;2(1):79-90.
24. Johansson ML, Molin G, Jeppsson B, et al. Administration of different Lactobacillus strains in fermented oatmeal soup: in vivo colonization of human intestinal mucosa and effect on the indigenous flora. *Appl Environ Microbiol*. 1993 Jan;59(1):15-20.
25. van Bokhorst-van de Veen H, et al. Congruent strain specific intestinal persistence of Lactobacillus plantarum in an intestine-mimicking in vitro system and in human volunteers. *PLoS One*. 2012;7(9):e44588.
26. Ghelardi E, Celandroni F, Salvetti S, et al. Survival and persistence of Bacillus clausii in the human gastrointestinal tract following oral administration as spore-based probiotic formulation. *J Appl Microbiol*. 2015 Aug;119(2):552-9.
27. Kelesidis T, Pothoulakis C. Efficacy and safety of the probiotic Saccharomyces boulardii for the prevention and therapy of gastrointestinal disorders. *Therap Adv Gastroenterol*. 2012 Mar;5(2):111-25.
28. Waller PA, Gopal PK, Leyer GJ, et al. Dose-response effect of Bifidobacterium lactis HN019 on whole gut transit time and functional gastrointestinal symptoms in adults. *Scand J Gastroenterol*. 2011 Sep;46(9):1057-64.
29. Larsen CN, Nielsen S, Kaestel P, et al. Dose-response study of probiotic bacteria Bifidobacterium animalis subsp lactis BB-12 and Lactobacillus paracasei subsp paracasei CRL-341 in healthy young adults. *Eur J Clin Nutr*. 2006 Nov;60(11):1284-93.
30. Evrard B, Coudeyras S, Dosgilbert A, et al. Dose-dependent immunomodulation of human dendritic cells by the probiotic Lactobacillus rhamnosus Lcr35. *PLoS One*. 2011;6(4):e18735.
31. Mañé J, Pedrosa E, Lorén V, et al. A mixture of Lactobacillus plantarum CECT 7315 and CECT 7316 enhances systemic immunity in elderly subjects. A dose-response, double-blind, placebo-controlled, randomized pilot trial. *Nutr Hosp*. 2011 Jan-Feb;26(1):228-35.
32. Tompkins TA, Mainville I, Arcand Y. The impact of meals on a probiotic during transit through a model of the human upper gastrointestinal tract. *Benef Microbes*. 2011 Dec 1;2(4):295-303.
33. Fredua-Agyeman M, Gaisford S. Comparative survival of commercial probiotic formulations: tests in biorelevant gastric fluids and real-time measurements using microcalorimetry. *Benef Microbes*. 2015 Mar;6(1):141-51.
34. Blanquet-Diot S, Denis S, Chalancon S, et al. Use of artificial digestive systems to investigate the biopharmaceutical factors influencing the survival of probiotic yeast during gastrointestinal transit in humans. *Pharm Res*. 2012 Jun;29(6):1444-53.
35. Wang J, Zhong Z, Zhang W, et al. Comparative analysis of the gene expression profile of probiotic Lactobacillus casei Zhang with and without fermented milk as a vehicle during transit in a simulated gastrointestinal tract. *Res Microbiol*. 2012 Jun;163(5):357-65.
36. Lo Curto A, Pitino I, Mandalari G, et al. Survival of probiotic lactobacilli in the upper gastrointestinal tract using an in vitro gastric model of digestion. *Food Microbiol*. 2011 Oct;28(7):1359-66.
37. Fedorak RN, Madsen KL. Probiotics and the management of inflammatory bowel disease. *Inflamm Bowel Dis*. May 2004;10(3):286-299.
38. Griffiths JK, Daly JS, Dodge RA. Two cases of endocarditis due to Lactobacillus species: antimicrobial susceptibility, review, and discussion of therapy. *Clin Infect Dis*. Aug 1992;15(2):250-255.
39. Antony SJ, Stratton CW, Dummer JS. Lactobacillus bacteremia: description of the clinical course in adult patients without endocarditis. *Clin Infect Dis*. Oct 1996;23(4):773-778.
40. Chomarat M, Espinouse D. Lactobacillus rhamnosus septicemia in patients with prolonged aplasia receiving ceftazidime-vancomycin. *Eur J Clin Microbiol Infect Dis*. Jan 1991;10(1):44.
41. Haghighat L, Crum-Cianflone NF. The potential risks of probiotics among HIV-infected persons: Bacteraemia due to Lactobacillus acidophilus and review of the literature. *Int J STD AIDS*. 2015 Jun 30. pii: 0956462415590725.
42. Patel R, Cockerill FR, Porayko MK, Osmon DR, Ilstrup DM, Keating MR. Lactobacillemia in liver transplant patients. *Clin Infect Dis*. Feb 1994;18(2):207-212.
43. Didari T, Solki S, Mozaffari S, Nikfar S, Abdollahi M. A systematic review of the safety of probiotics. *Expert Opin Drug Saf*. 2014 Feb;13(2):227-39.
44. Kowlgi NG, Chhabra L. D-lactic acidosis: an underrecognized complication of short bowel syndrome. *Gastroenterol Res Pract*. 2015;2015:476215.

45.   Lord RS, Bralley JA. Clinical applications of urinary organic acids. Part 2. Dysbiosis markers. *Altern Med Rev*. 2008 Dec;13(4):292-306.

46.   Hove H, Mortensen PB. Colonic lactate metabolism and D-lactic acidosis. *Dig Dis Sci*. 1995 Feb;40(2):320-30.

47.   Lu J, Zello GA, Randell E, et al. Closing the anion gap: contribution of D-lactate to diabetic ketoacidosis. *Clin Chim Acta*. 2011 Jan 30;412(3-4):286-91.

48.   Talasniemi JP, Pennanen S, Savolainen H, et al. Analytical investigation: assay of D-lactate in diabetic plasma and urine. *Clin Biochem*. 2008 Sep;41(13):1099-103.

49.   Munakata S, Arakawa C, Kohira R, et al. A case of D-lactic acid encephalopathy associated with use of probiotics. *Brain Dev*. 2010 Sep;32(8):691-4.

50.   Deepika Priyadarshani, W. M. and Rakshit, S. K. Screening selected strains of probiotic lactic acid bacteria for their ability to produce biogenic amines (histamine and tyramine). *International Journal of Food Science & Technology* 2011; 46: 2062–2069.

51.   Gao C, Major A, Rendon D, et al. Histamine H2 Receptor-Mediated Suppression of Intestinal Inflammation by Probiotic Lactobacillus reuteri. *MBio*. 2015 Dec 15;6(6):e01358-15.

52.   Leuschner RG, Heidel M, Hammes WP. Histamine and tyramine degradation by food fermenting microorganisms. *Int J Food Microbiol*. 1998 Jan 6;39(1-2):1-10.

Supporting the Barrier Function of the Gut

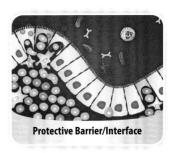

Protective Barrier/Interface

It is often difficult to conceive of the gut lumen as being "outside" the body, but there is an intricate set of barriers designed to ensure it remains so. Therefore, the barrier/permeability functions of the gut represent one of the most important interfaces between a person and the external environment. However, we should not imagine this barrier function as simply a means to keep things out, but as a sophisticated system to communicate with, and allow selective entry of, certain contents from the gut lumen into the body. This requires a tightly controlled, but thin barrier of tissues and secretions *intentionally designed for close proximity to the gut lumen*. This proximity permits the absorption of available nutrients and physiological interaction with trillions of non-human microbes and their metabolites and signals, but also creates a vulnerability to those same microbes, toxins and immunologically reactive components from the gut lumen. In this section, we will briefly overview the main features of the gut barrier, the functions and dysfunction of intestinal permeability, and how breaches in barrier function contributes to various GI dysfunctions and diagnostic phenomena. We will also review ways in which the barrier function of the gut can be measured and supported in patients with these conditions.

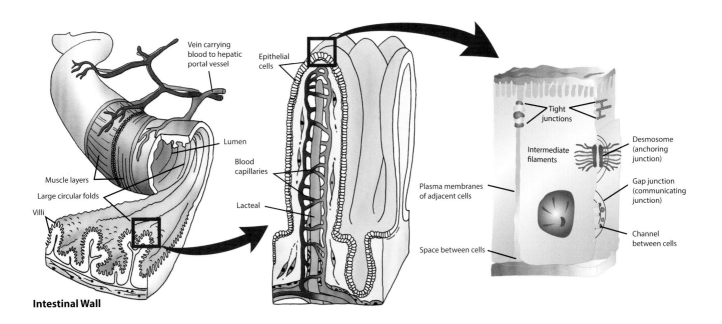

Intestinal Wall

Figure 29: Expanding Surface Area of the GI tract. The intestinal wall uses large folded surfaces containing many individual villi (center). These villi are lined with a single layer of epithelial cells with access to both the blood supply (capillaries) and the lymphatic system (lacteal). Each epithelial cell is joined to the adjacent cell by the formation of tight junctions, preventing particles from the gut lumen from passing between the epithelial cells.

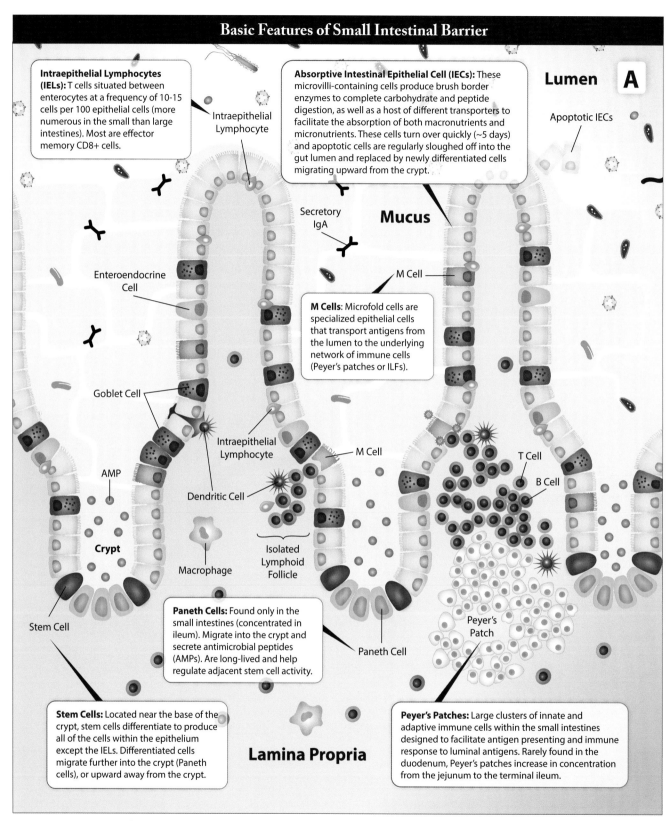

Figure 30: Basic Features of Small (A) and Large (B) Intestinal Barrier. Shown here are the basic cells and architecture of the gut barrier in both small and large intestines. Note that the large intestines lacks villi (and microvilli), but contains an additional thick layer of mucus. The associated circulatory and lymphatic systems are not shown. See text for more details.

Basic Features of Large Intestinal Barrier

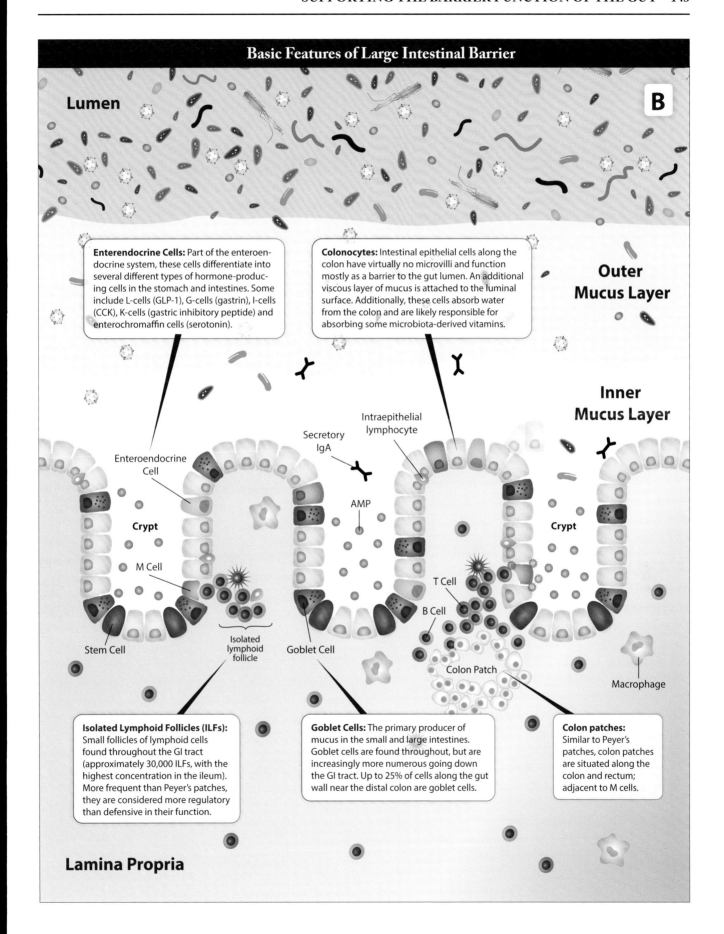

Lumen

B

Enterendocrine Cells: Part of the enteroendocrine system, these cells differentiate into several different types of hormone-producing cells in the stomach and intestines. Some include L-cells (GLP-1), G-cells (gastrin), I-cells (CCK), K-cells (gastric inhibitory peptide) and enterochromaffin cells (serotonin).

Colonocytes: Intestinal epithelial cells along the colon have virtually no microvilli and function mostly as a barrier to the gut lumen. An additional viscous layer of mucus is attached to the luminal surface. Additionally, these cells absorb water from the colon and are likely responsible for absorbing some microbiota-derived vitamins.

Outer Mucus Layer

Inner Mucus Layer

Intraepithelial lymphocyte

Secretory IgA

Enteroendocrine Cell

AMP

Crypt

Crypt

M Cell

T Cell

B Cell

Stem Cell

Isolated lymphoid follicle

Goblet Cell

Colon Patch

Macrophage

Isolated Lymphoid Follicles (ILFs): Small follicles of lymphoid cells found throughout the GI tract (approximately 30,000 ILFs, with the highest concentration in the ileum). More frequent than Peyer's patches, they are considered more regulatory than defensive in their function.

Goblet Cells: The primary producer of mucus in the small and large intestines. Goblet cells are found throughout, but are increasingly more numerous going down the GI tract. Up to 25% of cells along the gut wall near the distal colon are goblet cells.

Colon patches: Similar to Peyer's patches, colon patches are situated along the colon and rectum; adjacent to M cells.

Lamina Propria

The Anatomy of the Gut Barrier(s)

Similar to other barriers that interface with the external environment, the GI mucosal barrier is made of several physical and chemical barriers heavily penetrated with immune system surveillance and function.[1] The basic feature of this barrier depends on a single layer of columnar cells that create the foundational interface between the gut lumen and the underlying lamina propria, capillaries, lymphatic system (lacteals) and smooth muscle tissues (see Figure 29). Each of these columnar epithelial cells (described below) differentiates from stem cells located at the edge of the crypt, migrating to create a three-dimensional structure that increases the surface area of the lumen interface. The intestinal epithelium is renewed about every five days due to rapid differentiation and apoptosis of these cells. Figure 30 shows the basic architectural differences between the small intestines (containing both crypts and villi), which are designed to maximize the absorptive and enzymatic capacity of microvilli-containing enterocytes; and the colon (containing only crypts), which is designed to maximize microbial fermentation and limit lumen/colonocyte contact.

There are four basic types of epithelial cells formed from the stem cells located near the crypts: absorptive enterocytes (or colonocytes), goblet cells, enteroendocrine cells, and Paneth cells. These cells produce and secrete many different protective compounds (mucus, antimicrobial peptides, etc.) that, along with compounds formed elsewhere (pancreatic enzymes, stomach acid, bile, sIgA etc.), make up the chemical components of the gut barrier function. The paracellular space between these columnar cells is sealed by tight junctions, though adherence junctions and desmosomes are also important in the communication and special arrangement between these cells. As we shall see, the proteins that regulate tight junctions are very important to the integrity of the intestinal barrier, and when not functioning correctly, create vulnerability for increased permeability to harmful agents from the lumen. The final basic layer of the intestinal barrier includes the cells, signals and secretions of the immune system that are in close proximity to the entire gastrointestinal tract, usually referred to as the gastrointestinal-associated lymphoid tissue (GALT–see page 151).

As we have discussed in the previous section, there are many micro-environments within the lumen of the gastrointestinal tract; both longitudinally from stomach to rectum, but also along the architecture of both the small and large intestines (see Figures 18 and 19 on pages 93 and 19). These different micro-environments are mostly created by the differences in the types and amounts of barrier functions that exist along the gut, the types of cells found along different portions of the gut, and the secretions and metabolic capacities of these cells. Figure 30 describes the variety of cell types that make up the columnar cell lining of the gastrointestinal tract, their main functions and where they are concentrated. Note the vast differences in the concentration of both specific epithelial and immune cells along the whole GI tract. The different concentrations of these cells and the architecture and secretions they form, greatly influences the localization of GI function (e.g., digestion in the proximal small intestines vs. fermentation in the colon).

Mucus: A Critical Front-line Barrier

One of the most basic, and overlooked, features of the mucosal barrier in the gut is also one of its first lines of defense: the layer(s) of mucus secreted from and coating the cells lining the gastrointestinal tract.[2,3,4] Gastrointestinal mucus proteins are mostly produced by mucus neck cells in the stomach gastric glands and goblet cells within the small and large intestines, though some mucus proteins can also be secreted by enterocytes/colonocytes. Mucus is a highly viscous polymeric structure that is formed when large, highly glycosylated protein structures (mucins) are secreted into the gastrointestinal tract and become hydrated (mucus is ~98% water). This layer of mucus (200-300 μm thick) is also saturated with secreted proteins (sIgA, antimicrobial proteins) and chemicals (bicarbonate) that further protect the epithelial cells from specific harmful contents of the lumen.

There are two different layers or types of mucus: a highly dense matrix of mucus that is partially tethered to the epithelial cells and is difficult to aspirate, and a loose layer of mucus that is not tethered to the epithelium and is easily aspirated (see Figure 19 on page 98 and Figure 30 on page 142). The loose mucus layer is more easily penetrated by components of the lumen (bacteria, toxins, nutrients etc.) and is slowly eroded by the passage of the lumen contents. The dense layer is very compact and difficult to penetrate, forming a nearly sterile environment next to the epithelium. Both layers of mucus are formed within the stomach and large intestinal mucosa, while only the loose mucus layer is present in the small intestines. Interestingly, the thickness of this loose layer is extremely thin or absent where immune system Peyer's patches interface with M cells for immune surveillance of the gut lumen contents.

In order to form these different types of mucus, there are two basic types of mucin proteins: secretory mucin (mostly composed of MUC2, but include MUC5 and MUC6) and transmembrane mucins (e.g., MUC1, MUC3, MUC4, MUC13, MUC17). The transmembrane mucins are secreted by goblet cells or other epithelial cells and are embedded into the apical membrane to form a network into which secretory mucins also incorporate. The density of this mucus network is dependent on the types, glycosylation and amounts of the various transmembrane mucins secreted. Research investigating the role of mucins has shown genetic polymorphisms within mucin genes are associated with increased risk of gut-related outcomes such as IBD, colorectal and gastric cancers and susceptibility for certain gastrointestinal infection such as *H.pylori.*, further demonstrating the importance of the specific matrix created by these different mucins.[5,6,7] In addition, chemical, enzymatic or microbial disturbance of the mucus layers from the lumen, or cell signals that cause changes in mucin gene expression, can create a vulnerability that leads to barrier disruption. We will discuss some of these factors as they pertain to barrier function outcomes in this chapter, while also covering some specifics in other chapters as well.

Tight Junctions: Managing Paracellular Permeability

The paracellular space between each gastrointestinal epithelial cell is connected to the adjacent cells with three different transmembrane protein complexes: desmosomes, adherent junctions and tight junctions. Of the three, the tight junction is tasked with regulating paracellular transport of small ions while acting as a barrier to larger macromolecules. Tight junctions should not be viewed as static barriers between epithelial cells, but as a dynamic complex of proteins forming a fence to large particles and a network of pores (gates) for small ions (~3.5 kDa and smaller) and water. As Figure 31 shows, tight junctions form several tightly sealed layers around the entire cell between the apical and basolateral sides (tight junctions form mostly near the apical side).

Tight junctions (TJs) are composed of several different transmembrane proteins consisting mostly of occludin, claudins (at least 24 different kinds), and junctional adhesion molecule (JAM) proteins.[8] The extracellular portions of these proteins interact with similar proteins expressed on adjacent cells to form the interlocking junction (see Figures 31 and 32). The intracellular portions of these transmembrane proteins are tethered to intracellular actin/myosin filaments by linker or scaffolding proteins, most commonly zonula occludens (ZO) proteins. The TJ can be modulated by the expression pattern of the various proteins involved (some claudins form pores while others form tight barriers), as well as the phosphorylation pattern of these

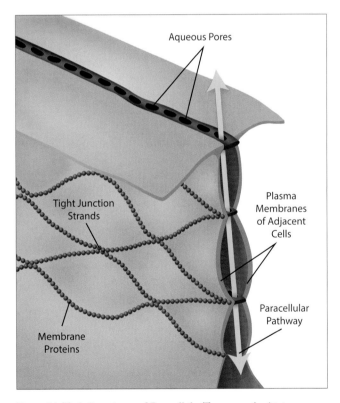

Figure 31: Tight Junctions and Paracellular Transport: As this image shows, tight junctions form a zipper-like network of proteins that link adjacent enterocytes at their apical ends (other types of junctions not shown here). The amounts and types of each protein that forms the tight junction allows for the formation of tiny pores to allow very small molecules to pass through the paracellular space.

proteins or of the myosin light chain.[9,10] For instance, myosin light chain phosphorylation triggers the contraction of the myosin light chain which, in turn, results in the opening of the paracellular pores in the TJ.[11] We will discuss other beneficial and detrimental alterations to TJ modulation below.

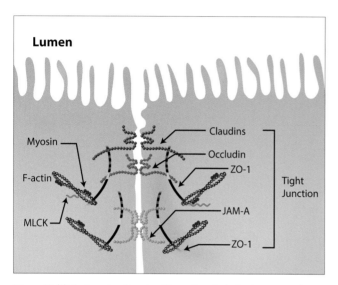

Figure 32: Tight Junction Proteins. Shown here is the basic transmembrane and intracellular proteins that form a tight junction unit. See text for more details. ZO-1:zonula occludins 1, JAM-A: junctional adhesion molecule-A, MLCK: myosin light-chain kinase.

Disrupting Barrier Function by Tight Junction Modulation

Since there are many ways to assemble/disassemble and modulate the integrity of the TJ complexes, there are also many ways to alter gut permeability through TJ modulation. It is well known that many pathogenic organisms trigger a variety of phosphorylation events that lead to alterations in TJ assembly that result in increased intestinal permeability.[12] These pathogenic or pathobiont organisms disrupt the barrier function of the TJ through signals initiated by directly binding to the gastrointestinal cell or by secreting toxins. Some of the organisms known to trigger TJ disruption include *Vibrio cholera*, Enteropathogenic *E. coli*, Enterohemorrhagic *E. coli*, *Clostridium spp.*, *H. pylori*, HepC, HIV and several other viruses (mostly disturbing TJ in non-GI barriers).[13,14,15,16,17]

While these microbial signals from the lumen are one pathophysiological factor that can affect the integrity of the tight junction assembly and lead to intestinal hyperpermeability (i.e., leaky gut), signals from within the enterocyte or from adjacent immune system cells can also lead to similar changes. In particular, inflammatory mediators and other cytokines can trigger the same sorts of phosphorylation of TJ proteins or myosin light chain that leads to increases in TJ pore size or partial disassembly.[18] In fact, phosphorylation-mediated mechanisms have been discovered for quite a range of cytokines, several which are known to be elevated in subjects with intestinal permeability-related inflammatory bowel disorders. They include interferon-γ (IFN-γ), tumor necrosis factor-α (TNF-α), IL-1β, IL-4, IL-6, and IL-13. However, other cytokines have been shown in cell-culture studies to decrease TJ permeability by increasing the expression of TJ proteins or by inhibiting the effects of other cytokine signals. Some of these cytokines include IL-10, IL-17, transforming growth factor-β (TGF-β) and epidermal growth factor (EGF).

Zonulin and Barrier Disruption

The discovery of the protein zonulin, and its relationship to the modulation of intestinal permeability, has been of great interest over the past decade. Alessio Fasano and his team, when looking for a human analog to the zonula occludens toxin (Zot) produced by *V. cholera*, discovered a ~45 kDa protein produced in the human gut that could mimic the Zot-induced TJ modulations and subsequent increase in intestinal permeability.[19] This protein, which they called zonulin, was later discovered to be the unprocessed precursor of the hemoglobin-binding protein haptoglobin-2 (pre-HP2). Zonulin/pre-HP2 is now thought to play an important role in mediating the increased intestinal permeability and immunological reactivity of celiac disease and other autoimmune conditions.[20,21,22]

Zonulin is released from cells of the gastrointestinal epithelium and lamina propria in response to a trigger encountered from the gastrointestinal lumen. The two best-described triggers are luminal bacteria and gliadin. Once zonulin is secreted into the gut lumen, it binds to receptors on the epithelial cells that triggers a cascade of secondary signals, leading to the phosphorylation of TJ proteins or the myosin light chain, and resulting in the destabilization of the TJ and increased intestinal permeability. Why such a signaling mechanism exists for self-induced TJ destabilization is not yet known, though some speculate the capacity to increase the paracellular space may be an adaptive mechanism to allow the immune system greater access to the gut lumen for temporary host benefits.

Gliadin, the protein found in wheat gluten and the related prolamins found in barley (hordein) and rye (secalin) is known to trigger the release of zonulin from the gastrointestinal mucosal tissues, a process mediated by its binding to the CXCR3 receptor. Fasano et al. have shown that subjects with active celiac disease express higher levels of gut epithelial CXCR3 receptor mRNA and zonulin than non-celiac subjects or celiac subjects on a strict gluten-free diet.[23] The role of gliadin consumption and zonulin-induced intestinal permeability is being explored in more subjects, though more research is needed to clearly define the role of gliadin consumption in non-celiac subjects who have gluten-sensitivity and those who do not.

Testing for Celiac Disease and Gluten Sensitivity

While little controversy exists regarding the need for gluten avoidance in subjects with celiac disease, there is an ongoing debate about the extent to which gluten ingestion is a trigger in subjects without celiac disease and its role in altering intestinal permeability in healthy subjects. We will not attempt to settle this debate here, though we will make some basic observations to help clinicians navigate these issues as they attempt to discern the role gluten ingestion/elimination plays in their therapeutic strategy.

As most are already aware, celiac disease is a potent immunological reaction to the peptide gliadin found in the gluten of wheat and related grains. Celiac disease appears to have a strong genetic link and is triggered by events that induce intestinal permeability mediated through the protein zonulin. The intense inflammatory response following gluten ingestion in subjects with celiac disease results in small intestinal villous atrophy that can be confirmed through biopsy, the gold standard for diagnosis. While support strategies designed to improve nutrient intake (digestive enzymes, multivitamin/minerals) or to reduce inflammation and heal the gut lining are often helpful, the life-long elimination of gluten from the diet must be the foundational therapeutic strategy.

For decades, anecdotal evidence has repeatedly shown GI symptom improvements in many non-celiac patients upon commencing a gluten-free diet.[1] These anecdotes were often not taken seriously by conventional gastroenterologists, but research has now confirmed that, indeed, biomarkers suggestive of an immune reaction to gluten can occur in non-celiac patients. This phenomenon is generally referred to as non-celiac gluten-sensitivity and differs from an allergic reaction to wheat proteins (induced by IgE antibodies).[2,3,4,5] Regardless of the names given to various non-celiac gluten reactions, it is critical for clinicians to rule out the role of gluten in subjects with symptoms suggestive of functional gastrointestinal disorders (e.g., IBS) and to determine the need for the patient to avoid gluten in the diet.[6]

While the diagnosis of celiac disease using laboratory testing of genetics, serum biomarkers and biopsy is now fairly straightforward, positive diagnostic criteria for non-celiac gluten sensitivity is a bit more challenging. First, it usually requires excluding both celiac disease and wheat allergy (skin prick test). In these assays, labs can evaluate several biomarkers such as total IgA antibody (non-specific), IgG and/or IgA anti-gliadin antibodies, anti-transglutaminase (tTG) antibodies and anti-endomysial (EMA) antibodies (from serum sample). Using this information as well as the presence/absence of specific genetic markers (HLA DQ2 or DQ8 genes), a diagnosis of celiac disease can be confirmed or ruled out. A variety of diagnostic algorithms have been proposed to help identify patients with non-celiac immunological reactions to gluten/gliadin based on the presence or absence of various serological markers.

Testing for Celiac Disease and Gluten Sensitivity (Continued)

Figure A shows a basic algorithm using both negative and positive serological markers for non-celiac gluten sensitivity, though we should note only about 50% of subjects with increased symptoms after consuming a blinded sample of gluten have been shown to have elevated anti-gliadin antibodies.[7,8] Please note, this test does not detect wheat, rye or barley allergies (IgE-mediated). Some laboratories test saliva or stool samples for anti-gliadin antibody levels. While these tests may be suggestive of an immunological response to gluten exposure, they should not be used to diagnose celiac disease or gluten sensitivity; the criterion for this requires the use of serum antibodies.

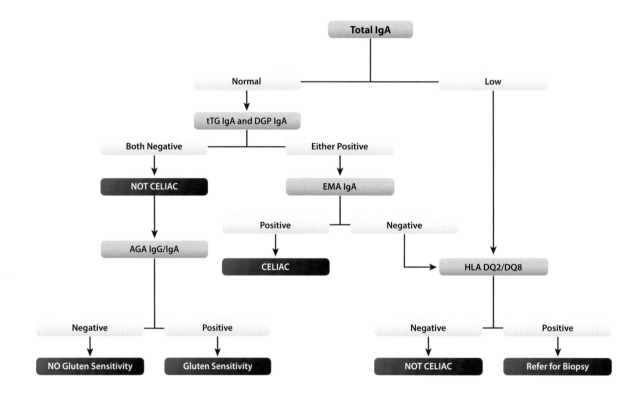

Figure A: A Typical Diagnostic Algorithm Used for Celiac/Gluten Sensitivity. Due to the prevalence of IgA deficiency in patients with celiac disease, the first step is an assessment of total IgA levels. If the IgA levels are within the age-adjusted reference range, the most appropriate second level of testing, given their sensitivity and specificity, are threshold detection of IgA antibodies against tissue transglutaminase (tTG) and deamidated gliadin peptides (DGP). If a patient is negative for both antibodies, the patient almost certainly does not have celiac disease, but the presence of anti-gliadin antibodies (AGA—either IgG or IgA) suggests an ongoing immunological reaction to gliadin/gluten and suggests the patient has "gluten sensitivity"- a condition that may require some level of gluten-restriction from the diet (elimination/re-challenge will determine the level of restriction needed). If a patient is positive for tTG or DGP antibodies, the additional presence of anti-endomysial antibodies (EMA) is almost certain to be diagnostic for celiac disease. Many clinicians may still want to confirm the diagnosis by positive genetic confirmation (HLA DQ2/DQ8) and/or biopsy, but the presence of EMA IgA with one of the other antibodies has a positive predictive value >98%. If EMA IgA is negative, the patient should be tested for the presence of the HLA DQ2/DQ8 genes; presence of either allele is diagnostic for celiac disease, absence rules out celiac disease (test with AGA antibodies to suggest gluten sensitivity). Individuals with low IgA will need genetic testing to determine celiac status (Modified from Genova Diagnostics).

References

1.   Biesiekierski JR, Newnham ED, Irving PM, et al. Gluten causes gastrointestinal symptoms in subjects without celiac disease: a double-blind randomized placebo-controlled trial. *Am J Gastroenterol.* 2011 Mar;106(3):508-14
2.   Elli L, Roncoroni L, Bardella MT. Non-celiac gluten sensitivity: Time for sifting the grain. *World J Gastroenterol.* 2015 Jul 21;21(27):8221-6.
3.   Lebwohl B, Ludvigsson JF, Green PH. Celiac disease and non-celiac gluten sensitivity. *BMJ.* 2015 Oct 5;351:h4347.
4.   Ludvigsson JF, Leffler DA, Bai JC et al. The Oslo definitions for coeliac disease and related terms. *Gut* 2013;62:43–52.
5.   Sapone A, Bai JC, Ciacci C et al. Spectrum of gluten-related disorders: consensus on new nomenclature and classification. *BMC Med* 2012;10:13.
6.   Makharia A, Catassi C, Makharia GK. The Overlap between Irritable Bowel Syndrome and Non-Celiac Gluten Sensitivity: A Clinical Dilemma. *Nutrients.* 2015 Dec 10;7(12):10417-26.
7.   Volta U, Tovoli F, Cicola R, et al. Serological tests in gluten sensitivity (nonceliac gluten intolerance). *J Clin Gastroenterol.* 2012 Sep;46(8):680-5.
8.   Infantino M, Manfredi M, Meacci F, et al. Diagnostic accuracy of anti-gliadin antibodies in Non Celiac Gluten Sensitivity (NCGS) patients: A dual statistical approach. *Clin Chim Acta.* 2015 Dec 7;451(Pt B):135-41

Measuring Intestinal Permeability

Before we discuss many of the lifestyle factors that can increase or decrease intestinal permeability, it is important to overview how intestinal permeability is measured in the research and clinical studies reporting these findings. Since there is no way to directly measure the gut permeability of an individual's entire GI tract, a variety of *ex vivo* procedures and surrogate markers have been used to find relative differences in gut permeability.[24] In some cases, more than one measurement, along with other biomarkers indicative of changes in intestinal permeability (cytokines, zonulin, etc.), may be used to strengthen the connection between the signal being measured (e.g., gliadin, stress, probiotics, etc.) and its effect on intestinal permeability.

Ex vivo tissue measurements

Much of what is known about intestinal permeability, TJs and the passage of various substances across the gut epithelium (e.g., drugs) has been done using either biopsied gut tissue or the formation of a layer of cultured cells (e.g., Caco2 cells) upon an artificial membrane. When these cells are polarized to orient the apical from the basolateral side, they form a monolayer similar to that formed in the gut. The Ussing chamber, originally invented in 1946 by the Danish physiologist Hans Henriksen Ussing, is designed to allow researchers to form such a monolayer of gut epithelium, allowing them to measure the flow of ions and other substances from one chamber to the other through the monolayer of cells.[25]

Today, researchers use modified cell culture plates to form two chambers with a monolayer of cells resting on the membrane between the two chambers. One of the most basic measures of an intact barrier using these two-chambered systems is a test of the trans-epithelial electrical resistance (TEER). A stable resistance to electrical resistance shows the proper formation and orientation of the monolayer and a limited flow of ions between the cells. A reduction in the TEER occurs when the paracellular space allows larger ions to flow from one chamber to the other, and this reduction is considered an objective measure of intestinal permeability. These systems can also be used to measure the flow of any substance from one chamber to the other; whether the substance moves through cellular pores, passive diffusion, receptor-mediated transport or paracellular passage.

In general, there are two ways that these two-membrane chambers are used in the study of intestinal permeability (using TEER or other measures of cell permeability). The first is simply to use biopsied tissue from various subjects (animals or humans) and compare the permeability of that tissue with tissue obtained from other (i.e., control) subjects. For example, Fasano et al. have demonstrated that tissue biopsied from celiac patients consuming gluten has a much lower average TEER (higher permeability) than tissue from celiac patients on a gluten-free diet.[26] Obviously, these sorts of measurements are invasive and many healthy subjects are reluctant to volunteer their tissue for such research. Also, since this tissue is removed from its biological context, other factors that are likely to affect permeability coming from immune cells, the enteric nervous system or the gut lumen; or subtle differences from the actual location of the biopsy could not by easily evaluated in such an experiment. Nonetheless, this is a helpful way to measure the relative differences in gut permeability between subjects based on their own tissue.

The second way in which such two-chambered systems are helpful is in the use of a standard cell line monolayer (e.g., Caco-2), which can be tested for changes in permeability when various agents or cells are added to one side of the monolayer. This is a common test for evaluating the possible gut permeability effects of certain food components such as macronutrients, micronutrients, phytonutrients or allergens. In addition, such studies are used to investigate potential mechanisms related to changes in gut permeability by measuring changes in mRNA expression, protein levels, enzyme activities or metabolites in the cells or media after adding the substance of interest. One such study showed that when zinc, quercetin, butyrate, indole or berberine were added to Caco-2 cell monolayers in such a system, each was able to improve gut permeability in a dose-dependent manner by measuring the TEER.[27] In addition, they were able to show specific changes in TJ protein expression (measuring protein and mRNA levels) as part of the mechanism accounting for these changes. The use of both *ex vivo* measures of biopsied tissue and the *in vitro* measure of standardized cell monolayers are still being used to understand the mechanisms and actions of a variety of signals that have the potential to alter gut permeability, many of which we will discuss in this and other chapters.

Lactulose/Mannitol and Related *In Vivo* Tests

If the two-chambered system is the gold standard for measuring the permeability of a monolayer of epithelial cells, then the lactulose/mannitol test is the gold standard functional test for estimating small intestinal permeability in human subjects. The use of two different sized sugar molecules that are not readily metabolized in the gut or serum, and are excreted in the urine in a manner that reflects their absorption from the gut, allows for a fairly reliable measure of gut permeability. The smaller mannitol molecule is thought to freely cross the gut barrier through the epithelial cells and is considered a general measure of small intestinal surface area; while the larger lactulose molecule is thought only to cross through the paracellular route if the pores are enlarged or cells are damaged in some way. Hence, the lactulose/mannitol ratio gives a rough estimate of small intestinal hyper-permeability (i.e., leaky gut), and is commonly elevated in subjects with IBS, IBD and celiac disease.[28,29,30,31,32]

For the most part, the lactulose/mannitol test is a fairly straight-forward and reliable test to help clinicians gauge the relative intestinal permeability of an individual. However, like all laboratory tests, there is the potential for sampling errors or misinterpretation of the result because of specific patient characteristics.[33] For instance, since mannitol absorption is related to the available surface area of the gut, intestinal inflammation that reduces its surface area (villous atrophy) can significantly alter the lactulose/mannitol ratio (by reducing the denominator) even when there is little increase in the lactulose absorption. Therefore, it is important to consider both the absolute levels of the absorption of each sugar in addition to the ratio of both. Also, since bowel transit time and colonic fermentation of lactulose by commensal microbiota can influence the timing (and amount) of the absorption of these sugars, urine sampling must be timed correctly for best interpretation of these biomarkers. Clinicians need to emphasize the importance of following the laboratory instructions on overnight fasting and abstaining from the consumption of foods and other substances during the testing period that would interfere with the test results.

Similar tests using different molecules (rhamnose, PEG of different size, etc.) or radiolabeled molecules have been used in clinical research to measure relative intestinal permeability with similar results as the lactulose/mannitol test described above.[34,35,36,37] Many of these tests are being refined to decrease the contamination of the sample with sugars consumed in the diet that were not part of the test solution. Clinicians should stay current with the available laboratory tests for measuring *in vivo* intestinal permeability, recognizing some laboratories may offer different tests as research confirms their clinical utility.

Other Measures of Intestinal Permeability

A number of other tests and assays have been considered as being indicative of intestinal permeability, though many are indirect measures requiring some interpretation. Measures of increased bacteria-related metabolites in the blood/urine (e.g., endotoxin, D-lactate) or an increase level of bacteria within the inner (dense) layer of mucus within biopsied tissue can be an indication of diminished intestinal barrier function. Biomarkers of intestinal cell integrity or gastrointestinal immune cell activation may also be indicative of intestinal barrier disruption. For instance, reduced plasma levels of citrulline, which is produced by small intestinal cells from glutamine, or increased levels of enterocyte fatty acid binding proteins are sensitive measure of gut permeability or enterocyte cell damage, as are measures of fecal calprotectin, a reliable measure of gut immune inflammation.[38,39,40] Some of these are currently being used in critical care settings, and/or to confirm associations with other diagnostic schemes (e.g., IBD).

Immune Surveillance and the Gut Barrier Function

Our previous book, *Supporting Immune Function: A Lifestyle and Nutrient Approach* (Point Institute, 2014), lists ten basic principles for building overall immune health. Not surprisingly, the first two of these principles are directly related to the core functions of the GI tract described in this book. Namely, maintaining and protecting barrier function and creating a commensal friendly environment.

Since the GI tract is designed to break down and absorb large amounts of nutrients in a relatively short time, architectural features in the form of folds and fingers, called villi, greatly expand the surface area of the GI tract, especially the small intestines where most nutrient absorption occurs. However, this expansive surface area, about the size of a tennis court, is only one cell-layer thin, and therefore represents a highly vulnerable interface with the antigen-rich environment of the gut lumen. This vulnerability requires a highly coordinated cooperation between the GI epithelial cells and the adjacent cells of the immune system. In fact, as is often pointed out, 70 to 80% of immune cells reside in the GI tract.[1] (see also Figure 30 for description of immune system features along the GI tract).

The innate and adaptive immune systems are critical components of the barrier function of the gut. Approximately 100 to 150 mesenteric lymph nodes are distributed throughout the gut to create numerous "stations" for concentrated interactions between antigens, antigen-presenting cells, regulatory cells and effector cells. This specialized feature of the immune system is often referred to as the gut-associated lymphoid tissue (GALT), a subcategory of the mucosa-associated lymphoid tissues (MALT) found throughout other mucosal barriers: eyes, mouth, lungs, breast, vagina, skin, etc. Another special feature of the GALT is the 100 to 200 Peyer's patches found primarily along the mucosa of the ileum.[2] These Peyer's patches include a large concentration of B cells surrounded by T cells and antigen-presenting cells—mostly dendritic cells—that interface directly with the gut lumen through the activities of special gut epithelial cells called M cells (microfold cells).[3] These M cells are designed to allow the controlled passage of antigens

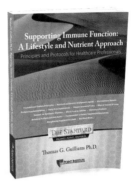

Supporting Immune Function: A Lifestyle and Nutrient Approach
A Guide for Healthcare Professionals
Thomas G. Guilliams Ph.D.

Ten Basic Principles For Building Overall Immune Health:

- Maintaining and Protecting Barrier Functions
- Creating a Commensal-Friendly Environment
- Maintaining Appropriate Hygiene Practices
- Avoiding Antigens and Allergens in Adulthood
- Building Micronutrient and Antioxidant Reserve
- Maintaining and Building Cellular (Mitochondrial) Energy
- Maintaining Adequate Detoxification Capacity
- Diminishing Stress and Cortisol-Induced Immune Suppression
- Reducing Chronic Inflammatory Triggers/Mediators
- Using Immune-Modulating Agents to Create Balance and Strengthen Immune Function

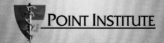

(commensal bacteria, pathogenic bacteria, viruses, fungi, food particles, etc.) from the gut lumen, where they can be delivered safely to antigen-presenting cells in the lamina propria that, in turn, present them to both mature and naïve T cells.[4]

A larger number of smaller aggregates of lymphoid cells similar to Peyer's patches, called isolated lymphoid follicles (ILFs), are dispersed throughout the GI tract. In fact, some 30,000 ILFs line the lamina propria of the human GI tract, reaching their highest concentration in the ileum, where there is approximately one ILF for every 28 villi.[5] Also, specialized memory T-lymphocytes, called intraepithelial lymphocytes (IELs), are located in the space between mucosal epithelial cells at a rate of approximately 10-15 IELs for every 100 epithelial cells. IELs are critical components in the first-line adaptive immune response (as dendritic cells are for the innate immune response), and directly communicate to adjacent epithelial cells to modulate barrier function.[6,7,8]

One of the unique features of the adaptive immune response within the GALT, as in most other mucosal tissues, is the abundance of antibody-secreting B cells, called plasma cells, which produce antibodies of the secretory IgA class (sIgA). This form of antibody is capable of passing into the lumen of the gut, as it does in breast milk, saliva, tears, etc., to interact with antigens while they are still "outside" the body. Antigens sampled via the M cells are presented to T helper cells and B cells and, when an appropriate cross-reactivity is triggered, B cells are activated to secrete the corresponding sIgA. Research now shows sIgA expression against both pathogenic and commensal organisms is a key regulatory aspect of the intestinal barrier itself.[9,10,11] Also, there is a well-documented relationship between increased HPA-axis stress and reduced sIgA levels.[12] Laboratory measurements of sIgA levels are often used as one of many markers of mucosal immune health and/or HPA axis stress-induced immune suppression, and specific sIgA levels measured in a stool or saliva sample can indicate a particular antigenic challenge.[13]

In addition to the M cell-mediated antigen sampling, specialized dendritic cells are capable of changing their morphology to permit direct surveillance of the gut lumen by an extension protruding between the gut epithelial cells. This allows the dendritic cell to use its many pattern-recognition receptors to begin reacting to changes within the "pattern" of pathogens in the gut before specific antigens are presented to the adaptive immune cells. This process of immune surveillance is considered to be an important part of the "education" and maturation of the immune system, and also provides an early warning of a potential pathogenic agent in the gut, allowing for a preemptive response.[14] The ultimate goal is to mount appropriate and timely immune responses to harmful and foreign antigens, while creating an active tolerance against harmless or self-antigens.

Intestinal Permeability: Testing Immune Resilience and Control

Breaches in the gut barrier as a result of hyper-permeability of the paracellular tight junctions or damage to the epithelium are one of the most potent challenges to the immune system. These breaches permit unprocessed antigens, or even intact organisms from the gut lumen, entry to the lamina propria without being processed through the specialized GI epithelial M cells. These unprocessed antigens are capable of triggering a vigorous acute immune response and, furthermore, increasing the susceptibility to autoimmune cross-reactivity. In fact, one of the leading theories for the genesis of autoimmune diseases is the immune exposure to unprocessed non-self-antigens that have breached the intestinal barrier (e.g., gliadin and zonulin; see main text).[15]

Once the mucosal immune system of the gut is triggered to respond to a potential threat (regardless of the source), the inflammatory process will be engaged and may persist well after the original trigger is neutralized.[16] Prolonged or inappropriate inflammatory responses by the immune system can, in turn, lead to signals that promote further intestinal permeability- leading to a chronic cycle of inflammatory bouts. This cycle is thought to be at the heart of inflammatory bowel diseases.[17] Therefore, it is imperative to consider all intestinal barrier issues as having an immune/

inflammatory component; which means therapies designed to improve intestinal barrier function should also include immune-supporting and anti-inflammatory components. For a complete review of immune system modulation and natural ingredients that can be used as anti-inflammatory agents, see our comprehensive discussion of these topics in our book, *Supporting Immune Function: A Lifestyle and Nutrient Approach* (Point Institute, 2014). For specific agents that have been used for IBD, see pages 174-184.

References

1.   Mason KL, Huffnagle GB, Noverr MC, Kao JY. Overview of gut immunology. *Adv Exp Med Biol.* 2008;635:1-14.
2.   Mowat AM, Agace WW. Regional specialization within the intestinal immune system. *Nat Rev Immunol.* 2014 Oct;14(10):667-85.
3.   Reboldi A, Cyster JG. Peyer's patches: organizing B-cell responses at the intestinal frontier. *Immunol Rev.* 2016 May;271(1):230-45.
4.   Mabbott NA, Donaldson DS, Ohno H, Williams IR, Mahajan A. Microfold (M) cells: important immunosurveillance posts in the intestinal epithelium. *Mucosal Immunol.* 2013 Jul;6(4):666-77.
5.   Moghaddami M, Cummins A, Mayrhofer G. Lymphocyte-filled villi: comparison with other lymphoid aggregations in the mucosa of the human small intestine. *Gastroenterology.* 1998 Dec;115(6):1414-25.
6.   Vitale S, Picascia S, Gianfrani C. The cross-talk between enterocytes and intraepithelial lymphocytes. *Mol Cell Pediatr.* 2016 Dec;3(1):20.
7.   Qiu Y, Yang Y, Yang H. The unique surface molecules on intestinal intraepithelial lymphocytes: from tethering to recognizing. *Dig Dis Sci.* 2014 Mar;59(3):520-9.
8.   Qiu Y, Yang H. Effects of intraepithelial lymphocyte-derived cytokines on intestinal mucosal barrier function. *J Interferon Cytokine Res.* 2013 Oct;33(10):551-62.
9.   Mantis NJ, Rol N, Corthésy B. Secretory IgA's complex roles in immunity and mucosal homeostasis in the gut. *Mucosal Immunol.* 2011 Nov;4(6):603-11.
10. Mathias A, Pais B, Favre L, Benyacoub J, Corthésy B. Role of secretory IgA in the mucosal sensing of commensal bacteria. *Gut Microbes.* 2014;5(6):688-95.
11. Brandtzaeg P. Gate-keeper function of the intestinal epithelium. *Benef Microbes.* 2013 Mar 1;4(1):67-82.
12. Campos-Rodríguez R, Godínez-Victoria M et al. Stress modulates intestinal secretory immunoglobulin A. *Front Integr Neurosci.* 2013 Dec 2;7:86.
13. Cole MF. Detection and quantitation of antifungal sIgA antibodies in body fluids. *Methods Mol Biol.* 2009;499:9-16.
14. Bekiaris V, Persson EK, Agace WW. Intestinal dendritic cells in the regulation of mucosal immunity. *Immunol Rev.* 2014 Jul;260(1):86-101.
15. Fasano A. Leaky gut and autoimmune diseases. *Clin Rev Allergy Immunol.* 2012 Feb;42(1):71-8.
16. Sánchez de Medina F, Romero-Calvo I, et al. Intestinal inflammation and mucosal barrier function. *Inflamm Bowel Dis.* 2014 Dec;20(12):2394-404.
17. Lee SH. Intestinal permeability regulation by tight junction: implication on inflammatory bowel diseases. *Intest Res.* 2015 Jan;13(1):11-8.

Improving Intestinal Permeability

Maintaining or improving the integrity of the gut barrier is foundational for preserving our overall health. Breaches in this barrier function will lead to gastrointestinal symptoms, but will further burden the immune system with a heavy antigenic/allergenic load and increase the number of toxins requiring detoxification and elimination. Here we list a number of lifestyle signals, mostly nutrients or food-containing compounds, known to affect one or more measures of intestinal permeability. We will focus mostly on those that have been tested in human clinical trials, or that have been used traditionally with known mechanisms that suggest how they might function. For the most part, they fall into five different categories:

·   Remove signals that damage gastrointestinal cells or promote intestinal permeability. This can be anything that increases gut inflammation such as allergens, inflammatory or immunogenic foods, stress signals, pathogens and their toxins, NSAIDS, etc.

·   Increase the intake of anti-inflammatory signals in the diet. These are mostly contained in plants, as many phytonutrients are reported to reduce inflammatory burden. Some of these agents also act as genomic signaling agents to improve enterocyte integrity/tight junction assembly.

·   Provide nutrients that specifically help the gastrointestinal cells build metabolic reserve. This helps maintain their capacity to rapidly divide and continue to form and secrete the necessary components to create and maintain barrier function. This might mean providing precursors for mucus production or fuel for enterocytes (directly) and colonocytes (indirectly, by feeding commensal organisms).

·   Provide receptor-mediated or genomic signals that stimulate the cells along the gastrointestinal tract is another way to improve barrier function. These might be signals that improve tight junction formation, changes in phosphorylation pathways of tight junction proteins, alterations in mucin production or changes in immune function signaling from the lumen.

·   Build immune system and detoxification metabolic reserve. Since these are the systems vulnerable to intestinal barrier failure, they should always be supported when intestinal permeability is compromised. Please see our Standard Road map, *Supporting Immune Function: A Lifestyle and Nutrient Approach* (Point Institute, 2014) for more details for immune system support.

Dietary Factors

Dietary components (foods, beverages, dietary supplements, etc.) are known to impact intestinal permeability in both positive and negative ways; and through direct (cell signaling) and indirect (microbiome alteration) mechanisms.[41,42] Much of what we know comes either from animal studies or Ussing chamber-like assays of cell culture monolayers; though some of these components have been used in clinical trials that measure intestinal permeability.

Western Diet, Obesity and Type 2 Diabetes

The Western or American diet is often used as a model for chronic disease and is mimicked in animal studies using various high fat and high simple sugar diets. When these sorts of diets are used in rodents (typically used as a model for inducing obesity, diabetes and related disorders), they have been shown to increase measures of intestinal permeability and gut dysbiosis. In one mouse model, chronic consumption of 30% fructose solution for eight weeks led to decreased levels of duodenal tight junction proteins occludin and ZO-1, leading to an increase in bacterial endotoxinemia.[43]

While these types of feeding studies have not been directly performed in humans, increases in the measures of intestinal permeability have been reported in obese subjects and those with type 2 diabetes and fatty liver disease.[44,45,46] This is not at all surprising since these metabolic disorders are noted to be associated with significant alterations in the gut microbiota, increased inflammatory signaling and, often, reduced nutrient absorption. In fact, several studies have shown obese subjects and newly diagnosed type 2 diabetic patients have higher concentrations of zonulin, often directly connected to the composition of their gut microbiota.[47,48,49,50]

Specifics are currently lacking on exactly which features of the Western dietary pattern are most influential in reducing gut barrier function,

and intervention study outcomes using intestinal permeability as an end-point are still lacking. Nonetheless, there are numerous reasons to make the recommendation to reduce processed foods typical of the Western dietary pattern and, instead, recommend a healthy dietary pattern (e.g., Mediterranean diet). See also our recommendations concerning diet and microbiome on pages 104 and specifics listed below.

Macronutrients

There is very limited evidence to conclude whether specific macronutrients directly affect intestinal permeability in human subjects, though many have been tested for such effects in the laboratory. **Long-chain omega-3 fatty acids** such as eicosapentaenoic acid (EPA) and docosahexaenoic acid (DHA) have been shown to improve some measures of gastrointestinal barrier function when tested in animal studies, and have been shown to limit the inflammatory-mediated effects on tight junction proteins in Caco-2 cell culture assays.[51,52] **Short-chain fatty acids (SCFAs)** from certain fermented foods, or more often from the colonic fermentation of fermentable fibers, have been shown to improve barrier function. SCFAs, such as acetate (acetic acid), propionate (propionic acid) and butyrate (butyric acid) are important for normal intestinal cell function, including cell division and barrier function.[53] Recall that most of the cells in the intestine turn over in approximately five days, a feat that requires an abundance of cellular energy. Butyrate, in particular, has been shown to improve measures of intestinal barrier function *in vitro*, and is likely an important mediator in the benefits derived from the consumption of prebiotics (and some probiotics).[54] In one study, healthy subjects were fed inulin-enriched pasta (or un-enriched pasta) for five weeks (n=20, crossover design) and tested for changes in their intestinal permeability.[55] Compared to the control pasta, the inulin-enriched pasta resulted in a significantly lower lactulose/mannitol ratio, a measure of overall paracellular hyper-permeability, as well as decreased levels of serum zonulin, a measure of intestinal tight junction disassembly. These limited data suggest the ingestion of **prebiotic/fermentable fibers** may improve intestinal barrier function through the increased fermentation of SCFA, though not all subjects with gastrointestinal dysfunction benefit equally from including such fibers in their diets (see FODMAPs dietary restrictions on page 236). Supplemental butyrate salts (e.g., sodium, calcium, magnesium) are also available and may provide some benefit for colon health if they are enteric-coated or microencapsulated for delivery to the colon, though limited data is currently available for specific changes in the measures of intestinal permeability.[56,57]

Micronutrients

Inadequate intake of any essential vitamin or mineral is likely to have some detrimental effect on gut barrier function. Therefore, clinicians should always assess the need for multivitamin/mineral supplementation in patients with suspected intestinal permeability issues. However, a few micronutrients have been investigated as potential therapeutic agents to help improve intestinal barrier function, especially the water-soluble vitamins A and D.

Vitamin A (retinol) is an important regulator of immune function, and deficiencies are a major worldwide epidemiological burden. Children with vitamin A deficiency develop a number of gastrointestinal infections and have increased measures of intestinal permeability, both of which can be improved through vitamin A supplementation.[58,59] While gross deficiencies of retinol or beta carotene are not routinely seen in Western countries, the percentage of Americans consuming less than the estimated average requirement (EAR) of vitamin A in their diet is quite high (>70%), a level that is reduced when fortification and supplementation is added (still >30%).[60]

The role of vitamin D in gut barrier function was discovered in animal and cell culture studies. Animals lacking the vitamin D receptor (VDR knockout mice) show intestinal barrier defects and cell culture studies show a direct enhancement of TJ and adherens junction proteins after vitamin D treatment.[61] Additional studies have shown inhibition of myosin light chain phosphorylation (cell culture) and improved intestinal barrier function (animal model) after the "supplementation" of vitamin D.[62,63] A recent study comparing biopsied tissue from patients with ulcerative colitis (both inflamed and non-inflamed portions of the colon of each subject), showed that the addition of vitamin D to the incubation medium altered the TJ protein expression to a favorable (less permeable) status, while also reducing inflammatory mediators.[64] While the role of vitamin D supplementation for intestinal permeability outcomes has not been rigorously studied in human subjects, we highly recommend clinicians test the vitamin D3 status of all patients with suspected intestinal hyper-permeability and recommend adequate supplementation when their status is insufficient. For a discussion of vitamin D supplementation for IBD, see page 176. (For our view of vitamin D testing, adequate serum levels and supplementation, see our Standard Road map, *Supplementing Dietary Nutrients: A Guide for Healthcare Professionals* [Point Institute 2014]).

Deficiencies of both iron and zinc are known to increase gastrointestinal infections and intestinal permeability, as measured by lactulose absorption in undernourished children; supplementation is known to improve these outcomes.[58,65,66] While zinc supplementation is commonly recommended to improve immune system resilience, its role in barrier function is not always an outcome measured in clinical studies of presumably well-nourished subjects.[67] It should be noted, however, that subjects with known intestinal hyperpermeability such as those with celiac disease or inflammatory bowel disease, are vulnerable to low zinc status.[68] Research has shown that supplementation of zinc improves both zinc status and intestinal permeability in such patients.[69] In one study that induced intestinal permeability with heavy exercise in healthy subjects, 14 days of zinc carnosine (37.5 mg providing 8 mg of zinc) was able to statistically improve intestinal barrier function using lactulose/mannitol absorption ratios (as well as a number of *in vitro*/cell culture measures of intestinal barrier integrity (TEER, TJ proteins, etc.)).[70] Generally, we recommend long-term zinc supplementation should not exceed 40 mg per day, in the context of a multivitamin/mineral supplement or as part of a product designed to improve gut integrity. Iron supplementation should only be recommended for subjects specifically identified with iron deficiency.

Glutamine and Other Amino Acids

The nutrient most commonly recommended for improving intestinal barrier function is glutamine (GLN), a non-essential amino acid that is a primary energy source for intestinal epithelial cells and integral to a host of cellular functions involved in maintaining the intestinal barrier function. Mechanisms linking glutamine with intestinal barrier functions include:[71]

· GLN is needed for the development of the gut epithelium during early life and supplementation is used to help neonates improve gut barrier function.[72]

- GLN is a critical substrate for a wide-range of metabolites within enterocytes including ATP, glutathione and DNA/RNA.[73,74]

- GLN is an important secondary signaling molecule within enterocytes, affecting critical metabolic and proliferative pathways in the cell.[75,76,77]

- GLN has been shown to modulate TJ proteins, phosphorylation and assembly, using both GLN deprivation and supplementation studies.[78,79,80]

- GLN contributes to favorable alterations in the gut microbiota.[81]

- GLN maintains intestinal structure and function during aging.[82]

- GLN promotes sIgA secretion via direct (immunomodulatory) and indirect (microbiota) signals.[83]

- GLN modulates the gastrointestinal permeability effects of HPA axis stress (i.e., CRF).[84]

- GLN modulates the gastrointestinal permeability effects of intensive exercise.[85,86]

Ironically, while the research into the mechanisms for how glutamine helps to maintain intestinal barrier function is vast (using cell culture and animal models, mostly swine), the number of published clinical trials in human subjects with intestinal hyper-permeability has only recently begun to grow. Even so, most of these studies have been performed in undernourished children or in subjects who are critically ill with acute or traumatic alterations in intestinal permeability.[87,88,89] For instance, glutamine supplementation alone or in combination with zinc and vitamin A, improved measures of intestinal permeability in "shanty town" children in Brazil, known to have intestinal hyper-permeability.[90] However, several recent studies may be useful to help inform the clinician in the use of glutamine in patients with intestinal hyper-permeability related to more common GI dysfunctions.

Thirty patients with Crohn's disease (in remission) with elevated lactulose/mannitol ratio were randomly assigned glutamine supplementation or a whey-protein supplement and tested two months later for changes in intestinal permeability.[91] The dose of glutamine (or whey protein) was 0.5g/kg of their ideal body weight per day, a substantial dose (40 grams for 80 kilo/176 lbs.) compared to previous studies. After two months, the lactulose/mannitol ratio was substantially improved in both groups, as was the villous to crypt ratio (from examining biopsy tissue, a measure that was also improved in an aged animal study using glutamine).[92] While a Cochrane review of this and a second study using glutamine in subjects with Crohn's disease suggests that these data are too limited to make specific recommendations for the use of glutamine for the treatment of Crohn's disease, it does suggest that the use of glutamine is safe and potentially beneficial for IBD-related intestinal permeability dysfunction.[93] Ironically, the availability of glutamine to the cells in the colon from oral intake may be hindered by the rapid absorption of glutamine in the small intestines.

As previously discussed, athletes who train intensively are prone to increased infectious illnesses, increased HPA activation and decreased measures of barrier function. A study was performed in 24 trained athletes, half of which were assigned to placebo and half of which were given 10 g of oral glutamine once daily for six weeks.[94] While they did not measure intestinal permeability in this study, glutamine supplementation was able to significantly improve measures of training-induced immune cell numbers and function, as compared to placebo.

One of the limitations of this, and many other studies evaluating glutamine, is the fact that most of these studies are evaluations as monotherapies, testing the role of glutamine alone. In many cases, subjects with and without acute inflammation are grouped together, as are subjects with varying degrees of glutamine dietary intake—making it difficult to assess the independent role of glutamine in these subjects (some studies suggest that inflammation is a necessary mediator for the role of GLN in altering measures of intestinal permeability).[95] So, while we believe more research is needed to make specific recommendations about the benefits of glutamine in subjects with measurable (or suspected) intestinal hyper-permeability, when combined with the basic science linking glutamine with intestinal barrier biology, we still strongly recommend the use of oral glutamine in such subjects. A dose of 4 to 8 g is commonly recommended, though more may be needed in some patients. Since these doses are difficult to consume as capsules or tablets, glutamine products are often available in flavored powders that can be mixed with water (often with other ingredients intended for gut health), or as part of a comprehensive protein-based product intended to help support gut and anti-inflammatory therapies.

Other amino acids and peptides have been tested for their ability to modify measures of intestinal barrier function in cell culture or animal studies. **Tryptophan** supplementation has been shown, in some models, to improve intestinal barrier function, though other studies (in piglets) suggest it may have a negative impact.[96,97] Interestingly, **5-HTP**, a tryptophan metabolite and precursor to serotonin, may improve barrier function in healthy subjects, but may actually increase intestinal permeability in subjects with IBS. In one study performed in 15 IBS subjects (Rome III criteria) and 15 healthy controls, subjects were given a single dose of 100 mg of 5-HTP or placebo (crossover design, seven-day washout) and then tested for changes in absorption of lactulose and mannitol (blood measures) and changes in TJ proteins.[98] They found that after consuming the 5-HTP, both healthy and IBS subjects were able to form secondary metabolites (5-HIAA and serotonin), but while they reported a decrease in lactulose absorption and improve TJ assembly in the healthy subjects, they saw an increase in lactulose absorption and no improvement in TJ assembly in the IBS subjects. They believe these data suggests that IBS subjects may have impairment in the serotonergic-mediated pathways affecting epithelial function.[99] While this study is small and based on a single dose of 5-HTP, clinicians should at least be cautious when using 5-HTP in subjects with IBS; at the same time, the use of 5-HTP may benefit non-IBS subjects with impaired intestinal permeability.

Phytonutrients

Within plant-based foods, spices, herbs and medicinal plants are thousands of different compounds generally called phytonutrients or phytochemicals. These compounds can have a number of physiological activities when they interact with the cells of the host or their microbiome. These activities are mediated through direct chemistry (e.g., antioxidant), receptor-mediated signaling, enzyme/protein modulation and, perhaps most importantly, genomic signaling (i.e., regulation of gene activity). Modern research techniques are making it easier to evaluate a wide variety of plant compounds for their ability to affect various measures of intestinal permeability. While the number of phytonutrient compounds with promising data continues to grow, there are a few with a more substantial base of evidence.

Flavonoids

Some 4,000 different flavonoid compounds (i.e., bioflavonoids) have been identified within the complex phytochemistry of the plant kingdom. Many of these have been extensively studied for their ability to affect a number of biological processes in humans and animals, including gastrointestinal-related pathophysiology (some have even been the basis for synthetic drug derivatives). While a complete review of these compounds is well beyond the scope of this Road map, several flavonoid compounds have been specifically tested for their ability to modulate intestinal permeability and/or regulate intestinal TJ integrity.[100]

One of the most researched flavonoids is the aglycone flavanol called quercetin. This yellow flavonoid, along with similar compounds such as myricetin and kaempferol, all appear to promote barrier integrity and stronger TJ assembly in cell culture models.[101,102,103,104] Similar benefits have been reported for other commonly used flavonoids including epigallocatechin gallate (EGCG- from green tea), genistein and daidzein (from soy), hesperetin, and naringenin.[105,106] Unfortunately, *in vivo* research on these ingredients using intestinal permeability (i.e., lactulose/mannitol absorption) is currently lacking.

Since most of these agents have already been shown to possess immune-modulating and/or anti-inflammatory activities, their ability to influence epithelial cell TJ formation adds one more way they can help to improve intestinal barrier function. In particular, the role mast cells play in altering intestinal permeability, motility and inflammation may be reduced when using natural mast cell stabilizers like quercetin.[107,108] We should note it is likely many other flavonoids have some ability to improve intestinal barrier function, even if there is limited available data. The flavonoids mentioned above are easy to obtain and commonly used in the research setting, and therefore should not be considered as the only, or even the most potent, flavonoids for such purposes. While we do recommend the addition of these flavonoids to products designed for improving gut barrier function, we also highly recommend the consumption of a diverse diet that includes abundant fresh fruits and vegetables, herbs and spices (dried spices are suitable in most cases) to maximize the amount and diversity of flavonoids and other phytonutrients.

Other Phytonutrients

As one would expect, any plant compound that has anti-inflammatory, immune-modulating, microbiome-altering effects or affects the signals that influence tight junctions is likely to have an effect on intestinal permeability. Compounds like curcumin (turmeric), boswellic acid (boswellia), caffeic acid phenethyl esters (CAPE- propolis), baicalein (Chinese skullcap), resveratrol (red grapes) and gingeroles (ginger) are some of the many compounds that may help to alter gut inflammation and should be considered when selecting a product that may help a patient improve barrier function. We have reviewed many of these compounds and their mechanisms in our previous Road map: *Supporting Immune Function: A Lifestyle and Nutrient Approach* (Point Institute, 2014).

Berberine, a bitter alkaloid derived from the root of *Coptis chinensis* and related plants, is also used for its antimicrobial activity, including its effect on the gut microbiota.[109] Research now shows berberine can modulate a number of pathways leading to improved tight junction assembly and reduced TEER in cell culture studies, as well as several animal models of intestinal permeability.[110,111,112,113,114] Interestingly, berberine is now mostly touted for its metabolic-enhancing benefits, especially in subjects with type 2 diabetes, now recognized as a condition with increased measures of intestinal permeability.[115,116] While no human clinical trials using berberine have been reported with measures of intestinal permeability as an outcome, the dose used in clinical trials for type 2 diabetes are usually 1 gram/day. A single clinical trial using berberine (HCl- 400 mg/bid) in subjects with IBS-D has been published and shown to be well-tolerated and helpful in reducing symptoms.[117]

Colostrum-Related Compounds

For many years, animal research has demonstrated the role of colostrum intake with improved measured of intestinal barrier function, even suggesting it as a major promoter of early gastrointestinal maturation in the young animals (of the same or different species). Colostrum, or one of several colostrum concentrated components, is also used as a dietary supplement ingredient, mostly for their putative immune-enhancing activities. In fact, several clinical trials have been performed in human subjects to investigate the effects of colostrum on post-exercise changes in immune and intestinal barrier function. These trials have shown that colostrum supplementation may improve intestinal barrier function, though studies with negative results (worsening measures) have also been reported. In one study, twelve exercise-trained volunteers were given colostrum (20 g/day, product was 15 to 20% immunoglobulin) or an iso-macronutrient placebo for 14 days prior to strenuous exercise (crossover design, 14-day washout) and tested for intestinal permeability using lactulose/mannitol absorption at the beginning and end of each 14 day arm.[118] Predictably, intestinal permeability was worse (~2.5x more lactulose absorption) immediately following a 20-minute, 80% VO2max treadmill run, in subjects consuming the placebo, while this alteration was substantially ameliorated in those consuming colostrum (80% less increase in lactulose absorption). This same group reported a similar effect in an additional small group of subjects (n=8) using either colostrum (10 g bid) or zinc carnosine (37.5 mg bid); showing amelioration of the post-exercise induction of intestinal permeability (individually and together).[119]

Others have studied the effects of colostrum on exercise-induced alterations in gut permeability with no, or even negative, results as measured by lactulose/rhamnose absorption assays. This includes a study using 1.7 g/kg/day of bovine colostrum (15% IgG) for seven days[120] and another using 60 grams/day of bovine colostrum (% IgG not stated) for eight weeks in 30 healthy males.[121] These studies used notably higher doses of colostrum than the previous (positive) studies, suggesting that there may be a threshold above 20 g/day that negatively impacts any benefits seen at lower doses. In one study, the increased intestinal permeability induced by the NSAID indomethacin (threefold increase in lactulose absorption over seven days) was eliminated when subjects (n=7) were given bovine colostrum along with the NSAID (equivalent to 125 ml, tid).[122]

Lactoferrin, an iron-binding immune-modulating protein found in colostrum (highest concentration) has been independently tested for its ability to modulate intestinal permeability. In most cell culture and animal models tested, lactoferrin has been able to significantly improve measures of barrier function.[123,124,125] Human clinical studies on the intestinal permeability effects of lactoferrin is limited. One study showed a benefit using oral supplementation with a single bolus of lactoferrin (5 g of human recombinant lactoferrin) or lactoferrin with indomethacin (NSAID known to increase intestinal permeability) followed by a lactulose/mannitol absorption assay.[126] Though it is likely the immunoglobulin portion of colostrum (and perhaps even bovine serum) effects intestinal permeability as well, there are less data looking at this particular mechanism.[127]

Probiotics and Intestinal Permeability

The potential therapeutic benefits of probiotics are quite far reaching and, not surprisingly, have extended to the notion of improving intestinal barrier function. Since commensal organisms are known to modulate TJ formation, alter zonulin levels, and affect gut immune system signaling, probiotic organisms are likely to affect intestinal permeability by similar direct and indirect means.[128,129] In fact, a number of probiotic species have been shown to improve mechanisms related to intestinal barrier function including numerous species from multiple genera (e.g., *Lactobacillus*, *Bifidobacterium*, *Streptococcus* and *Saccharomyces*); along with many reported benefits of multi-strain combinations. While the numbers of cell-culture and animal model studies are many, we will review the most recent human clinical trials using probiotics and measures of intestinal barrier here to show the diversity, complexity and potential interpretive value of these studies.

Several studies have been performed to evaluate the potential intestinal barrier benefits of probiotics in subjects with colorectal cancer (postoperative changes). A meta-analysis of 17 studies (12/17 published in Chinese) concluded that, while probiotics appear to improve nearly all measures of intestinal barrier function, the heterogeneity of the studies (different strains, doses, etc.), makes it difficult to recommend specific probiotics even in these subjects.[130] A recent double-blind placebo-controlled trial evaluated serum zonulin levels and other measures of intestinal epithelial function when a mixed-strain probiotic was given for six days before and 10 days after surgery for colorectal cancer (n=150).[131] The probiotic was delivered in acid-resistant capsules containing 2 g of a mixture of *L. plantarum* ($>10^{11}$ FU/gram), *L. acidophilus* ($>7x10^{10}$ CFU/gram) and *B. longum* ($>5x10^{10}$ CFU/gram). In these subjects, probiotic therapy was able to significantly reduce postoperative bacterial translocation, changes in lactulose absorption and serum zonulin levels compared to placebo. By examining tissue samples from some of these subjects, they determined that probiotic therapy significantly reduced the levels of the enzyme p38-MAPK, an important mediator for changes in intestinal permeability. Another mixed probiotic was tested for changes in zonulin and markers of intestinal inflammation after intense exercise in trained men (n=23).[132] This study used a product that delivered

10 billion CFU of a mixture of *Bifidobacterium bifidum*, *Bifidobacterium lactis*, *Enterococcus faecium*, *Lactobacillus acidophilus*, *Lactobacillus brevis*, and *Lactococcus lactis* for 14 weeks. Measures of zonulin in fecal samples taken after 14 weeks of probiotic supplementation decreased into a normal physiological range and was significantly lower in the probiotic group compared to placebo (20% lower, p = 0.019).

Some of these probiotic species have previously been studied for their effect on intestinal barrier function. *L. plantarum* at a dose of 1 billion CFU was infused over 6 hours into the duodenum of seven healthy subjects prior to collecting tissue biopsies from the infused area (compared to a placebo solution of glucose and saline).[133] Obviously this doesn't mimic how probiotics normally encounter the intestinal mucosa, but the purpose was to look at genomic or other changes in the tissue samples. Indeed, they did find that cells within the tissues infused with this probiotic had more concentrated tight junction proteins within the TJ. The intestinal permeability effects of the yeast probiotic *Saccharomyces boulardii* was tested in subjects with Crohn's disease (n=35) using the lactulose/mannitol assay.[134] Patients were maintained on their standard pharmaceutical regimen and given either 400 million CFU of *S. boulardii* every eight hours (or placebo) and tested after one and three months of therapy. Crohn's patients given the probiotic had significantly reduced lactulose absorption compared to Crohn's subjects given placebo, though they did not reach the levels of normal (non-Crohn's) controls. As these data show, the potential for improved intestinal barrier function with probiotic therapy is in keeping with the known mechanisms of both commensal and probiotic organisms.

Therefore, since there are positive outcomes in a number of different patient-groups with known intestinal permeability issues (IBS, IBD, colorectal cancer, post-exercise, etc.), and the use of probiotic therapy is safe in virtually all patients, we do not hesitate to suggest that clinicians recommend the use of a probiotic in such subjects. Currently, since no particular strain, strain combination or dose has shown systematic superiority to others, we advise that clinicians begin by recommending a multi-strain probiotic containing 10 to 20 billion CFU/day. Higher doses may be needed to affect other outcomes, such as high-dose regimens for IBD. For an in-depth discussion of the use of probiotics, including dose recommendation, see pages 114-140 and additional therapeutic suggestions in each of the condition-specific sections.

Supporting Barrier Function: Summary

- Use lactulose/mannitol absorption test to measure *in vivo* intestinal permeability as a baseline (especially in subjects previously treated, but untested, for intestinal barrier issues).

- Retest using lactulose/mannitol absorption test periodically to make adjustments to therapies.

- Discover and avoid foods known to cause increased intestinal permeability.

  ○ May include: gluten, dairy/lactose, capsicum/spicy foods, FODMAPs, etc.

- Test for (and avoid) food allergens (IgE/Mast cell stimulation).

- Cease NSAID use, if possible.

- Assess HPA axis stressors and treat accordingly. Stress directly influences gut permeability.[135]

  ○ See our previous book, *The Role of Stress and the HPA Axis in Chronic Disease Management* (Point Institute, 2015).

- Avoid strenuous physical activity/exercise or pay special attention to supporting gut and immune health before and after such activities. Moderate exercise is helpful.

- Avoid processed foods with artificial colors and flavors.

- Eat abundant amounts of fresh fruits and vegetables to maximize the amount and diversity of phytonutrients.

- Consider the following nutrients for supplementation:

  ○ Omega-3 fatty acids, ALA, EPA, DHA (through diet and supplementation)

  ○ Glutamine (4 to 8 grams daily)

  ○ Vitamin D (1,000 IU minimum daily; best to test and dose to desired serum levels)

  ○ Probiotics (mixed strain combination 20-40 billion CFU; consider high doses for long-standing intestinal barrier issues or when associated with IBD)

  ○ Prebiotics (precursor for important short-chain fatty acids [may be contraindicated if FODMAPs are to be avoided])

  ○ Zinc (25 mg daily with other minerals)

  ○ Iron (only when iron deficiency is confirmed)

  ○ Flavonoids (for quercetin and related compounds, dose not as important as consistent daily consumption from foods and supplementation)

  ○ Colostrum/Lactoferrin/IgG (consider using combination [usually a concentrated colostrum product contains 15 to 40% IgG and some level of lactoferrin])

  ○ Berberine (consider adding 1 g/day when subject is obese, insulin-resistant or has type 2 diabetes)

- Consider comprehensive gut-healing products.

Several dietary supplement companies in the physician channel have developed comprehensive products designed to help deliver many of these gut-healing and anti-inflammatory ingredients together. These products are usually designed as ready-to-mix powders with a protein base. These products provide a convenient way to consume many of the suggested nutrients above, along with additional natural anti-inflammatory agents. Clinicians may need to add additional ingredients (e.g., glutamine, probiotics) as these may be absent or inadequately dosed for some subjects.

References

1. Mowat AM, Agace WW. Regional specialization within the intestinal immune system. *Nat Rev Immunol.* 2014 Oct;14(10):667-85.
2. Pelaseyed T, Bergström JH, Gustafsson JK, et al. The mucus and mucins of the goblet cells and enterocytes provide the first defense line of the gastrointestinal tract and interact with the immune system. *Immunol Rev.* 2014 Jul;260(1):8-20.
3. Johansson ME, Ambort D, Pelaseyed T, et al. Composition and functional role of the mucus layers in the intestine. *Cell Mol Life Sci.* 2011 Nov;68(22):3635-41.
4. Faderl M, Noti M, Corazza N, Mueller C. Keeping bugs in check: The mucus layer as a critical component in maintaining intestinal homeostasis. *IUBMB Life.* 2015 Apr;67(4):275-85.
5. Sheng YH, Hasnain SZ, Florin TH, McGuckin MA. Mucins in inflammatory bowel diseases and colorectal cancer. *J Gastroenterol Hepatol.* 2012 Jan;27(1):28-38.
6. Wen R, Gao F, Zhou CJ, Jia YB. Polymorphisms in mucin genes in the development of gastric cancer. *World J Gastrointest Oncol.* 2015 Nov 15;7(11):328-37.
7. Kim YS, Ho SB. Intestinal goblet cells and mucins in health and disease: recent insights and progress. *Curr Gastroenterol Rep.* 2010 Oct;12(5):319-30.
8. Suzuki T. Regulation of intestinal epithelial permeability by tight junctions. *Cell Mol Life Sci.* 2013 Feb;70(4):631-59.
9. Capaldo CT, Nusrat A. Claudin switching: Physiological plasticity of the Tight Junction. *Semin Cell Dev Biol.* 2015 Jun;42:22-9.
10. Turner JR, Buschmann MM, Romero-Calvo I, Sailer A, Shen L. The role of molecular remodeling in differential regulation of tight junction permeability. *Semin Cell Dev Biol.* 2014 Dec;36:204-12.
11. Shen L, Black ED, Witkowski ED, et al. Myosin light chain phosphorylation regulates barrier function by remodeling tight junction structure. *J Cell Sci.* 2006 May 15;119(Pt 10):2095-106.
12. Lu RY, Yang WX, Hu YJ. The role of epithelial tight junctions involved in pathogen infections. *Mol Biol Rep.* 2014 Oct;41(10):6591-610.
13. Guttman JA, Finlay BB. Tight junctions as targets of infectious agents. *Biochim Biophys Acta.* 2009 Apr;1788(4):832-41.
14. Zhang Q, Li Q, Wang C, Li N, Li J. Redistribution of tight junction proteins during EPEC infection in vivo. *Inflammation.* 2012 Feb;35(1):23-32.
15. Caron TJ, Scott KE, Fox JG, Hagen SJ. Tight junction disruption: Helicobacter pylori and dysregulation of the gastric mucosal barrier. *World J Gastroenterol.* 2015 Oct 28;21(40):11411-27.
16. Tawar RG, Colpitts CC, Lupberger J, et al. Claudins and pathogenesis of viral infection. *Semin Cell Dev Biol.* 2015 Jun;42:39-46.
17. Assimakopoulos SF, Dimitropoulou D, Marangos M, Gogos CA. Intestinal barrier dysfunction in HIV infection: pathophysiology, clinical implications and potential therapies. *Infection.* 2014 Dec;42(6):951-9.
18. Capaldo CT, Nusrat A. Cytokine regulation of tight junctions. *Biochim Biophys Acta.* 2009 Apr;1788(4):864-71.
19. Lu R, Wang W, Uzzau S, Vigorito R, Zielke HR, Fasano A. Affinity purification and partial characterization of the zonulin/zonula occludens toxin (Zot) receptor from human brain. *J Neurochem.* 2000 Jan;74(1):320-6.
20. Fasano A. Zonulin, regulation of tight junctions, and autoimmune diseases. *Ann N Y Acad Sci.* 2012 Jul;1258:25-33.
21. Fasano A. Leaky gut and autoimmune diseases. *Clin Rev Allergy Immunol.* 2012 Feb;42(1):71-8.
22. Tripathi A, Lammers KM, Goldblum S, et al. Identification of human zonulin, a physiological modulator of tight junctions, as prehaptoglobin-2. *Proc Natl Acad Sci U S A.* 2009 Sep 29;106(39):16799-804.
23. Lammers KM, Lu R, Brownley J, Lu B, et al. Gliadin induces an increase in intestinal permeability and zonulin release by binding to the chemokine receptor CXCR3. *Gastroenterology.* 2008 Jul;135(1):194-204.e3.
24. Galipeau HJ, Verdu EF. The complex task of measuring intestinal permeability in basic and clinical science. *Neurogastroenterol Motil.* 2016 Jul;28(7):957-65.
25. Kirk L. Hamilton. Ussing's "Little Chamber": 60 Years+ Old and Counting. *Front Physiol.* 2011; 2: 6.
26. Hollon J, Puppa EL, Greenwald B, et al. Effect of gliadin on permeability of intestinal biopsy explants from celiac disease patients and patients with non-celiac gluten sensitivity. *Nutrients.* 2015 Feb 27;7(3):1565-76.
27. Valenzano MC, DiGuilio K, Mercado J, et al. Remodeling of Tight Junctions and Enhancement of Barrier Integrity of the CACO-2 Intestinal Epithelial Cell Layer by Micronutrients. *PLoS One.* 2015 Jul 30;10(7):e0133926.
28. Bischoff SC, Barbara G, Buurman W, et al. Intestinal permeability--a new target for disease prevention and therapy. *BMC Gastroenterol.* 2014 Nov 18;14:189.
29. Camilleri M, Madsen K, Spiller R, Greenwood-Van Meerveld B, Verne GN. Intestinal barrier function in health and gastrointestinal disease. *Neurogastroenterol Motil.* 2012 Jun;24(6):503-12.
30. Michielan A, D'Incà R. Intestinal Permeability in Inflammatory Bowel Disease: Pathogenesis, Clinical Evaluation, and Therapy of Leaky Gut. *Mediators Inflamm.* 2015;2015:628157.
31. Shulman RJ, Jarrett ME, Cain KC, Broussard EK, Heitkemper MM. Associations among gut permeability, inflammatory markers, and symptoms in patients with irritable bowel syndrome. *J Gastroenterol.* 2014 Nov;49(11):1467-76.
32. Vilela EG, Torres HO, Ferrari ML, Lima AS, Cunha AS. Gut permeability to lactulose and mannitol differs in treated Crohn's disease and celiac disease patients and healthy subjects. *Braz J Med Biol Res.* 2008 Dec;41(12):1105-9.
33. Sequeira IR, Lentle RG, Kruger MC, Hurst RD. Standardising the lactulose mannitol test of gut permeability to minimise error and promote comparability. *PLoS One.* 2014 Jun 5;9(6):e99256.
34. van Wijck K, Bessems BA, van Eijk HM, et al. Polyethylene glycol versus dual sugar assay for gastrointestinal permeability analysis: is it time to choose? *Clin Exp Gastroenterol.* 2012;5:139-50.
35. Maxton DG, Bjarnason I, Reynolds AP, et al. Lactulose, 51Cr-labelled ethylenediaminetetra-acetate, L-rhamnose and polyethyleneglycol 400 [corrected] as probe markers for assessment in vivo of human intestinal permeability. *Clin Sci (Lond).* 1986 Jul;71(1):71-80.
36. Grover M, Camilleri M, Hines J, et al. (13) C mannitol as a novel biomarker for measurement of intestinal permeability. *Neurogastroenterol Motil.* 2016 Jul;28(7):1114-9.
37. Blomquist L, Bark T, Hedenborg G, Norman A. Evaluation of the lactulose/mannitol and 51Cr-ethylenediaminetetraacetic acid/14C-mannitol methods for intestinal permeability. *Scand J Gastroenterol.* 1997 Aug;32(8):805-12.
38. Piton G, Capellier G. Biomarkers of gut barrier failure in the ICU. *Curr Opin Crit Care.* 2016 Apr;22(2):152-60.
39. van Vliet MJ, Tissing WJ, Rings EH, et al. Citrulline as a marker for chemotherapy induced mucosal barrier injury in pediatric patients. *Pediatr Blood Cancer.* 2009 Dec 15;53(7):1188-94.
40. Papadia C, Sherwood RA, Kalantzis C, et al. Plasma citrulline concentration: a reliable marker of small bowel absorptive capacity independent of intestinal inflammation. *Am J Gastroenterol.* 2007 Jul;102(7):1474-82.
41. Guzman JR, Conlin VS, Jobin C. Diet, microbiome, and the intestinal epithelium: an essential triumvirate? *Biomed Res Int.* 2013;2013:425146.
42. De Santis S, Cavalcanti E, Mastronardi M, Jirillo E, Chieppa M. Nutritional Keys for Intestinal Barrier Modulation. *Front Immunol.* 2015 Dec 7;6:612.
43. Spruss A, Kanuri G, Stahl C, Bischoff SC, Bergheim I. Metformin protects against the development of fructose-induced steatosis in mice: role of the intestinal barrier function. *Lab Invest.* 2012 Jul;92(7):1020-32.
44. Teixeira TF, Collado MC, Ferreira CL, et al. Potential mechanisms for the emerging link between obesity and increased intestinal permeability. *Nutr Res.* 2012 Sep;32(9):637-47.
45. Scarpellini E, Lupo M, Iegri C, et al. Intestinal permeability in non-alcoholic fatty liver disease: the gut-liver axis. *Rev Recent Clin Trials.* 2014;9(3):141-7.
46. Frazier TH, DiBaise JK, McClain CJ. Gut microbiota, intestinal permeability, obesity-induced inflammation, and liver injury. *JPEN J Parenter Enteral Nutr.* 2011 Sep;35(5 Suppl):14S-20S.
47. Zak-Gołąb A, Kocełak P, Aptekorz M, et al. Gut microbiota, microinflammation, metabolic profile, and zonulin concentration in obese and normal weight subjects. *Int J Endocrinol.* 2013;2013:674106.
48. Mokkala K, Röytiö H, Munukka E, et al. Gut Microbiota Richness and Composition and Dietary Intake of Overweight Pregnant Women Are Related to Serum Zonulin Concentration, a Marker for Intestinal Permeability. *J Nutr.* 2016 Jul 27. pii: jn235358. [Epub ahead of print]

49.   Moreno-Navarrete JM, Sabater M, Ortega F, et al. Circulating zonulin, a marker of intestinal permeability, is increased in association with obesity-associated insulin resistance. *PLoS One*. 2012;7(5):e37160.

50.   Zhang D, Zhang L, Zheng Y, et al. Circulating zonulin levels in newly diagnosed Chinese type 2 diabetes patients. *Diabetes Res Clin Pract*. 2014 Nov;106(2):312-8.

51.   Zhao J, Shi P, Sun Y, et al. DHA protects against experimental colitis in IL-10-deficient mice associated with the modulation of intestinal epithelial barrier function. *Br J Nutr*. 2015 Jul;114(2):181-8.

52.   Beguin P, Errachid A, Larondelle Y, Schneider YJ. Effect of polyunsaturated fatty acids on tight junctions in a model of the human intestinal epithelium under normal and inflammatory conditions. *Food Funct*. 2013 Jun;4(6):923-31.

53.   Ríos-Covián D, Ruas-Madiedo P, Margolles A, et al. Intestinal Short Chain Fatty Acids and their Link with Diet and Human Health. *Front Microbiol*. 2016 Feb 17;7:185.

54.   Peng L, He Z, Chen W, Holzman IR, Lin J. Butyrate enhances the intestinal barrier by facilitating tight junction assembly via activation of AMP-activated protein kinase in Caco-2 cell monolayers. *J Nutr*. 2009 Sep;139(9):1619-25.

55.   Russo F, Linsalata M, Clemente C, et al. Inulin-enriched pasta improves intestinal permeability and modifies the circulating levels of zonulin and glucagon-like peptide 2 in healthy young volunteers. *Nutr Res*. 2012 Dec;32(12):940-6.

56.   Di Sabatino A, Morera R, Ciccocioppo R, et al. Oral butyrate for mildly to moderately active Crohn's disease. *Aliment Pharmacol Ther*. 2005 Nov 1;22(9):789-94.

57.   Krokowicz L, Stojcev Z, Kaczmarek BF, et al. Microencapsulated sodium butyrate administered to patients with diverticulosis decreases incidence of diverticulitis--a prospective randomized study. *Int J Colorectal Dis*. 2014 Mar;29(3):387-93.

58.   Chen P, Soares AM, Lima AA, et al. Association of vitamin A and zinc status with altered intestinal permeability: analyses of cohort data from northeastern Brazil. *J Health Popul Nutr*. 2003 Dec;21(4):309-15.

59.   Quadro L, Gamble MV, Vogel S, et al. Retinol and retinol-binding protein: gut integrity and circulating immunoglobulins. *J Infect Dis*. 2000 Sep;182 Suppl 1:S97-S102.

60.   Fulgoni VL 3rd, Keast DR, Bailey RL, Dwyer J. Foods, fortificants, and supplements: Where do Americans get their nutrients? *J Nutr*. 2011 Oct;141(10):1847-54.

61.   Kong J, Zhang Z, Musch MW, et al. Novel role of the vitamin D receptor in maintaining the integrity of the intestinal mucosal barrier. *Am J Physiol Gastrointest Liver Physiol*. 2008 Jan;294(1):G208-16.

62.   Du J, Chen Y, Shi Y, et al. 1,25-Dihydroxyvitamin D Protects Intestinal Epithelial Barrier by Regulating the Myosin Light Chain Kinase Signaling Pathway. *Inflamm Bowel Dis*. 2015 Nov;21(11):2495-506.

63.   Zhao H, Zhang H, Wu H, et al. Protective role of 1,25(OH)2 vitamin D3 in the mucosal injury and epithelial barrier disruption in DSS-induced acute colitis in mice. *BMC Gastroenterol*. 2012 May 30;12:57.

64.   Stio M, Retico L, Annese V, Bonanomi AG. Vitamin D regulates the tight-junction protein expression in active ulcerative colitis. *Scand J Gastroenterol*. 2016 Oct;51(10):1193-9.

65.   Goto K, Chew F, Torún B, Peerson JM, Brown KH. Epidemiology of altered intestinal permeability to lactulose and mannitol in Guatemalan infants. *J Pediatr Gastroenterol Nutr*. 1999 Mar;28(3):282-90.

66.   Roy SK, Behrens RH, Haider R, et al. Impact of zinc supplementation on intestinal permeability in Bangladeshi children with acute diarrhoea and persistent diarrhoea syndrome. *J Pediatr Gastroenterol Nutr*. 1992 Oct;15(3):289-96.

67.   Mocchegiani E, Romeo J, et al. Zinc: dietary intake and impact of supplementation on immune function in elderly. *Age (Dordr)*. 2013 Jun;35(3):839-60.

68.   Wang X, Valenzano MC, Mercado JM, Zurbach EP, Mullin JM. Zinc supplementation modifies tight junctions and alters barrier function of CACO-2 human intestinal epithelial layers. *Dig Dis Sci*. 2013 Jan;58(1):77-87.

69.   Santucci NR, Alkhouri RH, Baker RD, Baker SS. Vitamin and zinc status pretreatment and posttreatment in patients with inflammatory bowel disease. *J Pediatr Gastroenterol Nutr*. 2014 Oct;59(4):455-7.

70.   Davison G, Marchbank T, March DS, et al. Zinc carnosine works with bovine colostrum in truncating heavy exercise-induced increase in gut permeability in healthy volunteers. *Am J Clin Nutr*. 2016 Aug;104(2):526-36.

71.   Wang B, Wu G, Zhou Z, et al. Glutamine and intestinal barrier function. *Amino Acids*. 2015 Oct;47(10):2143-54.

72.   Neu J, DeMarco V, Weiss M. Glutamine supplementation in low-birth-weight infants: mechanisms of action. *JPEN J Parenter Enteral Nutr*. 1999 Sep-Oct;23(5 Suppl):S49-51.

73.   Curi R, Lagranha CJ, Doi SQ, et al. Molecular mechanisms of glutamine action. *J Cell Physiol*. 2005 Aug;204(2):392-401.

74.   Reeds PJ, Burrin DG, Stoll B, et al. Enteral glutamate is the preferential source for mucosal glutathione synthesis in fed piglets. *Am J Physiol*. 1997 Aug;273(2 Pt 1):E408-15.

75.   Marc Rhoads J, Wu G. Glutamine, arginine, and leucine signaling in the intestine. *Amino Acids*. 2009 May;37(1):111-22.

76.   Xi P, Jiang Z, Dai Z, et al. Regulation of protein turnover by L-glutamine in porcine intestinal epithelial cells. *J Nutr Biochem*. 2012 Aug;23(8):1012-7.

77.   Rhoads JM, Argenzio RA, Chen W, et al. L-glutamine stimulates intestinal cell proliferation and activates mitogen-activated protein kinases. *Am J Physiol*. 1997 May;272(5 Pt 1):G943-53.

78.   Li N, Neu J. Glutamine deprivation alters intestinal tight junctions via a PI3-K/Akt mediated pathway in Caco-2 cells. *J Nutr*. 2009 Apr;139(4):710-4.

79.   Wang B, Wu Z, Ji Y, Sun K, Dai Z, Wu G. L-Glutamine Enhances Tight Junction Integrity by Activating CaMK Kinase 2-AMP-Activated Protein Kinase Signaling in Intestinal Porcine Epithelial Cells. *J Nutr*. 2016 Mar;146(3):501-8.

80.   Bertrand J, Ghouzali I, Guérin C, et al. Glutamine Restores Tight Junction Protein Claudin-1 Expression in Colonic Mucosa of Patients With Diarrhea-Predominant Irritable Bowel Syndrome. *JPEN J Parenter Enteral Nutr*. 2015 May 13. pii: 0148607115587330.

81.   de Souza AZ, Zambom AZ, Abboud KY, et al. Oral supplementation with L-glutamine alters gut microbiota of obese and overweight adults: A pilot study. *Nutrition*. 2015 Jun;31(6):884-9.

82.   Beaufrère AM, Neveux N, Patureau Mirand P, et al. Long-term intermittent glutamine supplementation repairs intestinal damage (structure and functional mass) with advanced age: assessment with plasma citrulline in a rodent model. *J Nutr Health Aging*. 2014 Nov;18(9):814-9.

83.   Wu M, Xiao H, Liu G, Chen S, et al. Glutamine promotes intestinal SIgA secretion through intestinal microbiota and IL-13. *Mol Nutr Food Res*. 2016 Jul;60(7):1637-48.

84.   Wang H, Zhang C, Wu G, et al. Glutamine enhances tight junction protein expression and modulates corticotropin-releasing factor signaling in the jejunum of weanling piglets. *J Nutr*. 2015 Jan;145(1):25-31.

85.   Zuhl MN, Lanphere KR, Kravitz L, et al. Effects of oral glutamine supplementation on exercise-induced gastrointestinal permeability and tight junction protein expression. *J Appl Physiol* (1985). 2014 Jan 15;116(2):183-91.

86.   Zuhl M, Dokladny K, Mermier C, et al. The effects of acute oral glutamine supplementation on exercise-induced gastrointestinal permeability and heat shock protein expression in peripheral blood mononuclear cells. *Cell Stress Chaperones*. 2015 Jan;20(1):85-93.

87.   Tian X, Song GM. Enteral glutamine supplementation in critically ill patients. *Crit Care*. 2015 Nov 24;19:405.

88.   Lima AA, Anstead GM, Zhang Q, et al. Effects of glutamine alone or in combination with zinc and vitamin A on growth, intestinal barrier function, stress and satiety-related hormones in Brazilian shantytown children. *Clinics (Sao Paulo)*. 2014;69(4):225-33.

89.   Mottaghi A, Yeganeh MZ, et al. Efficacy of glutamine-enriched enteral feeding formulae in critically ill patients: a systematic review and meta-analysis of randomized controlled trials. *Asia Pac J Clin Nutr*. 2016;25(3):504-12.

90.   Lima AA, Anstead GM, Zhang Q, et al. Effects of glutamine alone or in combination with zinc and vitamin A on growth, intestinal barrier function, stress and satiety-related hormones in Brazilian shantytown children. *Clinics (Sao Paulo)*. 2014;69(4):225-33.

91.   Benjamin J, Makharia G, Ahuja V, et al. Glutamine and whey protein improve intestinal permeability and morphology in patients with Crohn's disease: a randomized controlled trial. *Dig Dis Sci*. 2012 Apr;57(4):1000-12.

92.   Beaufrère AM, Neveux N, Patureau Mirand P, et al. Long-term intermittent glutamine supplementation repairs intestinal damage (structure and functional mass) with advanced age: assessment with plasma citrulline in a rodent model. *J Nutr Health Aging*. 2014 Nov;18(9):814-9.

93.   Akobeng AK, Elawad M, Gordon M. Glutamine for induction of remission in Crohn's disease. *Cochrane Database Syst Rev*. 2016 Feb 8;2:CD007348.

94.   Song QH, Xu RM, Zhang QH. et al. Glutamine supplementation and immune function during heavy load training. *Int J Clin Pharmacol Ther*. 2015 May;53(5):372-6.

95.   Hulsewé KW, van der Hulst RW, et al. Inflammation rather than nutritional depletion determines glutamine concentrations and intestinal permeability. *Clin Nutr*. 2004 Oct;23(5):1209-16.

96.   Kim CJ, Kovacs-Nolan JA, Yang C, Archbold T, Fan MZ, and Mine Y. l-Tryptophan exhibits therapeutic function in a porcine model of dextran sodium sulfate (DSS)-induced colitis. *J Nutr Biochem* 2009; 21:468-475

97.   Tossou MC, Liu H, Bai M, Chen S, et al. Effect of High Dietary Tryptophan on Intestinal Morphology and Tight Junction Protein of Weaned Pig. *Biomed Res Int.* 2016;2016:2912418.

98.   Keszthelyi D, Troost FJ, Jonkers DM, et al. Serotonergic reinforcement of intestinal barrier function is impaired in irritable bowel syndrome. *Aliment Pharmacol Ther.* 2014 Aug;40(4):392-402.

99.   Pai VP, Horseman ND. Multiple cellular responses to serotonin contribute to epithelial homeostasis. *PLoS ONE* 2011; 6: e17028.

100. Suzuki T, Hara H. Role of flavonoids in intestinal tight junction regulation. *J Nutr Biochem.* 2011 May;22(5):401-8.

101. Chuenkitiyanon S, Pengsuparp T, Jianmongkol S. Protective effect of quercetin on hydrogen peroxide-induced tight junction disruption. *Int J Toxicol.* 2010 Jul;29(4):418-24.

102. Amasheh M, Schlichter S, Amasheh S, et al. Quercetin enhances epithelial barrier function and increases claudin-4 expression in Caco-2 cells. *J Nutr.* 2008 Jun;138(6):1067-73.

103. Suzuki T, Hara H. Quercetin enhances intestinal barrier function through the assembly of zonula [corrected] occludens-2, occludin, and claudin-1 and the expression of claudin-4 in Caco-2 cells. *J Nutr.* 2009 May;139(5):965-74.

104. Suzuki T, Tanabe S, Hara H. Kaempferol enhances intestinal barrier function through the cytoskeletal association and expression of tight junction proteins in Caco-2 cells. *J Nutr.* 2011 Jan;141(1):87-94.

105. Watson JL, Ansari S, Cameron H, et al. Green tea polyphenol (-)-epigallocatechin gallate blocks epithelial barrier dysfunction provoked by IFN-gamma but not by IL-4. *Am J Physiol Gastrointest Liver Physiol.* 2004 Nov;287(5):G954-61.

106. Noda S, Tanabe S, Suzuki T. Differential effects of flavonoids on barrier integrity in human intestinal Caco-2 cells. *J Agric Food Chem.* 2012 May 9;60(18):4628-33.

107. De Winter BY, van den Wijngaard RM, de Jonge WJ. Intestinal mast cells in gut inflammation and motility disturbances. *Biochim Biophys Acta.* 2012 Jan;1822(1):66-73.

108. Lee EJ, Ji GE, Sung MK. Quercetin and kaempferol suppress immunoglobulin E-mediated allergic inflammation in RBL-2H3 and Caco-2 cells. *Inflamm Res.* 2010 Oct;59(10):847-54.

109. Han J, Lin H, Huang W. Modulating gut microbiota as an anti-diabetic mechanism of berberine. *Med Sci Monit.* 2011 Jul;17(7):RA164-7.

110. Valenzano MC, DiGuilio K, Mercado J, et al. Remodeling of Tight Junctions and Enhancement of Barrier Integrity of the CACO-2 Intestinal Epithelial Cell Layer by Micronutrients. *PLoS One.* 2015 Jul 30;10(7):e0133926.

111. Li GX, Wang XM, Jiang T, Gong JF, Niu LY, Li N. Berberine Prevents Intestinal Mucosal Barrier Damage During Early Phase of Sepsis in Rat through the Toll-Like Receptors Signaling Pathway. *Korean J Physiol Pharmacol.* 2015 Jan;19(1):1-7.

112. Cao M, Wang P, Sun C, He W, Wang F. Amelioration of IFN-γ and TNF-α-induced intestinal epithelial barrier dysfunction by berberine via suppression of MLCK-MLC phosphorylation signaling pathway. *PLoS One.* 2013 May 3;8(5):e61944.

113. DiGuilio KM, Mercogliano CM, Born J, et al. Sieving characteristics of cytokine- and peroxide-induced epithelial barrier leak: Inhibition by berberine. *World J Gastrointest Pathophysiol.* 2016 May 15;7(2):223-34.

114. Yu C, Tan S, Zhou C, et al. Berberine Reduces Uremia-associated Intestinal Mucosal Barrier Damage. *Biol Pharm Bull.* 2016 Aug 9. [Epub ahead of print]

115. de Kort S, Keszthelyi D, Masclee AA. Leaky gut and diabetes mellitus: what is the link? *Obes Rev.* 2011 Jun;12(6):449-58.

116. Shan CY, Yang JH, Kong Y, et al. Alteration of the intestinal barrier and GLP2 secretion in Berberine-treated type 2 diabetic rats. *J Endocrinol.* 2013 Jul 29;218(3):255-62.

117. Chen C, Tao C, Liu Z, et al. A Randomized Clinical Trial of Berberine Hydrochloride in Patients with Diarrhea-Predominant Irritable Bowel Syndrome. *Phytother Res.* 2015 Nov;29(11):1822-7.

118. Marchbank T, Davison G, Oakes JR, et al. The nutriceutical bovine colostrum truncates the increase in gut permeability caused by heavy exercise in athletes. *Am J Physiol Gastrointest Liver Physiol.* 2011 Mar;300(3):G477-84.

119. Davison G, Marchbank T, March DS, Thatcher R, Playford RJ. Zinc carnosine works with bovine colostrum in truncating heavy exercise-induced increase in gut permeability in healthy volunteers. *Am J Clin Nutr.* 2016 Aug;104(2):526-36.

120. Morrison SA, Cheung SS, Cotter JD. Bovine colostrum, training status, and gastrointestinal permeability during exercise in the heat: a placebo-controlled double-blind study. *Appl Physiol Nutr Metab.* 2014 Sep;39(9):1070-82.

121. Buckley JD, Butler RN, Southcott E, Brinkworth GD. Bovine colostrum supplementation during running training increases intestinal permeability. *Nutrients.* 2009 Feb;1(2):224-34.

122. Playford RJ, MacDonald CE, Calnan DP, et al. Co-administration of the health food supplement, bovine colostrum, reduces the acute non-steroidal anti-inflammatory drug-induced increase in intestinal permeability. *Clin Sci (Lond).* 2001 Jun;100(6):627-33.

123. Garas LC, Feltrin C, Hamilton MK, et al. Milk with and without lactoferrin can influence intestinal damage in a pig model of malnutrition. *Food Funct.* 2016 Feb;7(2):665-78.

124. Wu J, Chen J, Wu W, et al. Enteral supplementation of bovine lactoferrin improves gut barrier function in rats after massive bowel resection. *Br J Nutr.* 2014 Aug 28;112(4):486-92.

125. Hirotani Y, Ikeda K, Kato R, et al. Protective effects of lactoferrin against intestinal mucosal damage induced by lipopolysaccharide in human intestinal Caco-2 cells. *Yakugaku Zasshi.* 2008 Sep;128(9):1363-8.

126. Troost FJ, Saris WH, Brummer RJ. Recombinant human lactoferrin ingestion attenuates indomethacin-induced enteropathy in vivo in healthy volunteers. *Eur J Clin Nutr.* 2003 Dec;57(12):1579-85.

127. Pérez-Bosque A, Miró L, Maijó M, et al. Dietary intervention with serum-derived bovine immunoglobulins protects barrier function in a mouse model of colitis. *Am J Physiol Gastrointest Liver Physiol.* 2015 Jun 15;308(12):G1012-8.

128. Ulluwishewa D, Anderson RC, et al. Regulation of tight junction permeability by intestinal bacteria and dietary components. *J Nutr.* 2011 May;141(5):769-76.

129. Ramakrishna BS. Probiotic-induced changes in the intestinal epithelium: implications in gastrointestinal disease. *Trop Gastroenterol.* 2009 Apr-Jun;30(2):76-85.

130. Liu D, Jiang XY, Zhou LS, Song JH, Zhang X. Effects of Probiotics on Intestinal Mucosa Barrier in Patients With Colorectal Cancer after Operation: Meta-Analysis of Randomized Controlled Trials. *Medicine (Baltimore).* 2016 Apr;95(15):e3342.

131. Liu Z, Qin H, Yang Z, et al. Randomised clinical trial: the effects of perioperative probiotic treatment on barrier function and post-operative infectious complications in colorectal cancer surgery - a double-blind study. *Aliment Pharmacol Ther.* 2011 Jan;33(1):50-63.

132. Lamprecht M, Bogner S, Schippinger G, et al. Probiotic supplementation affects markers of intestinal barrier, oxidation, and inflammation in trained men; a randomized, double-blinded, placebo-controlled trial. *J Int Soc Sports Nutr.* 2012 Sep 20;9(1):45.

133. Karczewski J, Troost FJ, Konings I, et al. Regulation of human epithelial tight junction proteins by Lactobacillus plantarum in vivo and protective effects on the epithelial barrier. *Am J Physiol Gastrointest Liver Physiol.* 2010 Jun;298(6):G851-9.

134. Garcia Vilela E, De Lourdes De Abreu Ferrari M, et al. Influence of Saccharomyces boulardii on the intestinal permeability of patients with Crohn's disease in remission. *Scand J Gastroenterol.* 2008;43(7):842-8.

135. Kelly JR, Kennedy PJ, Cryan JF, et al. Breaking down the barriers: the gut microbiome, intestinal permeability and stress-related psychiatric disorders. *Front Cell Neurosci.* 2015 Oct 14;9:392.

Antibiotic and *Clostridium Difficile-*Associated Diarrhea

By most measures, the incidence of diarrhea unintentionally induced by the use of antibiotics (AAD) is on the rise in nations where broad-spectrum antibiotics are used for various clinical reasons (whether necessary or not).[1] In many cases, a positive overgrowth of the pathobiont organism *Clostridium difficile* (aka *C. diff.*) is known to be associated with the AAD, and is often simply referred to as an infection of *C. difficile* (CDI) or *C. difficile-*associated diarrhea (or CDAD, see Figure 33 for growing rates).[2] While there are other dysbiotic conditions related to antibiotic use, many of which alter bowel transit time and induce diarrhea, the major focus in the area of AAD research of late has been directly associated with CDAD.[3] (See additional discussion on the effects of antibiotics on the microbiome on page 110).

Diarrhea associated with post-antibiotic infections are a growing concern in hospital and long-term care settings, especially in the elderly, young children and those with weakened immune systems. In general, pediatric AAD and CDI have a more rapid onset of symptoms, a shorter duration of disease and fewer CDI complications (requiring surgery or extended hospitalizations) than in adults.[4,5] Children experience more community-associated CDI and are associated with smaller outbreaks than adult cases of CDI. Children and adults share some similar risk factors, but adults have more complex risk factor profiles associated with more co-morbidities, types of disruptive factors, and a wider range of exposures to *C. difficile* in the healthcare environment. Children with other gastrointestinal disorders (e.g., IBD) are at higher risk for CDI.[6] The treatment of pediatric and adult AAD is similar (discontinuing or switching the inciting antibiotic), but other treatment strategies for AAD have not been established. Pediatric CDI responds better to metronidazole, while adult CDI typically responds better to vancomycin.

Additionally, the continued use of broad-spectrum antibiotics selectively enhances vulnerable environments with strains that are antibiotic-resistant, making these infections more difficult to treat and more likely to spread from patient to patient. According to the Centers for Disease Control and Prevention, CDIs were estimated to cause almost a half million infections in the United States in 2011, and 29,000 deaths as a result within 30 days of the initial diagnosis.[7] The best preventative strategy is to limit the types and duration of antibiotic use, limit the time in hospital or similar environments where *C. difficile* infections are common, the use of diluted bleach or bleach wipes on surfaces thought to contain *C. difficile* or its spores and, most importantly, to maintain (or re-establish) a healthy gut microbiota (see the use of fecal microbiota transplants or probiotic therapies below).

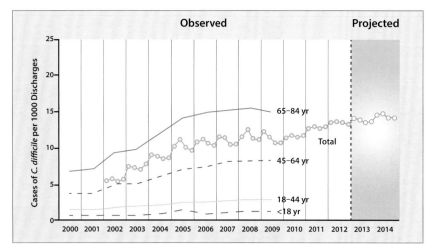

Figure 33: Rates of *Clostridium difficile* infection among hospitalized patients, by age group—National Hospital Discharge Survey, United States, 1996–2009 from Centers for Disease Control and Prevention. Morb Mortal *Wkly Rep (MMWR)* 2011;60(34):1171.

Clostridium Difficile Infections

Clostridium difficile is considered a pathobiont/pathogen, and appears to be of little consequence when there is a balance of healthy commensal organisms to keep it in check. However, the dysbiosis created by the use of broad-spectrum oral antibiotics forms an environment in which the organism and other pathobiont organisms can gain a metabolic advantage, leading to serious consequences for the host. Clostridium difficile synthesizes several toxins, two of which (TcdA and TcdB) are taken up by colonic epithelial cells, by a yet to be identified receptor, where they target the Rho/Ras superfamily of GTPases by irreversible glucosylation. Because these cellular GTPases are important regulatory proteins, this inactivation creates a dysregulation of tight junction integrity, damages the epithelial cells, and leads to cell death. Symptoms can range from mild-to-severe diarrhea to fulminant and often-fatal pseudomembranous colitis (PMC).[8] In addition to these toxins, other virulence factors (e.g., flagella) play an important role in the pathogenesis of C. difficile.[9,10]

Specific strains (or ribotypes) are known to affect the clinical outcomes and risk of recurrence. Ribotype 027 (i.e., BI/NAP1/027) is particularly virulent and has been associated with many fatal outbreaks, though many new strains are being discovered with a range of virulence capacities.[11,12]

While this species was named for its difficulty in culturing, clinicians are finding the aptly-named species is very difficult to treat and the incidence of recurrent CDIs is rising.[13] In fact, recent studies suggest 15 to 35% of subjects treated for CDI will have a recurrence after discontinuing their first antibiotic treatment, either as a relapse of the initial infection or a new infection of the same or different strain. Guideline recommendations for the treatment of CDI differ, though there are many similarities. As this guidebook is not intended to review these therapies in detail, we give only a basic summary of these guidelines here. Clinicians should review the latest guidelines and recommendations from trusted agencies or the hospital/clinic in which they practice.

Basic Summary of Guideline Protocols for CDI[14,15]

- Testing of stool should be used to confirm CDI (for organism/ribotype or toxin), though some guidelines recommend that treatment based on suspicion of severe CDI may commence prior to confirmation.

- Discontinue the inciting antimicrobial agent as soon as possible.

- The drugs of choice for first occurrence in most guideline recommendations is either metronidazole (mild/moderate- 500 mg TID) or vancomycin (severe-125 mg QID) for 10 to14 days. Vancomycin should be used in cases of metronidazole allergy or failure to respond to metronidazole after five to seven days (the American College of Gastroenterology recommends vancomycin use over metronidazole for pregnant/nursing women).

- Most guidelines recommend the first recurrent bout of CDI be first treated with the same antimicrobial

used for initial therapy. The use of vancomycin is recommended when recurrence is severe regardless of initial antimicrobial and for secondary or subsequent recurrences.

- The specific recommendation for the antimicrobial agent fidaxomicin is not given in these guidelines, though its efficacy appears to exceed vancomycin in many studies (and it is FDA-approved for recurrent CDI). The cost of this drug is extremely high and is considered only to be cost-effective when used against highly virulent strains.[16]

- Fecal Microbiota Transfers (or FMT, see page 110) are also now recommended after more than one reoccurrence of CDI.

- Most current guidelines do not include a recommendation for probiotic therapy (see our discussion on the use of probiotics for treating and/or preventing CDI on page 166).

Fecal Microbiota Transplantation (FMT)

The transfer of microbiota from one person (or animal) to another through fecal transplantation is being explored as a therapeutic strategy to re-establish a healthy microbiome. In humans, this technique primarily involves diluting donor feces in a manner to be infused into the recipient either through a retention enema, colonoscope, or nasogastric/nasoduodenal tube.[18] While FMT has been investigated for a range of microbiome-related conditions, the treatment of CDI is by far the most studied and successful indication. A recent meta-analysis of 18 studies (observational) using FMT in patients with recurrent CDI showed a remarkable "cure" rate of over 90%.[19] Failure to achieve a successful outcome is higher in women and higher in those with a hospital-acquired infection (or previously failed FMT).[20]

FMT research is moving quickly and clinicians considering using this technique should understand that regulatory and therapeutic guidelines are still emerging

Antibiotics Associated with CDAD[17]

- **Higher Risk**
  - Clindamycin
  - Advanced/broad spectrum cephalosporin-like antibiotics
  - Carbapenems
  - Flouroquinolones
  - Ampicillin

- **Moderate Risk**
  - Macrolides (azithromycin, erythromycin, clarithromycin, etc.)
  - Amoxicillin/clavulanic acid
  - Amoxicillin/campicillin
  - Tetracyclines
  - First-generation cephalosporins
  - Co-trimoxazole (Bactrim)

- **Lower Risk**
  - Vancomycin
  - Metronidazole
  - Penicillin
  - Aminoglycosides
  - Rifampin
  - Nitrofurantoin
  - Fusidic acid

to catch up with the research advances. Selecting the best candidate recipients and donors, screening donor feces for potential pathogens, choosing outcome and follow-up criteria, long-term safety and the need for ongoing treatments are issues that are still being discussed. In the United States, the FDA has published (March 2016) nonbinding comments saying they "*intend to exercise enforcement discretion under limited conditions, regarding the investigational new drug (IND) requirements for the use of fecal microbiota for transplantation (FMT) to treat Clostridium difficile (C. difficile) infection not responding to standard therapies.*"[21] Those limited conditions include getting the patient's proper consent, **not using** stool bank samples and proper screening and testing of the donor and their stool sample. The use of FMT for indications other than CDI would presumably require an IND prior to use. There is limited data on the use of FMT in children with CDI, though numerous case-studies suggest the success rate is similar in children, compared with adults.[22]

The use of FMT may prove to be an extremely helpful remedy for a number of important conditions for which dysbiosis is a major contributing factor. We encourage clinicians to investigate the most up-to-date methods, guidelines and regulations in order to ensure the use of this therapy maximizes the benefits to their patients.

Probiotics for AAD and CDI Prevention and Treatment

If the absence of a healthy commensal environment is a critical intermediate between antibiotic-use and the overgrowth and invasive activity of *C. difficile*, then the use of probiotics has the potential to mitigate this activity.[23] And, since both CDI and probiotics are both important research trends, it is not surprising that well over 100 clinical trials have been performed to investigate the potential benefits of probiotic therapies for AAD and/or CDI.

In 2012, JAMA published a systematic review and meta-analysis of more than 80 studies using probiotics for the prevention or treatment of AAD.[24] Though these studies were generally small, and some of the specific probiotic strains were poorly documented, they concluded the "evidence suggests that probiotics are associated with a reduction in AAD." In fact, in the trials reporting on the number of patients with AAD, the relative risk was reduced by over 40% (RR 0.58). Of the trials used for the analysis, 57 of 82 included *Lactobacillus* alone or in combination (32/82 in combination with a *Bifidobacterium* strain). Sixteen of the studies used *Saccharomyces boulardii* alone, commonly used for AAD and *Clostridium difficile*-related diarrhea.[25] A more recent meta-analysis of 16 studies (of various sizes and quality) shows a significant benefit in most studies of AAD or CDAD after probiotic therapy.[26]

Overall, a wide range of probiotic strains, strain combinations and doses have been used in clinical research investigating the role of probiotic therapies and AAD/CDI (in the case of CDI, usually with concomitant antibiotic therapy). This heterogeneity of trial design and outcomes has prevented most organizations from making any probiotic recommendations within their AAD and CDI prevention and treatment guidelines (although most have not been updated since 2013), though numerous positive clinical trials have since suggested their overall efficacy and safety.[27] One notable exception to this positive trend was the PLACIDE trial, performed in hospitalized elderly patients in Wales and England. It is one of the largest studies to test probiotics for AAD prevention (n=2941).[28] In this study, researchers used a four-strain combination: two strains of *L. acidophilus* (CUL60 and CUL21), along with *B. bifidum* (CUL20) and *B. lactis* (CUL34), at a dose of 60 billion CFU/day (strain ratio not described). The probiotics were taken with food and, when possible, between antibiotic doses for 21 days and subjects were monitored for the occurrence of AAD within eight weeks and CDAD within 12 weeks of recruitment. There were no statistical differences in AAD or CDAD incidence between the treatment or placebo groups in this study. Interestingly, the number of subjects with confirmed AAD or CDAD (~10.6% and 1%, respectively) was much lower than is typically reported in other similar trials. This may suggest that this study design (or population) is less suitable for evaluating the benefits of probiotic prophylaxis of AAD/CDAD, though it reminds us more research is still needed to understand the role of probiotics for these conditions.

Nonetheless, while numerous strains of both *Lactobacilli* and *Bifidobacterium* species (or combinations) have been associated with positive clinical outcomes, one probiotic that does get mentioned in some guidelines (though with limited information)

is the yeast *S. boulardii*. In fact, a recent systematic review with meta-analysis confirms the efficacy of *S. boulardii* in reducing AAD in children and adults.[29] A range of doses have been used for this probiotic, mostly described as from 250 mg to 1,000 mg/day (generally this is equivalent to 5 to 20 billion CFU, though many trials do not specify a concentration). Because yeast strains are generally not affected by antibiotic use and *S. boulardii* has been both safe and effective for AAD and CDAD, we highly recommend the use of this particular probiotic for these conditions (alone or in combination with other probiotic species). Yogurt is unlikely to help therapeutically against either AAD or CDAD, though it can be safely consumed during the use of other probiotics.[30]

Higher Doses for AAD and CDAD

While there is limited evidence, higher doses of probiotics appear to be more effective at reducing the incidence of AAD or CDAD when compared to lower doses of the same formula. Two studies, using very different definitions of "high-dose" therapy, have evaluated dose effects in subjects using antibiotics and the risk for AAD or CDAD. The largest such study was performed using 503 Chinese subjects who were hospitalized for various diseases requiring antibiotic therapy.[31] Subjects were randomly assigned to one of three therapies: placebo, 4.2 billion CFU (low-dose) or 17.4 billion CFU (high-dose) of an encapsulated product containing equal proportions of *Lactobacillus acidophilus*, *Lactobacillus paracasei*, and two strains of *Bifidobacterium lactis*. Products were consumed during the use of the antibiotic therapy, and continued until seven days after discontinuing the antibiotic (dose taken two hours after antibiotic/breakfast). The incidence of AAD was highest in the placebo group (24.6%) and was statistically lower in the high-dose group (12.5%, p=0.005), while the low-dose realized a non-statistical reduction from placebo (19.6%). Overall, both doses of probiotics were also able to reduce the CDAD incidence compared to placebo (1.8% vs 4.8%, respectively), though only the higher dose reached statistical significance compared to placebo.

A similar study was previously performed in 255 hospitalized elderly Chinese subjects prescribed antibiotics for various diseases.[32] These subjects were randomly assigned to one of three therapies: placebo and either one capsule (50 billion CFU) or two capsules (100 billion CFU) of a probiotic containing *Lactobacillus acidophilus* and *Lactobacillus casei* (ratio not specified). Products were consumed during the use of the antibiotic therapy, and continued for five days after discontinuing the antibiotic (dose taken two hours after antibiotic/breakfast). Incidence of AAD was highest in the placebo group (44.1%), and statistically lower in both the 50 billion/low-dose (28.2%) and 100 billion/high dose (15.5%) groups. Dramatic reductions in the incidence of CDAD were also reported in both the high-dose and low-dose probiotic therapies (1.2% and 9.2%, respectively) compared to placebo (23.8%). The higher incidence of AAD and CDAD in this trial, compared to the previous study mentioned, were likely due to the higher number of elderly in this group.

General Recommendations

In agreement with our previous general recommendation for the use of probiotics with the use of any antibiotic (see page 134), we recommend that clinicians consider using a multi-strain probiotic that includes a minimum of 5 billion CFU of *S. boulardii* (see page 127 for our definition of multi-strain probiotic) in addition to other appropriate therapies for AAD or CDAD (e.g., antibiotics, FMT). Due to the safety and likely higher efficacy, clinicians should consider recommending products that deliver a total of at least 50 billion CFU/day of total probiotics (*Lactobacilli spp.* and *Bifidobacterium spp.*) along with the *S. boulardii* dose. This may be achieved by taking multiple capsules of a single product, or by consuming a separate *S. boulardii*-only product in addition to a high-dose multi-strain probiotic. (see page 135 for more information about probiotic use in children, including AAD and CDAD). **Clinicians should specify to the patients that the probiotic dose should be consumed at least two hours after any oral dose of antibiotics.**

References

1. Elseviers MM, Van Camp Y, Nayaert S, et al. Prevalence and management of antibiotic associated diarrhea in general hospitals. *BMC Infect Dis*. 2015 Mar 17;15:129.
2. Vindigni SM, Surawicz CM. C. difficile Infection: Changing Epidemiology and Management Paradigms. *Clin Transl Gastroenterol*. 2015 Jul 9;6:e99
3. Johanesen PA, Mackin KE, et al. Disruption of the Gut Microbiome: Clostridium difficile Infection and the Threat of Antibiotic Resistance. *Genes (Basel)*. 2015 Dec 21;6(4):1347-60.
4. Sammons JS, Toltzis P. Recent trends in the epidemiology and treatment of C. difficile infection in children. *Curr Opin Pediatr*. 2013;25:116–21.
5. McFarland LV, Ozen M, Dinleyici EC, Goh S. Comparison of pediatric and adult antibiotic-associated diarrhea and Clostridium difficile infections. *World J Gastroenterol*. 2016 Mar 21;22(11):3078-104. [Our text includes several sentences quoted directly or modified from this open access source].
6. Na JY, Park JM, Lee KS, et al. Clinical Characteristics of Symptomatic Clostridium difficile Infection in Children: Conditions as Infection Risks and Whether Probiotics Is Effective. *Pediatr Gastroenterol Hepatol Nutr*. 2014 Dec;17(4):232-8.
7. Lessa FC, Mu Y, Bamberg WM, et al. Burden of Clostridium difficile infection in the United States. *N Engl J Med*. 2015;372(9):825.
8. Martin JS, Monaghan TM, Wilcox MH. Clostridium difficile infection: epidemiology, diagnosis and understanding transmission. *Nat Rev Gastroenterol Hepatol*. 2016 Apr;13(4):206-16.
9. Stevenson E, Minton NP, Kuehne SA. The role of flagella in Clostridium difficile pathogenicity. *Trends Microbiol*. 2015 May;23(5):275-82.
10. Monaghan TM. New perspectives in Clostridium difficile disease pathogenesis. *Infect Dis Clin North Am*. 2015 Mar;29(1):1-11.
11. Valiente E, Cairns MD, Wren BW. The Clostridium difficile PCR ribotype 027 lineage: a pathogen on the move. *Clin Microbiol Infect*. 2014 May;20(5):396-404.
12. Janezic S, Rupnik M. Genomic diversity of Clostridium difficile strains. *Res Microbiol*. 2015 May;166(4):353-60.
13. Shields K, Araujo-Castillo RV, Theethira TG, Alonso CD, Kelly CP. Recurrent Clostridium difficile infection: From colonization to cure. *Anaerobe*. 2015 Aug;34:59-73.
14. https://www.cdc.gov/HAI/pdfs/cdiff/Cohen-IDSA-SHEA-CDI-guidelines-2010.pdf
15. Surawicz CM, Brandt LJ, Binion DG, et al. Guidelines for diagnosis, treatment, and prevention of Clostridium difficile infections. *Am J Gastroenterol*. 2013 Apr;108(4):478-98.
16. Bartsch SM, Umscheid CA, Fishman N, Lee BY. Is fidaxomicin worth the cost? An economic analysis. *Clin Infect Dis*. 2013 Aug;57(4):555-61.
17. Cimolai N. My difficulty with C. difficile. *BCMJ*, Vol. 53, No. 1, January, February, 2011.
18. Bakken JS, Borody T, Brandt LJ, et al. Treating Clostridium difficile Infection with Fecal Microbiota Transplantation. *Clin Gastroenterol Hepatol*. 2011 Dec; 9(12): 1044–1049.
19. Li YT, Cai HF, Wang ZH, et al. Systematic review with meta-analysis: long-term outcomes of faecal microbiota transplantation for Clostridium difficile infection. *Aliment Pharmacol Ther*. 2016 Feb;43(4):445-57.
20. Meighani A, Hart BR, Mittal C, Miller N, John A, Ramesh M. Predictors of fecal transplant failure. *Eur J Gastroenterol Hepatol*. 2016 Jul;28(7):826-30.
21. http://www.fda.gov/downloads/BiologicsBloodVaccines/GuidanceComplianceRegulatoryInformation/Guidances/Vaccines/UCM488223.pdf
22. Hourigan SK, Oliva-Hemker M. Fecal microbiota transplantation in children: a brief review. *Pediatr Res*. 2016 Jul;80(1):2-6.
23. Issa I, Moucari R. Probiotics for antibiotic-associated diarrhea: do we have a verdict? *World J Gastroenterol*. 2014 Dec 21;20(47):17788-95.
24. Hempel S et al. Probiotics for the prevention and treatment of antibiotic-associated diarrhea: a systematic review and meta-analysis. *JAMA*. 2012 May 9; 307(18):1959-69.
25. Berni Canani R, Cucchiara S, Cuomo R, Pace F, Papale F. Saccharomyces boulardii: a summary of the evidence for gastroenterology clinical practice in adults and children. *Eur Rev Med Pharmacol Sci*. 2011 Jul; 15(7):809-22.
26. Pattani R, Palda VA, Hwang SW, Shah PS. Probiotics for the prevention of antibiotic-associated diarrhea and Clostridium difficile infection among hospitalized patients: systematic review and meta-analysis. *Open Med*. 2013 May 28;7(2):e56-67.
27. Lau CS, Chamberlain RS. Probiotics are effective at preventing Clostridium difficile-associated diarrhea: a systematic review and meta-analysis. *Int J Gen Med*. 2016 Feb 22;9:27-37.
28. Allen SJ, Wareham K, Wang D, et al. Lactobacilli and bifidobacteria in the prevention of antibiotic-associated diarrhoea and Clostridium difficile diarrhoea in older inpatients (PLACIDE): a randomised, double-blind, placebo-controlled, multicentre trial. *Lancet*. 2013 Oct 12;382(9900):1249-57.
29. Szajewska H, Kołodziej M. Systematic review with meta-analysis: Saccharomyces boulardii in the prevention of antibiotic-associated diarrhoea. *Aliment Pharmacol Ther*. 2015 Oct;42(7):793-801.
30. Patro-Golab B, Shamir R, Szajewska H. Yogurt for treating antibiotic-associated diarrhea: Systematic review and meta-analysis. *Nutrition*. 2015 Jun;31(6):796-800.
31. Ouwehand AC, DongLian C, Weijian X, et al. Probiotics reduce symptoms of antibiotic use in a hospital setting: a randomized dose response study. *Vaccine*. 2014 Jan 16;32(4):458-63.
32. Gao XW, Mubasher M, Fang CY, et al. Dose-response efficacy of a proprietary probiotic formula of Lactobacillus acidophilus CL1285 and Lactobacillus casei LBC80R for antibiotic-associated diarrhea and Clostridium difficile-associated diarrhea prophylaxis in adult patients. *Am J Gastroenterol*. 2010 Jul;105(7):1636-41.

Inflammatory Bowel Disease

Inflammatory bowel disease (IBD) is comprised of various chronic inflammatory conditions that affect the large and small intestines. The most common forms of IBD, which account for the vast majority of patients with IBD, include Crohn's disease (CD) and ulcerative colitis (UC). Other forms of colitis are also considered IBD by some definitions. It is estimated that IBD affects around 1.5 million people in the United States (roughly divided in half between the two forms), and are most commonly diagnosed in adolescence and young adulthood, although they can affect people of any age.[1] The prevalence of IBD is much higher in non-Hispanic whites compared to other demographics (in the US) and appears to be growing in much of the developed world.[2,3]

While both CD and UC share many common symptoms, such as abdominal pain, diarrhea and weight loss, each has distinctive features (described below). Periods of remissions and exacerbations/relapses commonly occur with both. IBD patients can experience long asymptomatic periods, but acute attacks occur intermittently lasting from weeks to months. Since similar symptoms are seen in both of these forms, it is often difficult to distinguish one from the other, and numerous case studies have been published reporting both can be diagnosed in the same subject.[4] Endoscopy and laboratory tests are useful tools that can help assist clinicians with the exact diagnosis. As this section will make clear, while conventional diagnosis is helpful, determining the status of the core gastrointestinal functions outlined throughout this guidebook can direct the clinician to the root underlying cause(s) and form the basis of therapies designed to optimize GI health in patients with IBD.

Crohn's Disease and Ulcerative Colitis: Similar, but Different[5,6]

Crohn's disease (CD) is a relapsing and transmural (spanning the entire depth of the intestinal wall) inflammatory condition of the GI mucosa that can affect any portion of the GI tract from the mouth to anus, but mostly involves the terminal ileum and colon. Inflammation and ulceration seen in CD usually occur in "skip lesions," or areas of affected tissue interspersed with normal tissue. Clinical presentation depends mainly on disease location and can include abdominal pain, diarrhea, fever, weight loss, signs of bowel obstruction, and a right lower quadrant mass upon examination (due to an inflamed ileum). Other characteristics of CD include ulcers, fissures and strictures, as well as complications such as intestinal obstruction, abscess formation, fistulas, colon cancer and systemic manifestations. CD activity is often graded on one of several disease activity scores, most commonly the Crohn's Disease Activity Index (CDAI). CDAI scores below 150 are often considered to constitute remission, while various cut-off points are designated as mild (150 to 220), moderate (220 to 450) and severe (>450).[7]

Ulcerative colitis (UC) is a relapsing and non-transmural inflammatory condition that affects the inner lining of the colonic mucosa, resulting in continuous areas of ulceration and abscesses without skip lesions. Patients with UC usually present with bloody diarrhea or bowel movements accompanied with the passage of pus and/or mucus. Abdominal cramping, rectal bleeding and weight loss (severe cases) can also be seen in these patients. Hemorrhage is a frequent complication, and the colon may become dilated and perforate. UC increases the risk of colon cancer and other extra-colonic complications. Though there are several different criteria grades for UC (remission, mild, moderate and severe), there is no index or scoring system as with CD.[7]

Etiology and Risk Factors for the Development of IBD

Genetics

The exact etiology of IBD is unknown, but it is mostly categorized as an altered immune response (sometimes viewed as an autoimmune response) resulting from a combination of a subject's genetic susceptibility, environmental triggers, intestinal barrier status and gut microbiota.[8] Evidence shows a major genetic basis for IBD risk, including family clustering and racial and ethnic differences. Studies suggest that 10 to 20% of individuals diagnosed with IBD have a family history of IBD, with the highest risk among first-degree relatives. This familial link is a key risk factor for IBD; having a close relative with IBD increases a person's risk tenfold.[9] Large genome-wide association studies (GWAS) using data from 75,000 IBD patients have identified 163 different potential risk loci (~300 genes), 110 of which were associated with both CD and UC.[10] Mutations of the *CARD15* gene (also known as the *NOD2* gene) on chromosome 16 appear to have the most significant impact on the risk for developing CD. Specific polymorphisms in this gene lead to alterations in NF-κB signaling, which drives increased inflammatory cytokines, dysregulation of gut barrier function, a decreased production of antimicrobial peptides—resulting in decreased clearance of invasive luminal bacteria.[11,12]

Immune/Barrier Dysfunction[13]

Other genetic links have also confirmed alterations in both innate and adaptive immune function as part of the pathophysiology of IBD.[14] Normally, the mucosal immune system is responsible for the balance between pro- and anti-inflammatory mediators. This system helps to defend against luminal pathogens, as well as prevent an immune over-reaction against harmless luminal antigens (such as beneficial bacteria or food). In IBD, this immunological balance is impaired and shifted toward a more pro-inflammatory state, driven by the increased activation of effector immune cells through up-regulation of the NF-κB pathway. These immune cells produce high levels of pro-inflammatory cytokines (such as TNF-α, IL-6 and interferon-γ), resulting in mucosal inflammation and tissue damage.[15] While mucosal inflammation explains some of the intestinal permeability issues in IBD patients, other factors that affect gut barrier function have also been reported in these subjects. The mucin glycoprotein MUC2, and related genes in the synthesis and post-translational modification of mucins, are known to be affected in subjects with IBD, altering the thickness/viscosity of this important part of the mucosal barrier, though these alterations are different in UC compared to CD.[16] Not surprisingly, tight junction regulation is

	CROHN'S DISEASE	ULCERATIVE COLITIS
Location of lesions	Mostly affects the terminal ileum and colon, but can affect any portion of GI tract	Colon exclusively; from the rectum and extending proximally
Depth of pathology	Entire bowel wall	Mucosa and submucosa
Blood in stool	Usually absent	Frequently present
Weight loss/anorexia	Weight loss and anorexia are common	Weight loss in more severe cases
Diarrhea	Moderate	Present
Immune response	Th1 and Th17 pathways predominate	Th2 and Th17 pathways predominate
Complications	• Small bowel abscesses, obstruction, and fistulas • Perianal disease • Malabsorption • Toxic megacolon • Colon cancer	• Perforation • Hemorrhage • Toxic megacolon • Colon cancer

Table 7: General Differences between Crohn's Disease and Ulcerative Colitis

altered in subjects with IBD, increasing paracellular permeability.[17] However, since inflammation itself is a trigger for TJ modulation, it is difficult to know if these are a cause or effect. Zonulin, known to be triggered by gliadin and some intestinal bacteria has not been specifically implicated in IBD pathophysiology, though some have speculated on its involvement.[18]

Microbiome Disturbance

Alterations in the gut microbiota of IBD patients are well-studied.[19] True dysbiosis (alteration in the composition of bacteria in the lumen) and genetic dysbiosis (alteration in the host immune system identifying the microbiota) likely contribute to this dysfunction (see page 103 for discussion of these phenomena, and above for discussion of *CARD15* polymorphisms).[20] The exact nature of the resulting dysbiosis differs between studies, as different sampling methods are used (fecal samples vs. biopsies, active vs. remission) as are methods of identifying species. In general, both CD and UC are associated with reduced microbiota diversity.[21,22] This may be a result of specific immunological interactions with the gut microbiota, an alteration in bowel transit time and concomitant intakes of food and drugs.

One particular species of bacteria that has gained some interest is *Faecalibacterium prausnitzii*, which has been shown in several studies to be reduced in subjects with IBD.[23,24] This mucus-associated bacterium is thought to protect the host by secreting anti-inflammatory and gut-healing substances like butyrate.[25] In fact, other butyrate-producing species are also noted as being reduced in IBD subjects (see more information on *F. prausnitzii* on page 90).[26] Some bacteria species are also known to be elevated in IBD subjects, many of which are known pathobiont organisms like *Clostridium difficile*, but also pathogenic organisms like *Salmonella* spp., *Shigella* spp., and several pathogenic *E.coli* strains.[8] Data suggest that microbiota changes occur between remission and subsequent exacerbations, though these changes cannot be generalized and are quite patient specific.[27]

Not surprisingly, the microbiome-destabilizing effects of antibiotics are also linked to increased risk of IBD.[28,29] Since antibiotic use is often recommended for gastroenteritis, which can be caused by some of the organisms associated with IBD, this link is often difficult to pin down (is it the infection, or the antibiotics used to treat it?).[30] The use of antibiotics in children has been linked with the onset of CD.[31] In keeping with our usual recommendation, antibiotic therapy should be used only when it is absolutely necessary, and subjects should be given probiotics to limit potential microbiome alterations (see page 134 for more details).

Environmental and Lifestyle Factors

There is a strong association between various lifestyle and environmental factors in the pathogenesis of and risk for IBD.[32] It has been well-established that cigarette **smoking** increases the risk for developing CD, but ironically, may decrease the disease severity in some patients with UC.[33,34] Despite these well-described associations, the mechanism by which cigarette smoking affects IBD is not exactly known. Hypoxia, nicotine, and carbon monoxide have all been implicated as mediators of the effects of smoking on IBD and smoking cessation is known to affect changes in the microbiota.[35,36,37] Most IBD subjects are likely unaware of the connection between smoking and the course of their symptoms, even while smoking cessation is a critical therapeutic priority for CD patients (though it is controversial in UC patients, as it is often associated with flairs).[38,39] However, extra-intestinal symptoms in both CD and UC may be reduced after smoking cessation.[40]

Dietary factors play an important role in the development of, or protection from, IBD.[41] Common to most chronic diseases, the Western dietary pattern that includes refined and processed sugars and fats with an excessive amount of processed and fried animal proteins is linked with increased prevalence of IBD. Since this dietary pattern is known to affect the gut microbiota, increase inflammatory burden and increase measures of gastrointestinal permeability, this connection is not surprising. Currently, the strongest evidence seems to be the ability of the diet to alter the gut microbiome, which then affects immune function and intestinal permeability in genetically susceptible people.[42,43] While this dietary pattern is a predisposing factor, there are likely specific features of the diet that act as triggering agents for initial onset, and for disease flair-ups after remission. **Dietary fiber** intake is associated, inversely and dose-dependently, with the risk for both UC and CD (more strongly with CD).[44,45] This is likely due to the well-studied effects of dietary fibers on microbial abundance and metabolism (e.g., SCFA production) as well as the ability to moderate bowel transit. Furthermore, two studies have suggested that diets with increased refined sugar (particularly sucrose) intake and high overall carbohydrate intake may precede the development of CD.[46,47] In the large European EPIC trial, a diet described as "high sugar and soft drink pattern" significantly increased the risk of UC (RR 1.68 in highest vs. lowest quintile).[48]

The intake of **omega-3 fatty acids**, alone or in the context of omega-6 fatty acid intake has also been explored in subjects with IBD. Generally, the available data suggest higher intakes of omega-3 fatty acids in the diet (including ALA, EPA and DHA) are associated with lower incidence of IBD.[49,50,51,52] Generally, this is considered to be related to their anti-inflammatory properties.[53] Epidemiological studies suggest increased intake of omega-6 fatty acids increases the risk for IBD, but this is complicated by other dietary factors in these studies (i.e., red meat intake).[54,55,56] However, animal studies do suggest that replacing linolenic acid (omega-6) with EPA and DHA (omega-3) can ameliorate measures of colitis.[57] Also, in the Nurses' Health Study, greater consumption of long-chain omega-3 fatty acids and a higher ratio of omega-3 to omega-6 fatty acid intake showed protection against development of UC.[58] The role of omega-3 fatty acids in the therapeutic intervention of IBD will be covered below.

Consistent with the dietary relationship of almost all other chronic and/or inflammatory conditions, increased intake of **fruits and vegetables** is also associated with decreased IBD risk.[59,60,61] This relationship has been linked with increased intake of vitamins, minerals, dietary fiber and a host of phytochemicals.[62,63] Some of these compounds have been further explored as therapeutic agents and will be explored further below. Finally, we should note that the **Mediterranean dietary pattern**, the pattern we generally recommend as the basis upon which to build a dietary prevention and intervention strategy for chronic disease management, fulfills most of the basic requirements for IBD risk prevention.[64] Currently, there have been no large intervention trials using the Mediterranean diet, but UC patients saw significantly favorable changes in gut microbiota and genomic expression changes six weeks after switching to a Mediterranean diet.[65] In addition, increased consumption of omega-9 containing olive oil, a common ingredient in the traditional Mediterranean diet, is also noted with lower incidence of IBD.[66]

Other lifestyle factors are also known to impact risk for IBD. Stressors that trigger **HPA axis activation** (or other alterations in the gut/brain axis) can have an effect on nearly all parameters related to IBD pathophysiology (microbiota, intestinal permeability, GI transit, inflammation, immune modulation).[67,68] Therefore, HPA axis evaluation is advised in subjects with IBD as it is with any other chronic GI dysfunction. For a complete discussion of the role of the HPA axis in chronic disease and up-to-date discussions of laboratory testing, see our Standard Road map, *The Role of Stress and the HPA Axis in Chronic Disease Management* (Point Institute, 2015). We should note that the frequent use of corticosteroid therapy in subjects with IBD is directly related to suppression of HPA axis function and is dependent of both dose and duration of therapy.[69] Termed tertiary adrenal insufficiency, this phenomenon is not an "adrenal" issue directly, but a down-regulation of the ACTH production from the pituitary, which may eventually have negative consequences on adrenal physiology.

Biomarker Assessment for IBD

Currently, there is no single "gold standard" biomarker or functional test to diagnose IBD, or to distinguish CD from UC. Therefore, clinicians must rely upon a combination of symptoms, clinical examinations, laboratory biomarkers, and invasive endoscopic/histological assessments to make a diagnosis.[70,71] Since subjects with functional bowel disorders (e.g., IBS) often present with similar symptoms, it is estimated that up to half of these patients are referred for unnecessary endoscopic evaluation.[71] For these reasons, extensive research over the past few decades has been invested in developing non-invasive biomarkers to identify IBD from other gastrointestinal disorders and, more challenging, to distinguish CD from UC.

Most generic markers for IBD are biomarkers of inflammation such as C-reactive protein (CRP) and the erythrocyte sedimentation rate (ESR). Both of these markers are still used to monitor disease progression in subjects with IBD, though they are not specific to inflammation from the gut, cannot distinguish UC from IBD, and some studies suggest them to have poor predictive value.[72,73,74,75] Fecal biomarkers of inflammation (i.e., calprotectin and lactoferrin), however, have a much better specificity for gut-derived inflammation and have been successfully used to distinguish IBD from functional gastrointestinal disorders (i.e., IBS). Currently, calprotectin is the most sensitive (depending on the cut-off used) and specific biomarker for clinicians to use for this purpose.

Calprotectin is a calcium-binding protein mostly produced by neutrophils, and its measures in the stool reflects the amount of neutrophil invasion into the gut (i.e, inflammation).[76] Calprotectin has been shown to be a useful biomarker for distinguishing IBS from IBD, for differentiating states of remission from relapsing flairs, for predicting mucosal healing after therapy, and predicting relapse onset (Figure 34).[70,77] A meta-analysis concluded that the use of fecal calprotectin testing resulted in 67% fewer unnecessary endoscopy procedures in adults with a small risk (6%) of delayed diagnosis.[78] Nonetheless, fecal calprotectin cannot distinguish CD from UC.

A few biomarkers have been explored for distinguishing CD from UC, though these may not be readily available from most laboratories. They include measures of perinuclear antineutrophil cytoplasmic antibodies (pANCA) and anti-*Saccharomyces cerevisiae* antibodies (ASCA). pANCA levels are elevated almost exclusively in subjects with UC, while ASCA levels were highly specific (95%) to patients with CD. Together, the combination of pANCA+/ASCA-, and pANCA-/ASCA+ has been shown to be very specific for positively distinguishing one form of IBD from the other, though this combination still lacks sensitivity (many false negatives for both forms).[79]

Conventional Pharmacological Treatment of IBD[†]

The conventional medical treatment of IBD involves an approach that focuses on both symptomatic relief as well as controlling overstimulation of the immune system. Exacerbations and maintenance of remission of CD and UC are commonly treated with 5-aminosalicylic acid (5-ASA), which is the active ingredient found in the pharmaceutical preparations sulfasalazine and Mesalamine (mesalazine).[80,81] 5-ASA helps to reduce inflammation and tissue damage by neutralizing reactive oxygen molecules produced by neutrophils, inhibiting the production of pro-inflammatory mediators, which limits the infiltration of neutrophils into the

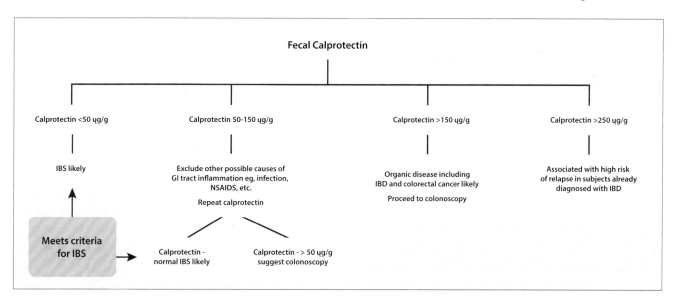

Figure 34: Fecal Calprotectin Diagnostic Tree. Fecal calprotectin levels can help rule out IBD, prioritize colonoscopy in at risk patients or be an early marker for IBD relapse.

† This overview of the conventional pharmacological treatment for IBD is very basic and not intended to be a complete guide to understanding the benefits, appropriate uses, contraindications or side-effects related to these therapies. In addition, we do not discuss surgical options for IBD in this guide. This brief discussion should not be viewed as an endorsement or a discouragement to use any of these therapies; they are merely designed to give some background to help further evaluate adjunct therapies that are often combined with (or compared to) one or more of these pharmacological therapies.

mucosa. Patients with CD are given the antimicrobials ciprofloxacin or metronidazole when complications such as infected abscesses or fistulas occur.

Corticosteroids (e.g., budesonide, prednisolone, hydrocortisone) are often employed for IBD patients presenting with moderate to severe disease, and are also an option for patients with mild symptoms who do not benefit from 5-ASA. Corticosteroids are also used for short-term therapy in IBD patients who experience acute exacerbations, which may reduce the side effect profile related to long-term use. Most of these medications have serious adverse effects in patients, which is a concern for many clinicians. 5-ASA has been known to commonly cause nausea, diarrhea, headaches, abdominal cramping, and occasionally, thrombocytopenia. Long-term use of corticosteroid therapy is associated with the development of cataracts, diabetes, osteoporosis, HPA axis dysfunction and other adverse effects.

In many patients, however, therapy with 5-ASA and corticosteroids simply fails to control the symptoms or are difficult for the patient to tolerate. In such cases, a growing number of immunosuppressive drugs (e.g., 6-mercaptopurine, azathioprine, methotrexate and cyclosporine) and biological agents (i.e., monoclonal antibody) have become available to reduce immune system function or block cytokine signaling (e.g., anti-TNF-α antibodies-infliximab, adalimumab and certolizumab).[82,83,84] Common serious side effects of immunosuppressive agents include increased risk of developing cancer, increased vulnerability for opportunistic infections, nausea or vomiting, abdominal pain, loss of appetite and other GI complaints.[85] The cost of these new biological drugs is extremely high, though the introduction of "biosimilars" may provide some cost reduction.[86]

A Functional Approach to IBD

While the clinician can decide whether the use of any (or all) of the conventional therapies previously mentioned is appropriate for their patients with IBD, it should be clear that none of these therapies address the causes and dysfunctions that are at the root of IBD pathophysiology. In fact, IBD is the quintessential example of a condition for which nearly every basic function of the GI tract has some disturbance (microbial imbalance, barrier dysfunction, inappropriate immune responses, pancreatic insufficiency, bowel transit issues, enteric nervous system dysregulation). Furthermore, a vicious cycle of inflammatory signaling continues to allow a small disturbance in one core function to further the dysfunction of the other functions leading to another relapse cycle and so on. The principles of the functional approach we describe here are designed to address these core foundational functions, while recognizing the need for symptom relief.

The 4R approach (outlined on page 22) is very well-suited for the IBD patient, as it deals with important strategies for rebuilding core GI functions. This section will show some of the main principles that should be considered when using the 4R approach to build a patient-specific protocol for treating IBD. We encourage clinicians to investigate the use of comprehensive stool analyses (CDA, CDSA™) when evaluating IBD patients. Along with measures of GI inflammation, they can assess the general status of other important core functions of the GI.

Remove

- Are there foods, allergens, toxins, stressors that need to be removed from the patient's environment or body?

- Rule out common GI infections and inflammatory conditions such as *C. difficile*, foodborne illnesses, celiac disease or gluten sensitivity.

- One of more common treatment approaches used in this step is an elimination (or rotation) diet focused on both the avoidance of common allergenic food groups and decreasing food toxins (pesticides, herbicides, additives, artificial ingredients, etc.).

- An elimination diet is often combined with a detoxification protocol that allows for removal of toxins stored in the body, and improves the process of the removal of toxins. (see page 70 for suggestions for detoxification protocols). One study looked at the effect of an elimination diet in 78 CD patients who achieved remission with an elemental diet. These patients were randomly assigned to corticosteroids or elimination diet. The corticosteroid group received 40 mg prednisone daily, which was tapered and stopped after 12 weeks; dietary advice and tips on healthy eating were given to this group as well. The diet group received a tapered placebo, and were recommended to introduce one new food daily (avoiding any food that was known to cause or aggravate symptoms). After treatment, the results showed the median remission time was 7.5 months in the diet group vs. 3.8 months in the corticosteroid group (both maintained >60% at two years).[87,88]

Replace
- Traditionally, this step involves the replacement of digestive enzymes or other factors needed to properly address the digestion and absorption of nutrients. Pancreatic insufficiency (as are other pancreatic disorders) is notably higher in subjects with IBD (lower measures of fecal elastase), especially those with more frequent loose stools.[89,90]

- Consider the use of digestive enzymes. Note: we are not aware of any published studies evaluating the benefits of such supplements (pancreatin/pancrelipase/fungal analogs) in subjects with IBD.

- Low exocrine pancreatic function may cause lower absorption of fat-soluble vitamins, for which supplementation is recommended with a comprehensive multivitamin/mineral formula. (see data for vitamin D supplementation below).

Re-establish [i.e., Re-inoculate] the ecosystem for a healthy microbiota.
- Diet is the most important factor in establishing and maintaining a healthy gut microbiome. See discussion above and also on page 104.

- Antibiotic therapies should be limited and always supported with the use of probiotics.

- Probiotic therapy can be helpful in IBD patients, though more positive outcomes have been reported in UC than CD (see details below).

- Prebiotic therapies (dietary or supplemental) have been helpful in subjects with IBD, though the low FODMAP diet (which limits most prebiotics) has been successful in some subjects with IBD.[91]

- Fecal Microbiota Transplants (FMTs) have been shown to be effective for C. difficile-associated diarrhea in IBD patients, but currently have shown limited efficacy specifically for long-term IBD remission.[92,93]

Repair
- Basically, this step involves the full healing of the intestinal mucosa. The three keys to repairing the integrity of the gut include: reducing inflammation, providing nutrients for specific GI cell growth, and strengthening immune and liver function. Here, we follow the principles laid out in our "Supporting Gut Barrier" section on pages (153-160). Details for some specific to subjects with IBD are listed below.

- Remove signals that damage gastrointestinal cells or increase intestinal permeability.

- Increase the intake of anti-inflammatory signals in the diet. These are mostly contained in plants, as many phytonutrients are reported to reduce inflammatory burden. Some of these agents also act as genomic signaling agents to improve enterocyte integrity/tight junction assembly.

- Provide nutrients that specifically help the gastrointestinal cells build metabolic reserve. This helps maintain their capacity to rapidly divide and continue to form and secrete the necessary components to create and maintain barrier function.

- Provide receptor-mediated or genomic signals that stimulate the cells along the gastrointestinal tract. These might be signals that improve tight junction formation, changes in phosphorylation pathways of tight junction proteins, alterations in mucin production or changes in immune function signaling from the lumen.

- Build immune system and detoxification metabolic reserve. Since these are the systems vulnerable to intestinal barrier failure, they should always be supported when intestinal permeability is compromised.

Supplementing Dietary Nutrients

It is essential that clinicians strongly consider supplementation of dietary nutrients in patients with IBD during the entire course of their treatment. Nutritional supplementation is used in IBD patients for two main reasons: supportive (to correct nutrient deficiencies) or primary (to help attain remission). A wide array of vitamin and mineral deficiencies exists in patients with IBD, with varying degrees of clinical significance.[94] Deficiencies that are common include iron, calcium, magnesium, vitamin D, vitamin K, vitamin B12, zinc, folic acid, vitamin B6, thiamin and vitamin A.[95] These deficiencies may be more common in CD than UC and more severe during active disease, compared to remission.[96] Clinicians should suspect a wide range of micronutrient insufficiencies/deficiencies (due to poor diet or poor digestion/absorption) in subjects with IBD and supplement accordingly. A quality multivitamin/mineral supplement at each meal would be a prudent start.

Elemental diets, composed of free-form amino acids, or semi-elemental diets (hydrolyzed proteins) have also been studied in IBD subjects, often as adjunctive therapies. Patients adhering to these diets realized some improvement, though compliance among patients on these diets are often difficult.[97, 98]

Glutamine

The gut healing potential for glutamine has been discussed extensively elsewhere (see page 155). Remarkably, several important mechanisms related to enterocyte metabolism and improved barrier function have been confirmed in a number of different cell culture and animal models of IBD (i.e. colitis) using glutamine.[99,100] However, as common as the recommendation for glutamine use in subjects with IBD is, few clinical trials confirming its efficacy for such subjects have been performed.[101] A recent Cochrane review found only two clinical trials with which to evaluate glutamine supplementation for the induction of remission in subjects with Crohn's disease.[102,103,104] They concluded that insufficient evidence is available to make any recommendations.

One study not reviewed in the above-mentioned Cochrane review included thirty patients with Crohn's disease (in remission), with elevated lactulose/mannitol ratio, randomly assigned glutamine supplementation or a whey protein supplement and tested two months later for changes in intestinal permeability.[105] The dose of glutamine (or whey protein) was 0.5 g/kg ideal body weight per day, a substantial dose (40 g for 80 kg/176 lbs.) compared to previous studies. After two months, the lactulose/mannitol ratio was substantially improved in both groups, as was the villous to crypt ratio (from examining biopsy tissue, a measure that was also improved in an aged animal study using glutamine).[106]

Based upon the very strong biological mechanisms linking glutamine to enterocyte function and integrity, the number of animal models showing oral glutamine supplementation as a protective therapy during models of colitis, and the consistent anecdotal evidence of numerous clinicians, we recommend clinicians consider the use of glutamine (4 to 8 g/day) as a safe, and potentially beneficial adjunct therapy for IBD subjects. Products designed to deliver higher doses of glutamine are usually flavored powders, since capsules or tablets rarely deliver more than 1 gram of glutamine.

Vitamin D

By now, most clinicians are familiar with the ubiquity of vitamin D deficiency and the growing understanding of the important role vitamin D plays in human health (beyond bone health). Unlike most other vitamins, vitamin D is a steroid nuclear regulator that modifies the expression of specific genes through the vitamin D receptor. Genes containing the vitamin D-response element (VDRE) are accessible on a wide range of cell types, and are especially common in both innate and adaptive immune cells.[107,108,109] Vitamin D is a key regulator of the immune system response in the gut by modulating the function of dendritic cells, considered the master conductor of the gut-immune system interface with the gut microbiota.[110,111] Dysregulation of dendritic cells are also considered to be part of the pathophysiology driving IBD.[112,113]

The role of vitamin D has been extensively studied in relation to inflammatory and auto-immune conditions, including both UC and CD (IBD is really more of an auto-inflammatory condition, than a classic autoimmune disorder).[114,115] Epidemiological data links low vitamin D status with higher prevalence of IBD, including studies suggesting that living in northern latitudes with low sunlight-induced vitamin D synthesis may contribute to higher incidence in certain global regions.[116,117] A recent meta-analysis of 14 studies, comprising 938 IBD cases and 953 controls, showed that subjects with IBD have a 64% higher likelihood of being vitamin D deficient than control subjects (defined as serum 25(OH)D level of ≤20 ng/mL); subjects with UC had an even higher odds of vitamin D deficiency (OR 2.28) compared to controls.[118] The relationship may be both cause and effect, in that low vitamin D status is likely to contribute to poor immune modulation and increased inflammation, while IBD pathophysiology likely contributes to poor absorption of any vitamin D from the diet.

For the clinician, two important and interrelated questions arise: 1) What is the need for vitamin D supplementation in IBD subjects, and what dose is likely to help them reach sufficient levels of serum 25(OH)D? and 2) Can vitamin D supplementation alter the course of disease in IBD patients, to reduce symptoms or extend remission times? Below are some clinical trials we will use to help answer these questions.

- 2,000 IU/day (oral) vitamin D3 for 3 months (winter) in CD patients (N=27).[119] Mean vitamin D levels went from 27.7 ng/dL to 36.6 ng/dL in the supplemented group (placebo group vitamin D levels fell from 20.7 to 16.1ng/dL). Intestinal permeability (as measured by lactulose/mannitol absorption) was maintained in the vitamin D group, while it was statistically worse in placebo group.

- 300,000 IU (single dose, intramuscular) vitamin D3 in UC patients (n=90) in remission.[120] Ninety days after injection, vitamin D3 rose from a mean of 33.3 ng/dL to 40.8 ng/dL (no change after saline injection). Both CRP and ESR (markers of inflammation) were significantly lower 90 days after the vitamin D injection.

- 1,100 IU/day (different forms used) in IBD subjects (N=167, 55 UC, 112 CD) self-supplementing vitamin D vs. subjects not supplementing.[121] Dose was not capable of changing the percent of subjects with vitamin D deficiency; the mean serum 25(OH)D levels in these subjects was 22.5 ng/mL during the winter.

- 800 IU/day (median of 400-1000 IU, form not specified) in IBD subjects (n=26; types not specified) supplemented cohort of larger study comparing vitamin D levels with quality of life scores in patients.[122] Dose was insufficient to alter vitamin D levels, compared to un-supplemented cohort. Overall study showed increasing quality of life scores as serum vitamin D status increased, highest at vitamin D levels of 50-59 ng/mL.

- 400 IU/day vs. 2,000 IU/day of oral vitamin D3 for six months in children with CD in remission (n=83).[123] Though both doses were able to raise serum vitamin D levels to >20 ng/mL, the 2000 IU dose was able raise serum 25(OH)D levels above 30ng/mL in 74% of subjects, while only 35% of subjects reached this level using the 400 IU/day dose. Disease activity was not significantly different between doses.

- Different regimens in children and adolescents (ages 5-21) with IBD (n=71, 41 CD, 27 UC, 3 other).[124] Subjects with serum 25(OH)D levels <20ng/ml were given oral supplementation (liquid) as 2000 IU/day vitamin D2, 2000 IU/day of vitamin D3, or 50,000 IU/week vitamin D2 for six weeks. Serum 25(OH)D levels rose by an average of 9.13, 16.4 and 25.4 ng/dL in the three groups, respectively. Vitamin D3 was statistically better at raising serum vitamin D levels compared to the same (2,000 IU/day) dose of vitamin D2. A 50,000 IU dose taken once per week (3 times the 2,000/day dose) appears to be a safe way to rapidly raise serum vitamin D levels and superior to 2,000 IU/day (at least over 6 weeks). A previous study by same group showed 2,000 IU/day of vitamin D2 could not maintain optimal serum vitamin D levels.[125]

- 5,000 or 10,000 IU of vitamin D3/10 kg of body weight per week for 6 weeks in children (ages 8-21) with IBD (N=32, 28 CD, 4 UC).[126] Maximum dose, per week, was 25,000 and 50,000 IU respectively. After eight weeks (two weeks after last weekly supplementation), mean serum 25(OH)D had risen from 23.7 ng/mL to 49.2 mg/dL in the higher dose, compared to a change from 24.0 to 41.5 ng/dL in the lower dose group. When both groups were tested at week 12 (six weeks without supplementation), both had significantly lower serum vitamin D levels compared to the eight-week measurement (35.1 ng/dL and 30.8 ng/dL, respectively).

- 1,200 IU/day oral vitamin D3 for 12 months compared to placebo in CD patients in remission (n=94).[127] After three months of supplementation, mean serum 25(OH)D levels rose from 27.6 ng/mL to 38.4 ng/mL and were maintained through the entire year (placebo group had slight, non-statistical increase during summer months). Interestingly, compared to the 29% of placebo-subjects experiencing a relapse over the year, only 13% of subjects in the vitamin D group experienced a relapse (58% reduced risk), though this was considered a non-statistical finding with a p=0.056!

Before rendering our conclusions and making our recommendations, we should note that the definition of "sufficient" serum levels of vitamin D in even healthy subjects is disputed. It is our view that minimum target serum levels should be 30 ng/ml (75 nmol/L) and may be optimal at 70 ng/ml (175 nmol/L), though 30 to 50 ng/ml are now commonly cited in the literature.[128] For perspective, a study calculating the optimal dose required to move healthy subjects into a target range of 30 to 88 ng/dL if they had baseline 25(OH)D levels of less than 22 ng/dl, found that a dose of 5,000 IU of vitamin D3 per day would be needed. Subjects with a baseline above 22 ng/dl would still need 3,800 IU to reach this target.[129] Notably, the clinical trials we list above, that use vitamin D supplementation in IBD subjects, do not alter the dose to reach specific target serum repletion levels based on baseline vitamin D levels, something that limits the interpretation of many of these trials.

What we conclude from the trials performed in IBD subjects is:

✓ IBD subjects should have their serum vitamin D levels tested regularly to evaluate status and the efficacy of vitamin D supplementation.

✓ Optimal serum levels of vitamin D in IBD subjects is likely to be >50 ng/dL. Though most trials did not achieve these levels, reports of improved quality of life in IBD subjects who had achieved these levels and based on other non-IBD trials, this level seems a reasonable target.

✓ The dose needed to maintain an optimal serum levels in adult IBD subjects is likely to exceed 5,000 IU/day and may require up to 10,000 IU/day.

✓ The use of 50,000 IU, once or twice per week to achieve optimal serum vitamin D levels (in adults) may be needed to combat poor bioavailability in IBD subjects.

✓ Vitamin D3 is superior to vitamin D2 for increasing serum 25(OH)D.

✓ While there are nuances in some studies, our recommendation for UC and CD are the same.

Essential Fatty Acids

While the dietary intake of omega-3 fatty acids appears to reduce the risk of IBD, the role of supplementation with concentrations of ALA, EPA and/or DHA (mostly as fish oil) is still under rigorous investigation. Dozens of clinical trials over the past three decades have evaluated a number of different combinations and doses of omega-3 fatty acid supplementation in both UC and CD (in subjects with active disease and in remission).

A recent systematic review published in the British Journal of Nutrition found 19 randomized clinical trials with which to evaluate omega-3 supplementation in IBD subjects (7 UC active, 4 UC remission, 2 CD active, 6 CD remission).[130] They conclude that, while several small trials show significant benefit, the number of negative results in large trials and the poor selection of placebo (i.e., olive oil or MCTs) in several trials, makes it difficult to recommend omega-3 fatty acids for the treatment of IBD. The fact that most studies did not measure patient omega-3 levels at baseline and after supplementation, and used fatty acid preparations known to have different bioavailability (TG, EE, FFA, enteric coated, etc.), increases the difficulty in making specific recommendations. Others have made similar conclusions.[131]

A departure from this trend is a study often excluded from systematic reviews because it was performed using children with CD (n=38).[132] These children (ages five to 16) had been given a diagnosis of CD, but were in remission for at least two months prior to the start of the trial. All subjects were treated with 5-ASA (50 mg/kg/day) and given either fish oil (3 gastro-resistant capsules/day containing 400 mg/day EPA, 200 mg/day DHA each) or olive oil capsules for 12 months. After 1 year, 95% of subjects in the "placebo" group treated with mesalazine and olive oil had relapsed, while only 61% had relapsed in the fish oil group, a statistically significant difference (p=0.0016).

Overall, the available clinical trials using omega-3 fatty acids as a therapeutic intervention for IBD have yet to corroborate the basic science, cell culture, animal and human epidemiological data. However, realizing the potential anti-inflammatory benefits of supplementing omega-3 fatty acids in all subjects and their role in decreasing markers of inflammation, clinicians should consider supplementing ALA, EPA and DHA in all subjects to reach an omega-3 index of at least 4 to 8%.[133] Those studies that did report improvements in disease or quality of life scores used doses between 2 and 4 g total EPA and DHA.[132,134,135]

Phosphatidylcholine (PC)

Recent evidence suggests that patients with UC have a very low level of phosphatidylcholine in colonic mucosal tissue, compared to CD patients and healthy controls.[136] The importance of PC for maintaining barrier function is not yet well understood, but it is hypothesized to play a role in maintaining hydrophobicity of the mucosal membrane and also as a signaling molecule within the phospholipid membrane of the enterocytes.[137] Supplementation with delayed-released PC delivering 500 mg of PC qid (2 g total) have shown great promise at initiating or maintaining remission in subjects with UC.[138,139] Ironically, a newer preparation designed to contain a highly purified PC (97%) compared to the previous mixtures (~30% PC with other phospholipids) showed a lower rate of efficacy, though it was the first multicenter trial for this preparation and was used in mesalazine-refractory subjects.[140] The authors claim that slow-release PC is needed to allow it to avoid absorption in the small intestines, allowing it to accumulate in the distal colon where UC inflammation and tissue damage occurs; the product (LT-02) has yet to complete Phase III clinical trials and is not currently available.

Probiotics

Since a variety of alterations in the gut microbiome are common in subjects with IBD and the microbiota-immune interface is considered a key pathophysiological mediator, it seems quite plausible that probiotic therapy would have a positive outcome on disease progression. However, the heterogeneity of the trials evaluating the role of probiotics in IBD subjects has created some confusion. Recently, several systematic reviews and meta-analyses have been published in the attempt to provide the clinician some clarity as to the potential benefits of certain species or doses of probiotics in patients with IBD.[141,142,143,144,145,146]

In general, there appears to be a substantial difference in the reported efficacy of probiotic therapy between the two forms of IBD, favoring UC. That is, few clinical trials using probiotics have been effective at inducing or extending the maintenance of remission (beyond concomitant therapy controls) in patients with Crohn's disease, while numerous clinical trials using probiotics have been successful in subjects with ulcerative colitis. It is unknown whether this is a fundamental difference in the immune-microbiome interface between these two conditions, the concentration of lesions in the distal colon in UC versus the many intermittent lesions in CD, or simply the quality of the trials performed. Nonetheless, these differences have been maintained over many years of trials using a variety of probiotic preparations. We will, therefore, review the information for both conditions separately.

Probiotics for Crohn's Disease

As mentioned above, the general consensus is that probiotic therapy has shown little benefit for CD subjects in controlled clinical trials. However, since probiotics are generally considered safe in CD patients, we briefly review the results of a few trials where positive outcomes were reported to inform the clinician in the event they intend to use probiotics in such patients (see review for all trials).[142] A few small studies performed with the probiotic yeast, *Saccharomyces boulardii*, have yielded improvements in symptom scores or prolonged relapses in CD patients in remission. In one very early double-blind placebo-controlled study (1993), twenty subjects with CD suffering from diarrhea and moderate complaints as measured by the BEST Index were treated with *Saccharomyces boulardii* (250 mg/tid, likely 15 billion CFU/day, though the study did not define concentration) for two weeks in addition to conventional treatment.[147] Patients saw a statistical reduction in both bowel movement frequency and disease index score. Ten of the subjects were then randomized to continue the treatment of *S. boulardii* (same dose), while seven were given placebo for an additional seven weeks. After 10 total weeks, the group given *S. boulardii* had further reduced bowel frequencies and disease index scores while both measures rose to near their original baseline values in the placebo group.

A second study (2000) evaluated the benefit of *S. boulardii* as an adjunct therapy with mesalamine in 32 CD patients in clinical remission for an average of 33 weeks.[148] Patients were treated for 6 months with either 3 grams per day of mesalamine (1 gram/tid) or 2 grams per day of mesalamine (1 gram/bid) with 1 g *S. boulardii* (given as two, 500 mg capsules in the morning; the concentration was not listed, but likely 20 billion CFU). Of the sixteen patients on mesalamine alone, six subjects experienced a clinical relapse, while only one subject in the mesalamine plus *S. boulardii* group experienced a relapse (p=0.04). Even in a more recent, larger trial (2013) that failed to show statistical benefits in relapse prevention using *S.boulardii* (1 g/day), there was an interaction between *S. boulardii* treatment and smoking status that was statistically significant. In post hoc analysis, nonsmokers given a placebo had more relapses (72.0%) than those treated with *S. boulardii* (34.5%). However, in smokers and former smokers, the proportion of relapse was not significantly different. When adjusting for stratification factor, nonsmokers treated with *S boulardii* were 82% less likely to relapse than those receiving placebo (OR, 0.18; P=0.006).

The only other species of probiotics to show marginal benefits in CD subject in a controlled trial is *Bifidobacterium longum* (400 billion CFU/day consumed as a synbiotic with inulin at 6 g/day).[149] However, a combination of *B. longum*, *B. breve* and *L. casei* (combined with psyllium) showed some improvement in an open-labeled, uncontrolled trial.[150] The high-dose combination product VSL#3, which has been used successfully in subjects with UC or pouchitis, has been tested with only limited reported success in subjects with CD.[151]

Based on the available evidence, there are limited data upon which to make a strong recommendation for the clinical treatment of CD using probiotics. The use of probiotics in such patients is generally recommended to help maintain a commensal-friendly environment, though they should not be relied upon to induce or extend remission. The use of *S. boulardii* at 1 g (20 billion CFU) may be an exception; clinicians should consider the use of this dose as a potential adjunct therapy in subjects with CD, or include *S. boulardii* in a mixed-strain probiotic.

Probiotics for Ulcerative Colitis

Unlike the situation for CD, the evidence supporting the successful use of probiotic therapy for UC is much more promising, though concentrated around a few strains or strain combinations. In three double-blind, placebo-controlled randomized clinical trials, researchers found that a non-pathogenic strain of *E. coli* (Nissle 1917) was equally effective as mesalazine in maintaining remission among UC patients. In one of these trials involving 120 patients, Kruis et al. reported that patients receiving this probiotic strain (50 billion CFU/day) had a similar relapse-free time (106± 5 d) compared to UC patients

who were given mesalamine (103± 4 d).[152] Similar outcomes were confirmed by Rembacken et al. in a trial involving 116 patients with UC. Relapse rates were 73% for the mesalazine group and 67% for the *E.coli* group (100 billion CFU/day), and the time to relapse was not significantly different between both groups.[153] In another larger clinical trial of 327 patients, researchers also found that *E.coli* (Nissle 1917) was effective and safe in maintaining remission equivalent to the gold standard mesalazine in patients with UC (dose 50 billion CFU/day).[154] The *E.coli* (Nissle 1917) strain, sold elsewhere in enteric-coated capsules as "Mutaflor®," is not currently available in the United States as it was not considered a dietary ingredient by FDA, nor has it been approved as a drug.[155]

The other major probiotic mixture used in subjects with UC is the eight-strain probiotic blend known as VSL#3. This probiotic preparation (containing 3 strains of *Bifidobacterium*, 4 strains of *Lactobacilli*, and 1 strain of *Streptococcus salivarius* ssp.) has been used in at least nine different clinical trials in UC patients, most of them at very high doses (see Figure 28, Page 131). A recent meta-analysis of 5 of these trials (n=441) has been published, showing a pooled remission rate of 49%.[156] When pooling together three studies in which subjects were given 3.6 trillion CFU/day of the probiotic blend (in patients also given 5-ASA and/or immunomodulators), they realized a >50% decrease in disease activity index in 44.6% of subject taking probiotics (placebo 25.1%, p=0.008), a response rate of 53.4% (placebo 29.3, p < 0.001), and a remission rate of 43.8% (placebo 24.8%, p = 0.006). Studies were short, generally eight weeks, and there were no serious adverse effects at these doses.

Compared to these two preparations, there are only a few other probiotic strains or strain combinations that have been tested for benefit in UC subjects such as *S. boulardii*, *L. rhamnosus GG*, *B. breve*, *B. bifidum*, *L. acidophilus*, *B. lactis*, *L. casei*, *L. reuteri*, and *B. longum*, though most of these trials were small pilot trials, uncontrolled, given rectally or open-label studies.[157,158,159,160] Unfortunately, systematic studies have not been performed on most strains of probiotics (or combinations of strains) at high doses to compare to VSL#3. This strain combination generally fits with our recommendation of a multi-strain probiotic, though there are no specific studies comparing this particular blend with other similar blends. While no clinical study has been published to compare, it is likely that similar strain combination given at similar doses may have similar results. Clinicians should choose products, typically provided in pouches or sachets, that allow for very high dosing, as doses of greater than 3 trillion CFU/day may be needed over a two-month period to realize benefits in patients with UC.

In light of these studies, the clinician must always remember that that the efficacy of a probiotic preparation is unlikely to be the same in all patients or in the same patient at different stages of disease. Successful treatment may also be dependent on several variables, such as characteristics of a patient (gender, lifestyle habits, smoking status, age), lesions in IBD (location, extent, type of gross lesion), and risk factors (genetic predisposition, familial history). Most studies on probiotics have included women as a significant portion of the cohort, and men have traditionally been underrepresented.

Prebiotics and IBD

The role of prebiotics as therapeutic agents for IBD is not well as studied as probiotics. In many cases, fiber products that have limited evidence as prebiotics (e.g., psyllium) are evaluated along with well-known prebiotics (e.g., inulin). Nonetheless, several of both types of fiber have shown some benefit in subjects with both UC and CD. (see page 108 for discussion of prebiotics and the microbiome)

Psyllium seeds were shown to benefit UC patients in remission (n=105) in a randomized clinical trial where subjects were given either 10 g of ground psyllium seeds twice daily, 500 mg mesalamine three times daily, or a combination of mesalamine and psyllium for 12 months.[161] The relapse rate for the psyllium group (37.1%) and the mesalamine group (35.1%) were statistically the same after one year; and while the combination therapy had a lower relapse rate (23.3%), it was not statistically different than the others. The authors suggest that psyllium may be symptomatically equivalent to mesalamine for maintaining remission in subjects with UC (a trial published 8 years prior showed psyllium to be superior to placebo for similar outcomes).[162] We are not aware of any studies evaluating the role of psyllium in CD patients.

In contrast, inulin and fructoligosaccharides (FOS), both traditional prebiotics, have been evaluated in both UC and CD subjects. Patients with active Crohn's disease consume lower amounts of inulin-type fructans than either healthy controls or Crohn's patients in remission.[163] This suggests that inulin or FOS supplementation may improve disease outcome in these subjects. When this hypothesis was tested in intervention trials, however, there have been mixed results. The largest of these studies enrolled 103 *active* Crohn's patients (Crohn's Disease Activity Index [CDAI] ≥220), randomizing 54 to receive 15 g/day of FOS and 49 to receive a non-prebiotic placebo (maltodextrin) for 4 weeks.[164] First of all, 26% of the FOS-treated patients withdrew before the end of the trial, while only 8% of the placebo group withdrew, and therefore, they saw no difference between the groups in terms of improvement of disease activity scores using an intent-to-treat analysis. In contrast, a small pilot study of 10 active CD patients given 15 g/day of FOS for three weeks showed a statistical reduction in disease score (Harvey-Bradshaw index) and improvements in measures of fecal bacteria and dendritic cell activities.[165] Ironically, there were no dropouts or reports of serious adverse events. While it is difficult to merge these two studies into a meaningful conclusion, we suggest that longer trials using lower doses may be more appropriate to approximate how such prebiotics would be encountered in the diet. While the microbiome can change over a three- to four-week period, an individual with active auto-inflammation driven by immune activation to luminal bacteria may not realize benefits from these changes, or respond negatively to these changes (gas, bloating, etc.).

A small study evaluating the tolerability of inulin in subjects with active UC (n=19), all treated with 3 g/day of mesalazine, has been performed.[166] These subjects were randomly assigned to receive 12 g/day of an oligofructose-enriched inulin (4 gram/tid) or similar placebo (maltodextrin) for 14 days. A total of four individuals dropped out of this short study: three from the active and one from the placebo group. After two weeks, there was a significant decrease in disease activity scores in both groups (not statistically different between groups); though, while all seven subjects consuming inulin reached clinical remission, two of the eight subjects consuming placebo still showed clinical activity. Furthermore, there was a statistical decrease in fecal calprotectin levels in the inulin group that was not realized by the placebo group. While this study is small in size and short in length, it suggests prebiotics may be a helpful adjunct to standard therapy for UC.

Another prebiotic that has shown benefit in UC patients and animal models with colitis is germinated barley foodstuff (GBF), which mainly consists of a protein-rich insoluble fiber naturally rich in the amino acid glutamine. Kanauchi et al. reported an increase in SCFA production, a reduction in frequency of bowel movements, amelioration of severe bloody diarrhea, and an attenuation of colonic mucosal damage when rats (in an experimental colitis model) were administered GBF.[167] Furthermore, a small (and short) clinical trial involving mild to moderate UC patients (n=18) randomly assigned GBF (20-30 g/day) along with baseline anti-inflammatory or anti-inflammatory therapy alone was performed.[168] After four weeks of adding GBF to their standard therapy, subjects realized a statistically lower clinical activity score, suggesting an attenuation of symptoms. Currently, it does not appear that GBF is commercially available in the US for therapeutic use.

Clinicians should consider the use of prebiotics in subjects with IBD as a potential means to maintain a healthy microbiome (especially to increase butyrate production), rather than as a therapeutic intervention for IBD. **Note:** Prebiotics are generally excluded on a low FODMAP diet (see low FODMAP diet on page 236).

Botanicals and Phytonutrients as IBD Therapeutics

The use of botanical preparations (herbs, herbal extracts, or concentrated phytochemicals) for the management of chronic diseases of the GI tract is both an ancient practice and a modern focus of investigative research. Also, since many botanical compounds have been shown to have immune-modulating and anti-inflammatory effects, many of these compounds have been investigated in animal models of IBD, and some have been tested in clinical trials in subjects with IBD.

We have discussed the immune-modulating and anti-inflammatory mechanisms of many such compounds in our Standard Road map: *Supporting Immune Function: A Lifestyle and Nutrient Approach* (Point Institute, 2014). These include curcumin, boswellic acid, caffeic-acid phenyl esters (CAPE-propolis), quercetin and related flavonoids, Chinese skullcap, ginger, devil's claw, cat's claw, omega-3 fatty

acids, and others. It is possible that a majority of these compounds may be helpful at reducing inflammation in subjects with IBD and subsequently reduce disease index scores, induce or extend remission times. However, while some of these compounds have been tested in animal models of IBD, only a few of these compounds have been tested in human subjects, which is our focus in this discussion.

Curcuminoids (Turmeric)

Turmeric is a well-known flavorful spice derived from the herb *Curcuma longa*, a member of the ginger family. Turmeric is often used as a major cooking spice in curry, found predominantly in South Asian cuisines. Besides being a food flavoring and coloring agent, turmeric has been used in Ayurvedic medicine for numerous health benefits since ancient times. Curcuminoids are the major active constituents found in turmeric, and include curcumin, demethoxycurcumin and bisdemethoxycurcumin. Given the recent interest of turmeric for many health benefits, many papers have been published showing its role in the treatment or prevention of many diseases – ranging from heart disease to cancer.[169,170,171,172,173]

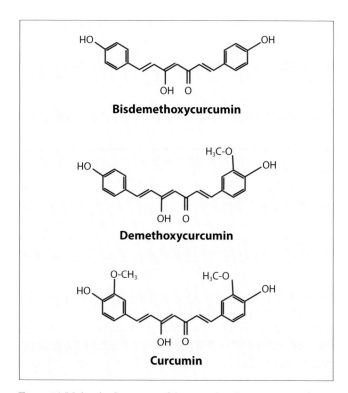

Figure 35: Molecular Structures of the most abundant curcuminoids found in turmeric root extracts. Together they are often known simply as "curcumin."

Curcumin is known to be a potent inhibitor of NF-κB, COX-2, LOX, as well as many other enzymes within the inflammatory pathway, many regulated through NF-κB.[174] Curcumin also reduces other inflammatory mediators such as IL-6, IL-1β, MCP-1 and metalloproteases in animal models.[175,176] Animal and cell culture studies have shown positive benefits for curcumin in diverse conditions such as ulcer prevention and healing, treating and preventing hepatotoxicity, direct anti-inflammatory studies (induced edema studies), reduction in advanced glycation end products (AGEs), antibacterial, antiviral and antitumor activities.[177] Perhaps most intriguing for its therapeutic potential for IBD is that several human clinical trials have shown that curcumin is a potent inhibitor of TNF-α signaling, considered to be a key regulator of the pathophysiology of IBD (and the reason for the use of anti-TNF-α biologic agents).[178,179]

While many studies have been performed in animal models of colitis, only a handful of clinical trials have been performed using curcumin in subjects with IBD. In an open-label pilot study, Holt and colleagues reported that curcumin reduced the inflammatory response in nine out of 10 patients with IBD (n=10, 5 UC, 5 CD).[180] The UC subjects were treated with 550 mg of curcumin (pure powder) twice daily for one month and then 550 mg three times daily for another month. The five CD patients were treated with 360 mg of curcumin (pure powder) three times daily for one month and then 360 mg four times daily for the remaining two months. Serological tests in all patients from both groups indicated a reduction of inflammation, and out of the 10 patients, nine reported an improvement in clinical symptoms (four of the five UC subjects decreased or eliminated pharmaceutical therapies).

Curcumin was evaluated for its ability to maintain remission among quiescent UC patients in a larger double-blind, randomized, placebo-controlled multicenter clinical trial.[181] In this trial, 89 UC patients were enrolled in one of two groups to either receive 1 g curcumin (powder in capsule) twice daily plus sulfasalazine (SZ) or mesalamine, or receive a placebo plus SZ or mesalamine. During this six-month trial, patients enrolled in the curcumin group experienced clinical improvement and a statistically significant decrease in the rate of relapse compared to placebo (4.65% vs. 20.5%). In these studies, curcumin was demonstrated to also have an excellent safety profile.

Recently, curcumin was tested as an adjunct to mesalamine for inducing remission in subjects with mild-moderate UC (n=50).[182] Subjects were already treated with mesalamine (optimized oral and topical) and randomized to receive one-month therapy of 3 g/day of curcumin (1.5 g bid, pure powder in capsules) or identical-looking placebo. After one month of therapy, 53.8% (14 of 26) of those taking the curcumin achieved remission while none of the 24 patients taking placebo achieved remission (p=0.01). Of those who consented to endoscopy prior to the start of the trial, 36.3% achieved endoscopic remission in the curcumin group, while none of the placebo group achieved remission (p=0.043).

In all studies to date, pure curcumin powder has been employed. While it is known that curcumin has poor bioavailability, and numerous curcumin preparations have become available designed to enhance absorption/bioavailability, these have yet to be evaluated in IBD subjects. Furthermore, while enhanced absorption may be a benefit for systemic inflammation, curcumin's role in the gut may actually be hindered by alterations that increase its bioavailability, making it less available to intestinal epithelial cells or the microbiota. It is also important to note that curcumin has been shown to modulate the gut microbiota in animal models of colitis, perhaps an important factor in its effect on IBD subjects.[183] Furthermore, each of the three curcuminoids is substantially metabolized into tetrahydrocurcumin by the gut microbiota, considered to be one of the more potent bioactive metabolites of curcumin.[184] Therefore, until studies of curcumin preparations with altered bioavailability are confirmed to be effective for inflammatory bowel disease or related GI applications, we can only recommend the use of highly concentrated curcumin extracts (~95%) at a dose of 1.5 to 3 g daily. These doses have shown to be tolerated in both adults and children.[185]

Boswellia
The resin of *Boswellia serrata* has been used for inflammatory conditions in Ayurvedic medicine for many years. The triterpene compounds, known as boswellic acids, are considered to be the main active compounds. Boswellic acids are strong inhibitors of 5-LOX and TNF-α induced metalloproteinase expression.[186,187] *Boswellia* is also known as an inhibitor of NF-κB, which helps to downregulate the pro-inflammatory cascade.[188] To date, there have been a few human studies showing

the efficacy of *Boswellia* preparations in subjects with IBD. *Boswellia* gum resin (350 mg/tid) was compared to sulfasalazine (SZ, 1 g/tid) during a six-week intervention trial among UC patients.[189] Patients that were administered *Boswellia* were found to have similar improvement (82% remission) as patients in the SZ group (75% remission). Following this trial, the same group of researchers conducted an interventional study involving 30 UC patients that were given *Boswellia* gum resin (900 mg daily, divided in three doses) or SZ (1 g/tid) for six weeks.[190] The primary goal of treatment was to attain remission. Secondary endpoints included changes in stool property, sigmoidoscopic scores, histopathology of colonic mucosa, and various laboratory markers of inflammation and anemia. Eighteen of the 20 patients in the *Boswellia* treatment group had improvement in at least one secondary endpoint, and 14 experienced remission. Conversely, six of the 10 patients in the SZ group had improvement in at least one secondary endpoint, and only four went into remission.

In a larger clinical trial in 22 centers throughout Germany, 108 patients with CD in remission were randomized to receive a soft gel preparation *Boswellia* resin extract (800 mg/tid) or matching placebo for 52 weeks.[191] After stopping the trial early for "insufficient discrimination of drug and placebo with regard to primary efficacy endpoint" they analyzed 66 patients for efficacy and found that 59.9% of subjects taking *Boswellia* remained in remission compared to 55.3% of those taking placebo. We should note that while this showed little benefit compared to placebo, this is an extremely high "placebo benefit." While this preparation was tolerated well, this study did not show any efficacy in this group of CD patients.

Boswellia serrata resin extracts may benefit IBD subjects, but more evidence will be needed to make specific recommendations, though some preparations may have more activity than others. In general, the use of curcumin appears to be the better choice over *Boswellia* preparations, though they may have some added benefit when combined.

Other Botanicals

A number of other botanical preparations, including a number of herbal combinations used in Traditional Chinese Medicine, have been used in clinical trials with IBD subjects, though rarely more than single small trials for each preparation. While some of these may be promising, more research is needed before specific recommendations can be given to clinicians. Some of them include: baicalin (from *Scuttelaria baicalensis*),[192] EGCG (green tea),[193] bilberry extract,[194] *Andrographis* extract,[195] wheat grass juice,[196] and several others not represented by commercially-available ingredients.

References

1. Kappelman MD, Rifas-Shiman SL, Kleinman K, et al. The prevalence and geographic distribution of Crohn's disease and ulcerative colitis in the United States. *Clin Gastroenterol Hepatol.* 2007 Dec;5(12):1424-9.
2. Nguyen GC, Chong CA, Chong RY. National estimates of the burden of inflammatory bowel disease among racial and ethnic groups in the United States. *J Crohns Colitis.* 2014 Apr;8(4):288-95.
3. Ananthakrishnan AN. Epidemiology and risk factors for IBD. *Nat Rev Gastroenterol Hepatol.* 2015 Apr;12(4):205-17.
4. Chen GI, Saibil F, Morava-Protzner I. Two for one: coexisting ulcerative colitis and Crohn's disease. *Can J Gastroenterol.* 2002 Jan;16(1):29-34.
5. Yadav V, Varum F, Bravo R, et al. Inflammatory bowel disease: exploring gut pathophysiology for novel therapeutic targets. *Transl Res.* 2016 May 6. pii: S1931-5244(16)30035-4.
6. Bamias G, Pizarro TT, Cominelli F. Pathway-based approaches to the treatment of inflammatory bowel disease. *Transl Res.* 2016 Jan;167(1):104-15.
7. Peyrin-Biroulet L, Panés J, Sandborn WJ, et al. Defining Disease Severity in Inflammatory Bowel Diseases: Current and Future Directions. *Clin Gastroenterol Hepatol.* 2016 Mar;14(3):348-354.e17.
8. Vindigni SM, Zisman TL, Suskind DL, Damman CJ. The intestinal microbiome, barrier function, and immune system in inflammatory bowel disease: a tripartite pathophysiological circuit with implications for new therapeutic directions. *Therap Adv Gastroenterol.* 2016 Jul;9(4):606-25.
9. Yamamoto-Furusho JK, Fonseca-Camarillo G. Genetic Markers Associated with Clinical Outcomes in Patients with Inflammatory Bowel Disease. *Inflamm Bowel Dis.* 2015 Nov;21(11):2683-95.
10. McGovern DP, Kugathasan S, Cho JH. Genetics of Inflammatory Bowel Diseases. *Gastroenterology.* 2015 Oct;149(5):1163-1176.e2.
11. Zanello G, Kevans D, Goethel A, et al. Genetics and innate and adaptive immunity in IBD. *Nestle Nutr Inst Workshop Ser.* 2014;79:41-55.
12. Cooney R, Jewell D. The genetic basis of inflammatory bowel disease. *Dig Dis.* 2009;27(4):428-42.
13. Michielan A, D'Incà R. Intestinal Permeability in Inflammatory Bowel Disease: Pathogenesis, Clinical Evaluation, and Therapy of Leaky Gut. *Mediators Inflamm.* 2015;2015:628157.
14. Geremia A, Biancheri P, Allan P, et al. Innate and adaptive immunity in inflammatory bowel disease. *Autoimmun Rev.* 2014 Jan;13(1):3-10.
15. Xu XR, Liu CQ, Feng BS1, Liu ZJ. Dysregulation of mucosal immune response in pathogenesis of inflammatory bowel disease. *World J Gastroenterol.* 2014 Mar 28;20(12):3255-64.
16. Boltin D, Perets TT, Vilkin A, Niv Y. Mucin function in inflammatory bowel disease: an update. *J Clin Gastroenterol.* 2013 Feb;47(2):106-11.
17. Lee SH. Intestinal permeability regulation by tight junction: implication on inflammatory bowel diseases. *Intest Res.* 2015 Jan;13(1):11-8.
18. Vanuytsel T, Vermeire S, Cleynen I. The role of Haptoglobin and its related protein, Zonulin, in inflammatory bowel disease. *Tissue Barriers.* 2013 Dec 1;1(5):e27321.
19. Miyoshi J, Chang EB. The gut microbiota and inflammatory bowel diseases. *Transl Res.* 2016 Jun 14. pii: S1931-5244(16)30095-0.
20. Takaishi H, Matsuki T, Nakazawa A, et al. Imbalance in intestinal microflora constitution could be involved in the pathogenesis of inflammatory bowel disease. *Int J Med Microbiol.* 2008 Jul;298(5-6):463-72.

21. Ott SJ, Musfeldt M, Wenderoth DF, et al. Reduction in diversity of the colonic mucosa associated bacterial microflora in patients with active inflammatory bowel disease. *Gut*. 2004 May;53(5):685-93

22. Manichanh C, Rigottier-Gois L, Bonnaud E, et al. Reduced diversity of faecal microbiota in Crohn's disease revealed by a metagenomic approach. *Gut*. 2006 Feb;55(2):205-11.

23. Lopez-Siles M, Martinez-Medina M, Abellà C, et al. Mucosa-associated Faecalibacterium prausnitzii phylotype richness is reduced in patients with inflammatory bowel disease. *Appl Environ Microbiol*. 2015 Nov;81(21):7582-92.

24. Sokol H, Seksik P, Furet JP, et al. Low counts of Faecalibacterium prausnitzii in colitis microbiota. *Inflamm Bowel Dis*. 2009 Aug;15(8):1183-9.

25. Sokol H, Pigneur B, Watterlot L, et al. Faecalibacterium prausnitzii is an anti-inflammatory commensal bacterium identified by gut microbiota analysis of Crohn disease patients. *Proc Natl Acad Sci U S A*. 2008 Oct 28;105(43):16731-6.

26. Machiels K, Joossens M, Sabino J, et al. A decrease of the butyrate-producing species Roseburia hominis and Faecalibacterium prausnitzii defines dysbiosis in patients with ulcerative colitis. *Gut*. 2014 Aug;63(8):1275-83.

27. Wills ES, Jonkers DM, Savelkoul PH, et al. Fecal microbial composition of ulcerative colitis and Crohn's disease patients in remission and subsequent exacerbation. *PLoS One*. 2014 Mar 7;9(3):e90981.

28. Bernstein, C. N. and Shanahan, F. Disorders of a modern lifestyle: reconciling the epidemiology of inflammatory bowel diseases. *Gut*. 2008; 57(9):1185-1191.

29. Lewis JD. A review of the epidemiology of inflammatory bowel disease with a focus on diet, infections and antibiotic exposure. *Nestle Nutr Inst Workshop Ser*. 2014;79:1-18.

30. Lee TW, Russell L, Deng M, Gibson PR. Association of doxycycline use with the development of gastroenteritis, irritable bowel syndrome and inflammatory bowel disease in Australians deployed abroad. *Intern Med J*. 2013 Aug;43(8):919-26.

31. Ungaro R, Bernstein CN, Gearry R, Hviid A, Kolho KL, Kronman MP, Shaw S, Van Kruiningen H, Colombel JF, Atreja A. Antibiotics associated with increased risk of new-onset Crohn's disease but not ulcerative colitis: a meta-analysis. *Am J Gastroenterol*. 2014;109:1728-1738.

32. Legaki E, Gazouli M. Influence of environmental factors in the development of inflammatory bowel diseases. *World J Gastrointest Pharmacol Ther*. 2016 Feb 6;7(1):112-25.

33. Lakatos, P. L., Szamosi, T. et al. Smoking in inflammatory bowel diseases: good, bad or ugly? *World J Gastroenterol*. 2007; 13(46):6134-6139.

34. Lunney PC, Kariyawasam VC, Wang RR, et al. Smoking prevalence and its influence on disease course and surgery in Crohn's disease and ulcerative colitis. *Aliment Pharmacol Ther*. 2015 Jul;42(1):61-70.

35. Cosnes, J. Tobacco and IBD: relevance in the understanding of disease mechanisms and clinical practice. *Best Pract Res Clin Gastroenterol*. 2004; 18(3):481-496.

36. Lunney PC, Leong RW. Review article: Ulcerative colitis, smoking and nicotine therapy. *Aliment Pharmacol Ther*. 2012 Dec;36(11-12):997-1008.

37. Biedermann L, Zeitz J, Mwinyi J, et al. Smoking cessation induces profound changes in the composition of the intestinal microbiota in humans. *PLoS One*. 2013;8(3):e59260.

38. Ducharme-Bénard S, Côté-Daigneault J, et al. Patients With Inflammatory Bowel Disease Are Unaware of the Impact of Smoking on Their Disease. *J Clin Gastroenterol*. 2016 Jul;50(6):490-7.

39. De Bie C, Ballet V, Hendriks N, et al. Smoking behaviour and knowledge of the health effects of smoking in patients with inflammatory bowel disease. *Aliment Pharmacol Ther*. 2015 Dec;42(11-12):1294-302.

40. Severs M, van Erp SJ, van der Valk ME, et al. Smoking is Associated With Extra-intestinal Manifestations in Inflammatory Bowel Disease. *J Crohns Colitis*. 2016 Apr;10(4):455-61.

41. Lee D, Albenberg L, Compher C, et al. Diet in the pathogenesis and treatment of inflammatory bowel diseases. *Gastroenterology*. 2015 May;148(6):1087-106.

42. Dolan KT, Chang EB. Diet, gut microbes, and the pathogenesis of inflammatory bowel diseases. *Mol Nutr Food Res*. 2016 Jun 27. doi: 10.1002/mnfr.201600129. [Epub ahead of print]

43. Dixon LJ, Kabi A, Nickerson KP, McDonald C. Combinatorial effects of diet and genetics on inflammatory bowel disease pathogenesis. *Inflamm Bowel Dis*. 2015 Apr;21(4):912-22.

44. Liu X, Wu Y, Li F, Zhang D. Dietary fiber intake reduces risk of inflammatory bowel disease: result from a meta-analysis. *Nutr Res*. 2015 Sep;35(9):753-8.

45. Ananthakrishnan AN, Khalili H, Konijeti GG, et al. A prospective study of long-term intake of dietary fiber and risk of Crohn's disease and ulcerative colitis. *Gastroenterology*. 2013 Nov;145(5):970-7.

46. Reif, S., Klein, I. et al. Pre-illness dietary factors in inflammatory bowel disease. *Gut*. 1997; 40(6):754-760.

47. Tragnone, A., Valpiani, D. et al. Dietary habits as risk factors for inflammatory bowel disease. *Eur J Gastroenterol Hepatol*. 1995; 7(1):47-51.

48. Racine A, Carbonnel F, Chan SS, et al. Dietary Patterns and Risk of Inflammatory Bowel Disease in Europe: Results from the EPIC Study. *Inflamm Bowel Dis*. 2016 Feb;22(2):345-54.

49. Chan SS, Luben R, Olsen A, et al. Association between high dietary intake of the n-3 polyunsaturated fatty acid docosahexaenoic acid and reduced risk of Crohn's disease. *Aliment Pharmacol Ther*. 2014 Apr;39(8):834-42.

50. Reifen R, Karlinsky A, Stark AH, Berkovich Z, Nyska A. α-Linolenic acid (ALA) is an anti-inflammatory agent in inflammatory bowel disease. *J Nutr Biochem*. 2015 Dec;26(12):1632-40.

51. Barbalho SM, Goulart Rde A, Quesada K, et al. Inflammatory bowel disease: can omega-3 fatty acids really help? *Ann Gastroenterol*. 2016 Jan-Mar;29(1):37-43.

52. John S., Luben R., Shrestha S.S., Welch A., Khaw K.T., and Hart A.R.: Dietary n-3 polyunsaturated fatty acids and the aetiology of ulcerative colitis: a UK prospective cohort study. *Eur. J. Gastroenterol. Hepatol*. 2010; 22: pp. 602-606.

53. Schwanke RC, Marcon R, Bento AF, Calixto JB. EPA- and DHA-derived resolvins' actions in inflammatory bowel disease. *Eur J Pharmacol*. 2016 Aug 15;785:156-64.

54. Tjonneland A, Overvad K, et al. Linoleic acid, a dietary n-6 polyunsaturated fatty acid, and the aetiology of ulcerative colitis: a nested case-control study within a European prospective cohort study. *Gut*. 2009;58:1606–11.

55. Hou JK, Abraham B, El-Serag H. Dietary intake and risk of developing inflammatory bowel disease: a systematic review of the literature. *Am J Gastroenterol*. 2011;106:563–73.

56. De Silva P.S., Olsen A., Christensen J., Schmidt E.B., Overvaad K., Tjonneland A., and Hart A.R.: An association between dietary arachidonic acid, measured in adipose tissue, and ulcerative colitis. *Gastroenterology* 2010; 139: pp. 1912-1917.

57. Tyagi A, Kumar U, Santosh VS, et al. Partial replacement of dietary linoleic acid with long chain n-3 polyunsaturated fatty acids protects against dextran sulfate sodium-induced colitis in rats. *Prostaglandins Leukot Essent Fatty Acids*. 2014 Dec;91(6):289-97.

58. Ananthakrishnan AN, Khalili H, Konijeti GG, et al. Long-term intake of dietary fat and risk of ulcerative colitis and Crohn's disease. *Gut*. 2014 May;63(5):776-84.

59. Hou JK, Abraham B, El-Serag H. Dietary intake and risk of developing inflammatory bowel disease: a systematic review of the literature. *Am J Gastroenterol*. 2011;106:563-573.

60. Amre DK, D'Souza S, Morgan K, Seidman G, Lambrette P, Grimard G, Israel D, Mack D, Ghadirian P, Deslandres C. Imbalances in dietary consumption of fatty acids, vegetables, and fruits are associated with risk for Crohn's disease in children. *Am J Gastroenterol*. 2007;102:2016-2025.

61. Li F, Liu X, Wang W, Zhang D. Consumption of vegetables and fruit and the risk of inflammatory bowel disease: a meta-analysis. *Eur J Gastroenterol Hepatol*. 2015 Jun;27(6):623-30.

62. Somani SJ, Modi KP, Majumdar AS, Sadarani BN. Phytochemicals and their potential usefulness in inflammatory bowel disease. *Phytother Res*. 2015 Mar;29(3):339-50.

63. Kaulmann A, Bohn T. Bioactivity of Polyphenols: Preventive and Adjuvant Strategies toward Reducing Inflammatory Bowel Diseases-Promises, Perspectives, and Pitfalls. *Oxid Med Cell Longev*. 2016;2016:9346470.

64. Bifulco M. Mediterranean diet: the missing link between gut microbiota and inflammatory diseases. *Eur J Clin Nutr*. 2015 Sep;69(9):1078.

65. Marlow G, Ellett S, Ferguson IR, et al. Transcriptomics to study the effect of a Mediterranean-inspired diet on inflammation in Crohn's disease patients. *Hum Genomics*. 2013 Nov 27;7:24.

66. de Silva PS, Luben R, Shrestha SS, et al. Dietary arachidonic and oleic acid intake in ulcerative colitis etiology: a prospective cohort study using 7-day food diaries. *Eur J Gastroenterol Hepatol*. 2014 Jan;26(1):11-8.

67. Reber SO. Stress and animal models of inflammatory bowel disease--an update on the role of the hypothalamo-pituitary-adrenal axis. *Psychoneuroendocrinology*. 2012 Jan;37(1):1-19.

68. Stasi C, Orlandelli E. Role of the brain-gut axis in the pathophysiology of Crohn's disease. *Dig Dis*. 2008;26(2):156-66.

69. Broersen LH, Pereira AM, Jørgensen JO, Dekkers OM. Adrenal Insufficiency in Corticosteroids Use: Systematic Review and Meta-Analysis. *J Clin Endocrinol Metab*. 2015 Jun;100(6):2171-80.

70. Viennois E, Zhao Y, Merlin D. Biomarkers of Inflammatory Bowel Disease: From Classical Laboratory Tools to Personalized Medicine. *Inflamm Bowel Dis.* 2015 Oct;21(10):2467-74.
71. Soubières AA, Poullis A. Emerging Biomarkers for the Diagnosis and Monitoring of Inflammatory Bowel Diseases. *Inflamm Bowel Dis.* 2016 Aug;22(8):2016-22.
72. Solem CA, Loftus EV Jr, Tremaine WJ, et al. Correlation of C-reactive protein with clinical, endoscopic, histologic, and radiographic activity in inflammatory bowel disease. *Inflamm Bowel Dis.* 2005 Aug;11(8):707-12.
73. Rodgers AD, Cummins AG. CRP correlates with clinical score in ulcerative colitis but not in Crohn's disease. *Dig Dis Sci.* 2007 Sep;52(9):2063-8.
74. Langhorst J, Elsenbruch S, Koelzer J, et al. Noninvasive markers in the assessment of intestinal inflammation in inflammatory bowel diseases: performance of fecal lactoferrin, calprotectin, and PMN-elastase, CRP, and clinical indices. *Am J Gastroenterol.* 2008 Jan;103(1):162-9.
75. Menees SB, Powell C, Kurlander J, Goel A, Chey WD. A meta-analysis of the utility of C-reactive protein, erythrocyte sedimentation rate, fecal calprotectin, and fecal lactoferrin to exclude inflammatory bowel disease in adults with IBS. *Am J Gastroenterol.* 2015 Mar;110(3):444-54.
76. Walsham NE, Sherwood RA. Fecal calprotectin in inflammatory bowel disease. *Clin Exp Gastroenterol.* 2016 Jan 28;9:21-9.
77. Sipponen T, Kolho KL. Fecal calprotectin in diagnosis and clinical assessment of inflammatory bowel disease. *Scand J Gastroenterol.* 2015 Jan;50(1):74-80.
78. van Rheenen PF, Van de Vijver E, Fidler V. Faecal calprotectin for screening of patients with suspected inflammatory bowel disease: diagnostic meta-analysis. *BMJ.* 2010 Jul 15;341:c3369.
79. Reese GE, Constantinides VA, Simillis C, et al. Diagnostic precision of anti-Saccharomyces cerevisiae antibodies and perinuclear antineutrophil cytoplasmic antibodies in inflammatory bowel disease. *Am J Gastroenterol.* 2006 Oct;101(10):2410-22.
80. Ham M, Moss AC. Mesalamine in the treatment and maintenance of remission of ulcerative colitis. *Expert Rev Clin Pharmacol.* 2012 Mar;5(2):113-23.
81. Sonu I, Lin MV, Blonski W, Lichtenstein GR. Clinical pharmacology of 5-ASA compounds in inflammatory bowel disease. *Gastroenterol Clin N Am.* 2010;39:559–599.
82. Zenlea T, Peppercorn MA. Immunosuppressive therapies for inflammatory bowel disease. *World J Gastroenterol.* 2014 Mar 28;20(12):3146-52.
83. Levin AD, Wildenberg ME, van den Brink GR. Mechanism of Action of Anti-TNF Therapy in Inflammatory Bowel Disease. *J Crohns Colitis.* 2016 Aug;10(8):989-97.
84. Danese S, Vuitton L, Peyrin-Biroulet L. Biologic agents for IBD: practical insights. *Nat Rev Gastroenterol Hepatol.* 2015 Sep;12(9):537-45.
85. Khanna R, Feagan BG. Safety of infliximab for the treatment of inflammatory bowel disease: current understanding of the potential for serious adverse events. *Expert Opin Drug Saf.* 2015 Jun;14(6):987-97.
86. Ben-Horin S, Casteele NV, Schreiber S, Lakatos P. Biosimilars in Inflammatory Bowel Disease: Facts and Fears of Extrapolation. *Clin Gastroenterol Hepatol.* 2016 May 20. pii: S1542-3565(16)30212-9.
87. Riordan, A. M., Hunter, J. O. et al. Treatment of active Crohn's disease by exclusion diet: East Anglian multicentre controlled trial. *Lancet.* 1993; 342(8880):1131-1134.
88. Giaffer, M. H., Cann, P. et al. Long-term effects of elemental and exclusion diets for Crohn's disease. *Aliment Pharmacol Ther.* 1991; 5(2):115-125.
89. Maconi G, Dominici R, Molteni M, et al. Prevalence of pancreatic insufficiency in inflammatory bowel diseases. Assessment by fecal elastase-1. *Dig Dis Sci.* 2008 Jan;53(1): 262-70.
90. Antonini F, Pezzilli R, Angelelli L, Macarri G. Pancreatic disorders in inflammatory bowel disease. *World J Gastrointest Pathophysiol.* 2016 Aug 15;7(3):276-82.
91. Gearry RB, Irving PM, Barrett JS, et al. Reduction of dietary poorly absorbed short-chain carbohydrates (FODMAPs) improves abdominal symptoms in patients with Inflammatory bowel disease-a pilot study. *J Crohns Colitis.* 2009 Feb;3(1):8-14.
92. Colman RJ, Rubin DT. Fecal microbiota transplantation as therapy for inflammatory bowel disease: a systematic review and meta-analysis. *J Crohns Colitis.* 2014 Dec;8(12): 1569-81.
93. Lopez J, Grinspan A. Fecal Microbiota Transplantation for Inflammatory Bowel Disease. *Gastroenterol Hepatol* (N Y). 2016 Jun;12(6):374-9.
94. Goh, J. and O'Morain, C. A. Review article: nutrition and adult inflammatory bowel disease. *Aliment Pharmacol Ther.* 2003; 17(3):307-320.
95. Owczarek D, Rodacki T, et al. Diet and nutritional factors in inflammatory bowel diseases. *World J Gastroenterol.* 2016 Jan 21;22(3):895-905.
96. Weisshof R, Chermesh I. Micronutrient deficiencies in inflammatory bowel disease. *Curr Opin Clin Nutr Metab Care.* 2015 Nov;18(6):576-81.
97. Kamata N, Oshitani N, Watanabe K, et al. Efficacy of concomitant elemental diet therapy in scheduled infliximab therapy in patients with Crohn's disease to prevent loss of response. *Dig Dis Sci.* 2015 May;60(5):1382-8.
98. Tsertsvadze A, Gurung T, Court R, Clarke A, Sutcliffe P. Clinical effectiveness and cost-effectiveness of elemental nutrition for the maintenance of remission in Crohn's disease: a systematic review and meta-analysis. *Health Technol Assess.* 2015 Mar;19(26):1-138.
99. Hou YC, Wu JM, Wang MY, et al. Glutamine supplementation attenuates expressions of adhesion molecules and chemokine receptors on T cells in a murine model of acute colitis. *Mediators Inflamm.* 2014;2014:837107.
100. Crespo I, San-Miguel B, Prause C, et al. Glutamine treatment attenuates endoplasmic reticulum stress and apoptosis in TNBS-induced colitis. *PLoS One.* 2012;7(11):e50407.
101. Buchman AL. Glutamine for the gut: mystical properties or an ordinary amino acid? *Curr Gastroenterol Rep.* 1999 Oct;1(5):417-23.
102. Akobeng AK, Elawad M, Gordon M. Glutamine for induction of remission in Crohn's disease. *Cochrane Database Syst Rev.* 2016 Feb 8;2:CD007348.
103. Ockenga J, Borchert K, Stüber E, et al. Glutamine-enriched total parenteral nutrition in patients with inflammatory bowel disease. *Eur J Clin Nutr.* 2005 Nov;59(11):1302-9.
104. Akobeng AK, Miller V, Stanton J, et al. Double-blind randomized controlled trial of glutamine-enriched polymeric diet in the treatment of active Crohn's disease. *J Pediatr Gastroenterol Nutr.* 2000 Jan;30(1):78-84.
105. Benjamin J, Makharia G, Ahuja V, et al. Glutamine and whey protein improve intestinal permeability and morphology in patients with Crohn's disease: a randomized controlled trial. *Dig Dis Sci.* 2012 Apr;57(4):1000-12.
106. Beaufrère AM, Neveux N, Patureau Mirand P, et al. Long-term intermittent glutamine supplementation repairs intestinal damage (structure and functional mass) with advanced age: assessment with plasma citrulline in a rodent model. *J Nutr Health Aging.* 2014 Nov;18(9):814-9.
107. Lin R. Crosstalk between Vitamin D Metabolism, VDR Signalling, and Innate Immunity. *Biomed Res Int.* 2016;2016:1375858.
108. Wei R, Christakos S. Mechanisms Underlying the Regulation of Innate and Adaptive Immunity by Vitamin D. *Nutrients.* 2015 Sep 24;7(10):8251-60.
109. Trochoutsou A, Kloukina V, Samitas K, Xanthou G. Vitamin-D in the Immune System: Genomic and Non-Genomic Actions. *Mini Rev Med Chem.* 2015;15(11):953-63.
110. Bscheider M, Butcher EC. Vitamin D immunoregulation through dendritic cells. *Immunology.* 2016 Jul;148(3):227-36.
111. Schiavi E, Smolinska S, O'Mahony L. Intestinal dendritic cells. *Curr Opin Gastroenterol.* 2015 Mar;31(2):98-103.
112. Rutella S, Locatelli F. Intestinal dendritic cells in the pathogenesis of inflammatory bowel disease. *World J Gastroenterol.* 2011 Sep 7;17(33):3761-75.
113. Niess JH. Role of gut-resident dendritic cells in inflammatory bowel disease. *Expert Rev Clin Immunol.* 2009 Jul;5(4):451-61.
114. Limketkai BN, Bechtold ML, Nguyen DL. Vitamin D and the Pathogenesis of Inflammatory Bowel Disease. *Curr Gastroenterol Rep.* 2016 Oct;18(10):52.
115. McGonagle D, McDermott MF. A proposed classification of the immunological diseases. *PLoS Med.* 2006 Aug;3(8):e297.
116. Limketkai BN, Bechtold ML, Nguyen DL. Vitamin D and the Pathogenesis of Inflammatory Bowel Disease. *Curr Gastroenterol Rep.* 2016 Oct;18(10):52.
117. Nerich V, Jantchou P, Boutron-Ruault MC, Monnet E, Weill A, Vanbockstael V, et al. Low exposure to sunlight is a risk factor for Crohn's disease. *Aliment Pharmacol Ther.* 2011;33:940–5.
118. Del Pinto R, Pietropaoli D, Chandar AK, Ferri C, Cominelli F. Association Between Inflammatory Bowel Disease and Vitamin D Deficiency: A Systematic Review and Meta-analysis. *Inflamm Bowel Dis.* 2015 Nov;21(11):2708-17.
119. Raftery T, Martineau AR, Greiller CL, et al. Effects of vitamin D supplementation on intestinal permeability, cathelicidin and disease markers in Crohn's disease: Results from a randomised double-blind placebo-controlled study. *United European Gastroenterol J.* 2015 Jun;3(3):294-302.
120. Sharifi A, Hosseinzadeh-Attar MJ, Vahedi H, Nedjat S. A randomized controlled trial on the effect of vitamin D3 on inflammation and cathelicidin gene expression in ulcerative colitis patients. *Saudi J Gastroenterol.* 2016 Jul-Aug;22(4):316-23.
121. Kojecky V, Adamikova A, Klimek P. Vitamin D supplementation in inflammatory bowel disease: the role of dosage and patient compliance. *Bratisl Lek Listy.* 2016;117(3):148-51.
122. Hlavaty T, Krajcovicova A, Koller T, et al. Higher vitamin D serum concentration increases health related quality of life in patients with inflammatory bowel diseases. *World J Gastroenterol.* 2014 Nov 14;20(42):15787-96.
123. Wingate KE, Jacobson K, Issenman R, et al. 25-Hydroxyvitamin D concentrations in children with Crohn's disease supplemented with either 2000 or 400 IU daily for 6 months: a randomized controlled study. *J Pediatr.* 2014 Apr;164(4):860-5.

124. Pappa HM, Mitchell PD, Jiang H, Kassiff S, et al. Treatment of vitamin D insufficiency in children and adolescents with inflammatory bowel disease: a randomized clinical trial comparing three regimens. *J Clin Endocrinol Metab*. 2012 Jun;97(6):2134-42.

125. Pappa HM, Mitchell PD, Jiang H, et al. Maintenance of optimal vitamin D status in children and adolescents with inflammatory bowel disease: a randomized clinical trial comparing two regimens. *J Clin Endocrinol Metab*. 2014 Sep;99(9):3408-17.

126. Simek RZ, Prince J, Syed S, et al. Pilot Study Evaluating Efficacy of 2 Regimens for Hypovitaminosis D Repletion in Pediatric Inflammatory Bowel Disease. *J Pediatr Gastroenterol Nutr*. 2016 Feb;62(2):252-8.

127. Jørgensen SP, Agnholt J, Glerup H, et al. Clinical trial: vitamin D3 treatment in Crohn's disease - a randomized double-blind placebo-controlled study. *Aliment Pharmacol Ther*. 2010 Aug;32(3):377-83.

128. Target Levels and Optimal Dosing of Vitamin D. Published Online at http://www.pointinstitute.org/wp-content/uploads/2012/10/Target-serum-levels-and-optimal-dosing-of-vitamin-D-paper.pdf

129. Aloia JF, Patel M, Dimaano R, et al. Vitamin D intake to attain a desired serum 25-hydroxyvitamin D concentration. *Am J Clin Nutr*. 2008 Jun;87(6):1952-8.

130. Cabré E, Mañosa M, Gassull MA. Omega-3 fatty acids and inflammatory bowel diseases - a systematic review. *Br J Nutr*. 2012 Jun;107 Suppl 2:S240-52.

131. Turner D, Shah PS, Steinhart AH, et al. Maintenance of remission in inflammatory bowel disease using omega-3 fatty acids (fish oil): a systematic review and meta-analyses. *Inflamm Bowel Dis*. 2011 Jan;17(1):336-45.

132. Romano C, Cucchiara S, Barabino A, et al. Usefulness of omega-3 fatty acid supplementation in addition to mesalazine in maintaining remission in pediatric Crohn's disease: a double-blind, randomized, placebo-controlled study. *World J Gastroenterol*. 2005 Dec 7;11(45):7118-21.

133. Li K, Huang T, Zheng J, Wu K, Li D. Effect of marine-derived n-3 polyunsaturated fatty acids on C-reactive protein, interleukin 6 and tumor necrosis factor α: a meta-analysis. *PLoS One*. 2014 Feb 5;9(2):e88103.

134. Belluzzi, A., Brignola, C. et al. Effect of an enteric-coated fish-oil preparation on relapses in Crohn's disease. *N Engl J Med*. 1996; 334(24):1557-1560.

135. Aslan, A. and Triadafilopoulos, G. Fish oil fatty acid supplementation in active ulcerative colitis: a double-blind, placebo-controlled, crossover study. *Am J Gastroenterol*. 1992; 87(4):432-437.

136. Braun A, Treede I, Gotthardt D, et al. Alterations of phospholipid concentration and species composition of the intestinal mucus barrier in ulcerative colitis: a clue to pathogenesis. *Inflamm Bowel Dis*. 2009 Nov;15(11):1705-20.

137. Ehehalt R, Braun A, Karner M, et al. Phosphatidylcholine as a constituent in the colonic mucosal barrier--physiological and clinical relevance. *Biochim Biophys Acta*. 2010 Sep;1801(9):983-93.

138. Stremmel W, Hanemann A, Braun A, et al. Delayed release phosphatidylcholine as new therapeutic drug for ulcerative colitis--a review of three clinical trials. *Expert Opin Investig Drugs*. 2010 Dec;19(12):1623-30.

139. Stremmel W, Ehehalt R, Autschbach F, Karner M. Phosphatidylcholine for steroid-refractory chronic ulcerative colitis: a randomized trial. *Ann Intern Med*. 2007 Nov 6;147(9):603-10.

140. Karner M, Kocjan A, Stein J, et al. First multicenter study of modified release phosphatidylcholine "LT-02" in ulcerative colitis: a randomized, placebo-controlled trial in mesalazine-refractory courses. *Am J Gastroenterol*. 2014 Jul;109(7):1041-51.

141. Ghouri YA, Richards DM, Rahimi EF, et al. Systematic review of randomized controlled trials of probiotics, prebiotics, and synbiotics in inflammatory bowel disease. *Clin Exp Gastroenterol*. 2014 Dec 9;7:473-87.

142. Lichtenstein L, Avni-Biron I, Ben-Bassat O. Probiotics and prebiotics in Crohn's disease therapies. *Best Pract Res Clin Gastroenterol*. 2016 Feb;30(1):81-8.

143. Lichtenstein L, Avni-Biron I, Ben-Bassat O. The current place of probiotics and prebiotics in the treatment of pouchitis. *Best Pract Res Clin Gastroenterol*. 2016 Feb;30(1):73-80.

144. Derikx LA, Dieleman LA, Hoentjen F. Probiotics and prebiotics in ulcerative colitis. *Best Pract Res Clin Gastroenterol*. 2016 Feb;30(1):55-71.

145. Chibbar R, Dieleman LA. Probiotics in the Management of Ulcerative Colitis. *J Clin Gastroenterol*. 2015 Nov-Dec;49 Suppl 1:S50-5.

146. Guandalini S, Cernat E, Moscoso D. Prebiotics and probiotics in irritable bowel syndrome and inflammatory bowel disease in children. *Benef Microbes*. 2015;6(2):209-17.

147. Plein K, Hotz J. Therapeutic effects of Saccharomyces boulardii on mild residual symptoms in a stable phase of Crohn's disease with special respect to chronic diarrhea--a pilot study. *Z Gastroenterol*. 1993 Feb;31(2):129-34.

148. Guslandi M, Mezzi G, Sorghi M, Testoni PA. Saccharomyces boulardii in maintenance treatment of Crohn's disease. *Dig Dis Sci*. 2000 Jul;45(7):1462-4.

149. Steed H, Macfarlane GT, Blackett KL, et al. Clinical trial: the microbiological and immunological effects of synbiotic consumption - a randomized double-blind placebo-controlled study in active Crohn's disease. *Aliment Pharmacol Ther*. 2010 Oct;32(7):872-83.

150. Fujimori S., Tatsuguchi A., Gudis K., Kishida T., Mitsui K., Ehara A., et al: High dose probiotic and prebiotic cotherapy for remission induction of active Crohn's disease. *J Gastroenterol Hepatol* 2007; 22: pp. 1199-1204.

151. Fedorak RN, Feagan BG, Hotte N, et al. The probiotic VSL#3 has anti-inflammatory effects and could reduce endoscopic recurrence after surgery for Crohn's disease. *Clin Gastroenterol Hepatol*. 2015 May;13(5):928-35.e2.

152. Kruis, W., Schutz, E. et al. Double-blind comparison of an oral Escherichia coli preparation and mesalazine in maintaining remission of ulcerative colitis. *Aliment Pharmacol Ther*. 1997; 11(5):853-858.

153. Rembacken, B. J., Snelling, A. M. et al. Non-pathogenic Escherichia coli versus mesalazine for the treatment of ulcerative colitis: a randomised trial. *Lancet*. 1999; 354(9179):635-639.

154. Kruis, W., Fric, P. et al. Maintaining remission of ulcerative colitis with the probiotic Escherichia coli Nissle 1917 is as effective as with standard mesalazine. *Gut*. 2004; 53(11):1617-1623.

155. https://www.regulations.gov/document?D=FDA-2012-S-1178-0014.

156. Mardini HE, Grigorian AY. Probiotic mix VSL#3 is effective adjunctive therapy for mild to moderately active ulcerative colitis: a meta-analysis. *Inflamm Bowel Dis*. 2014 Sep;20(9):1562-7.

157. Guslandi M, Giollo P, Testoni PA. A pilot trial of Saccharomyces boulardii in ulcerative colitis. *Eur J Gastroenterol Hepatol*. 2003 Jun;15(6):697-8.

158. Kato K, Mizuno S, Umesaki Y, et al. Randomized placebo-controlled trial assessing the effect of bifidobacteria-fermented milk on active ulcerative colitis. *Aliment Pharmacol Ther*. 2004 Nov 15;20(10):1133-41.

159. Oliva S, Di Nardo G, Ferrari F, et al. Randomised clinical trial: the effectiveness of Lactobacillus reuteri ATCC 55730 rectal enema in children with active distal ulcerative colitis. *Aliment Pharmacol Ther*. 2012 Feb;35(3):327-34.

160. Wildt S, Nordgaard I, Hansen U, et al. A randomised double-blind placebo-controlled trial with Lactobacillus acidophilus La-5 and Bifidobacterium animalis subsp. lactis BB-12 for maintenance of remission in ulcerative colitis. *J Crohns Colitis*. 2011 Apr;5(2):115-21.

161. Fernández-Bañares F, Hinojosa J, Sánchez-Lombraña JL, et al. Randomized clinical trial of Plantago ovata seeds (dietary fiber) as compared with mesalamine in maintaining remission in ulcerative colitis. Spanish Group for the Study of Crohn's Disease and Ulcerative Colitis (GETECCU). *Am J Gastroenterol*. 1999 Feb;94(2):427-33.

162. Hallert C, Kaldma M, Petersson BG. Ispaghula husk may relieve gastrointestinal symptoms in ulcerative colitis in remission. *Scand J Gastroenterol*. 1991 Jul;26(7):747-50.

163. Anderson JL, Hedin CR, Benjamin JL, et al. Dietary intake of inulin-type fructans in active and inactive Crohn's disease and healthy controls: a case-control study. *J Crohns Colitis*. 2015 Nov;9(11):1024-31.

164. Benjamin JL, Hedin CR, Koutsoumpas A, et al. Randomised, double-blind, placebo-controlled trial of fructo-oligosaccharides in active Crohn's disease. *Gut*. 2011 Jul;60(7):923-9.

165. Lindsay JO, Whelan K, Stagg AJ, et al. Clinical, microbiological, and immunological effects of fructo-oligosaccharide in patients with Crohn's disease. *Gut*. 2006 Mar;55(3):348-55.

166. Casellas F, Borruel N, Torrejón A, et al. Oral oligofructose-enriched inulin supplementation in acute ulcerative colitis is well tolerated and associated with lowered faecal calprotectin. *Aliment Pharmacol Ther*. 2007 May 1;25(9):1061-7.

167. Kanauchi, O., Iwanaga, T. et al. Dietary fiber fraction of germinated barley foodstuff attenuated mucosal damage and diarrhea, and accelerated the repair of the colonic mucosa in an experimental colitis. *J Gastroenterol Hepatol*. 2001; 16(2):160-168.

168. Kanauchi O, Suga T, Tochihara M, et al. Treatment of ulcerative colitis by feeding with germinated barley foodstuff: first report of a multicenter open control trial. *J Gastroenterol*. 2002 Nov;37 Suppl 14:67-72.

169. Kunnumakkara AB, Bordoloi D, Padmavathi G, et al. Curcumin, The Golden Nutraceutical: Multitargeting for Multiple Chronic Diseases. *Br J Pharmacol*. 2016 Sep 17. doi: 10.1111/bph.13621. [Epub ahead of print]

170. Kasi PD, Tamilselvam R, Skalicka-Woźniak K, et al. Molecular targets of curcumin for cancer therapy: an updated review. *Tumour Biol*. 2016 Jul 28. [Epub ahead of print]

171. Ghosh S, Banerjee S, Sil PC. The beneficial role of curcumin on inflammation, diabetes and neurodegenerative disease: A recent update. *Food Chem Toxicol*. 2015 Sep;83:111-24.

172. Shanmugam MK, Rane G, Kanchi MM, et al. The multifaceted role of curcumin in cancer prevention and treatment. *Molecules*. 2015 Feb 5;20(2):2728-69.

173. Gupta SC, Patchva S, Aggarwal BB. Therapeutic roles of curcumin: lessons learned from clinical trials. *AAPS J*. 2013 Jan;15(1):195-218.

174. Bengmark S. Curcumin, an atoxic antioxidant and natural NFkappaB, cyclooxygenase-2, lipooxygenase, and inducible nitric oxide synthase inhibitor: a shield against acute and chronic diseases. *JPEN J Parenter Enteral Nutr*. 2006; 30(1):45-51.

175. Parodi FE, Mao D, Ennis TL, Pagano MB, Thompson RW. Oral administration of diferuloylmethane (curcumin) suppresses proinflammatory cytokines and destructive connective tissue remodeling in experimental abdominal aortic aneurysms. *Ann Vasc Surg*. 2006; 20(3):360-8.

176. Swarnakar S, Ganguly K et al. Curcumin regulates expression and activity of matrix metalloproteinases 9 and 2 during prevention and healing of indomethacin-induced gastric ulcer. *J Biol Chem*. 2005; 280(10):9409-15.

177. Chattopadhyay I, Biswas K et al. Turmeric and curcumin: Biological actions and medicinal applications. *Current Science* 2004; 87(1): 44-53.

178. Sahebkar A, Cicero AF, Simental-Mendía LE, et al. Curcumin downregulates human tumor necrosis factor-α levels: A systematic review and meta-analysis of randomized controlled trials. *Pharmacol Res*. 2016 May;107:234-42.

179. Aggarwal BB, Gupta SC, Sung B. Curcumin: an orally bioavailable blocker of TNF and other pro-inflammatory biomarkers. *Br J Pharmacol*. 2013 Aug;169(8):1672-92.

180. Holt, P. R., Katz, S. et al. Curcumin therapy in inflammatory bowel disease: a pilot study. *Dig Dis Sci*. 2005; 50(11):2191-2193.

181. Hanai, H., Iida, T. et al. Curcumin maintenance therapy for ulcerative colitis: randomized, multicenter, double-blind, placebo-controlled trial. *Clin Gastroenterol Hepatol*. 2006; 4(12):1502-1506.

182. Lang A, Salomon N, Wu JC, et al. Curcumin in Combination With Mesalamine Induces Remission in Patients With Mild-to-Moderate Ulcerative Colitis in a Randomized Controlled Trial. *Clin Gastroenterol Hepatol*. 2015 Aug;13(8):1444-9.e1

183. McFadden RM, Larmonier CB, Shehab KW, et al. The Role of Curcumin in Modulating Colonic Microbiota During Colitis and Colon Cancer Prevention. *Inflamm Bowel Dis*. 2015 Nov;21(11):2483-94.

184. Tan S, Calani L, Bresciani L, et al. The degradation of curcuminoids in a human faecal fermentation model. *Int J Food Sci Nutr*. 2015;66(7):790-6.

185. Suskind DL, Wahbeh G, Burpee T, et al. Tolerability of curcumin in pediatric inflammatory bowel disease: a forced-dose titration study. *J Pediatr Gastroenterol Nutr*. 2013 Mar;56(3):277-9.

186. Ammon HP, Mack T, Singh GB, Safayhi H. Inhibition of leukotriene B4 formation in rat peritoneal neutrophils by an ethanolic extract of the gum resin exudate of Boswellia serrata. *Planta Med*. 1991; 57(3):203-7.

187. Roy S, Khanna S et al. Regulation of vascular responses to inflammation: inducible matrix metalloproteinase-3 expression in human microvascular endothelial cells is sensitive to antiinflammatory boswellia. *Antioxid Redox Signal*. 2006; 8(3-4):653-60.

188. Takada, Y., Ichikawa, H. et al. Acetyl-11-keto-beta-boswellic acid potentiates apoptosis, inhibits invasion, and abolishes osteoclastogenesis by suppressing NF-kappa B and NF-kappa B-regulated gene expression. *J Immunol*. 2006; 176(5):3127-3140.

189. Gupta, I., Parihar, A. et al. Effects of Boswellia serrata gum resin in patients with ulcerative colitis. *Eur J Med Res*. 1997; 2(1):37-43.

190. Gupta, I., Parihar, A. et al. Effects of gum resin of Boswellia serrata in patients with chronic colitis. *Planta Med*. 2001; 67(5):391-395.

191. Holtmeier W, Zeuzem S, Preiss J, Kruis W, et al. Randomized, placebo-controlled, double-blind trial of Boswellia serrata in maintaining remission of Crohn's disease: good safety profile but lack of efficacy. *Inflamm Bowel Dis*. 2011 Feb;17(2):573-82.

192. Yu FY, Huang SG, Zhang HY, et al. [Effect of baicalin on signal transduction and activating transcription factor expression in ulcerative colitis patients]. [Article in Chinese] *Zhongguo Zhong Xi Yi Jie He Za Zhi*. 2015 Apr;35(4):419-24.

193. Dryden GW, Lam A, Beatty K, Qazzaz HH, McClain CJ. A pilot study to evaluate the safety and efficacy of an oral dose of (-)-epigallocatechin-3-gallate-rich polyphenon E in patients with mild to moderate ulcerative colitis. *Inflamm Bowel Dis*. 2013 Aug;19(9):1904-12.

194. Biedermann L, Mwinyi J, Scharl M, Frei P, et al. Bilberry ingestion improves disease activity in mild to moderate ulcerative colitis - an open pilot study. *J Crohns Colitis*. 2013 May;7(4):271-9.

195. Sandborn WJ, Targan SR, Byers VS, et al. Andrographis paniculata extract (HMPL-004) for active ulcerative colitis. *Am J Gastroenterol*. 2013 Jan;108(1):90-8.

196. Ben-Arye E, Goldin E, Wengrower D, et al. Wheat grass juice in the treatment of active distal ulcerative colitis: a randomized double-blind placebo-controlled trial. *Scand J Gastroenterol*. 2002 Apr;37(4):444-9.

Irritable Bowel Syndrome (IBS) and Related Functional Bowel Disorders

In many ways, IBS is the hallmark functional gastrointestinal disorder (FGID); the investigation of which was one of the main reasons the Rome Foundation was initiated in the late 1980s.[1,2] Since then, various IBS diagnostic criteria (detailed below) have been used to conduct thousands of clinical trials for a variety of epidemiological, observational and interventional investigations, further refining the clinical definition and potential therapies for this prevalent GI malady. Within the list of FGIDs (see page 17), IBS is now one of six closely related functional bowel disorders defined by the Rome Foundation†. The list includes IBS, functional constipation, functional diarrhea, functional abdominal bloating/distention, unspecified functional bowel disorder, and opioid-induced constipation (though this is not technically a functional disorder).[3]

IBS is the most commonly diagnosed FGID and, depending on the definition used, has a worldwide prevalence of 10 to 20%, with the lowest reported prevalence in France (4 to 5%) and the highest (>20%) reported prevalence rates (in Western countries) in the United States, United Kingdom, Greece and Iceland (>30%).[4] Studies suggest most patients with IBS have not consulted with their physicians about their bowel disorder, though the vast majority of patients who do consult with a physician (in the United States) have the IBS-diarrhea subtype.[5] The rates of IBS in women are about 1.5 to threefold higher than in men, worldwide; IBS is generally more prevalent (and severe) in those younger than 50 years old.[4]

Defining Irritable Bowel Syndrome

For many years, IBS was considered a diagnosis of exclusion, when all other organic diseases were eliminated and no positive findings were noted after performing available laboratory tests. Today, while it is still important to rule out conditions with overlapping symptoms, the definition of IBS is now a positive diagnosis based on specific criteria. However, these IBS diagnostic criteria, like all the other FGID diagnostic criteria defined by the Rome Foundation, are still based primarily on symptoms rather than other laboratory

Rome III

Must include **both** of the following criteria:*

- Abdominal discomfort** or pain associated with two or more of the following at least 25% of the time:
  o Improvement with defecation
  o Onset associated with a change in frequency of stool
  o Onset associated with a change in form (appearance) of stool
- No evidence of an inflammatory, anatomic, metabolic, or neoplastic process that explains the subject's symptoms

Criteria fulfilled at least three days per month in the past 12 weeks.
**"Discomfort" means an uncomfortable sensation not described as pain.*

Rome IV

Recurrent abdominal pain, on average, at least one day per week in the last three months, associated with two or more of the following criteria:*

- Related to defecation
- Associated with a change in frequency of stool
- Associated with a change in form (appearance) of stool

Criteria fulfilled for the last three months with symptom onset at least six months before diagnosis.

---

† Since the Rome IV criteria were published as this Standard Road map was being prepared (2016), these criteria have not been critically examined outside the Rome Foundation group, and have yet to be used as the basis for clinical research. Rome III or II criteria are used for most of the studies discussed in this chapter.

biomarkers or physiological criteria.[1] The Rome III (2006) and Rome IV (2016) diagnostic criteria for IBS are different, and compared on page 189.

There are several notable changes in the IBS diagnostic criteria between Rome III and IV, both in the overall definition and also in the criteria used to define the four subtypes of IBS. First is the change from the use of the term "discomfort" (Rome III) to the term "pain" (Rome IV) as the main differentiator between IBS and other functional bowel disorders. The term "discomfort" was eliminated as being too ambiguous, especially across different cultures and languages. Abdominal pain must be present (see Figure 36); the absence of this symptom precludes the diagnosis of IBS (i.e.,

constipation without pain as a *predominant* feature is deemed functional constipation, even if all other criteria for IBS are met; see page 52 for more on constipation). Also, the term "improvement with defecation" was changed to "related to defecation," as many IBS patients experience no improvement in pain with defecation; some, in fact; have worsening pain. Likewise, the word "onset" was removed from each of the last two criteria, as pain may not coincide directly with these changes. The subtle difference between three days per month and one day per week is helpful to define the frequency of symptoms, especially for inclusion in clinical trials. Finally, subtle changes to help define subtypes of IBS were included in Rome IV (see below).

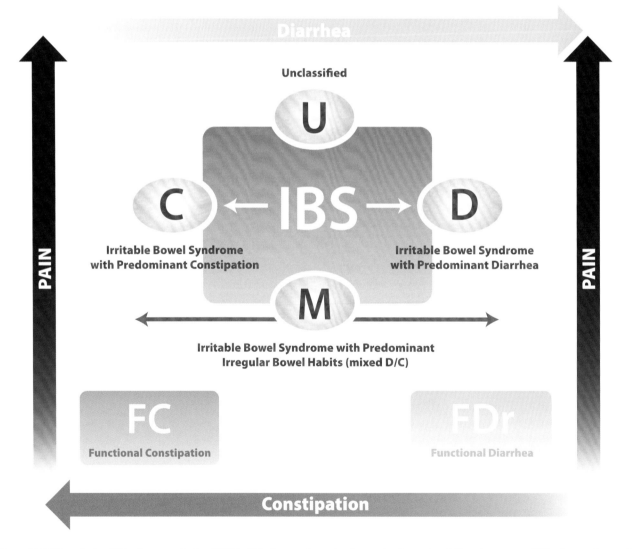

Figure 36: Differentiating IBS subtypes and other FGIDs. This diagram shows the diagnostic scheme that differentiates various IBS subtypes from each other (based on stool morphology and frequency), and from similar functional bowel disorders that are not associated with pain as a prominent distinguishing feature. See text for further information.

IBS Subtypes

IBS is associated with unpredictable bowel patterns and stool morphology. Therefore, the subtypes of IBS (constipation, diarrhea, mixed, and unclassified) are not considered distinct disorders, but exist along a spectrum of related symptoms and severities. Nonetheless, the use of subtyping can be helpful in understanding underlying dysfunctions and prioritizing helpful therapies. IBS subtypes are defined by the *predominant* bowel habits and stool form based on the Bristol Stool Form Scale (BSS; see page 52 for more details). Since IBS is associated with changing bowel patterns and morphology, subtyping is based on predominant bowel habits and stool morphology on the days with an abnormal bowel movement.[3] It is important to note that a patient is evaluated when they are off medication used to treat these symptoms (e.g., laxatives, loperimide, etc.).

IBS-C (Predominant Constipation)

More than one-fourth (>25%) of bowel movements with BSS types 1 or 2 and less than one-fourth (<25%) of bowel movements with BSS types 6 or 7. Alternative for clinical practice: Patient meets IBS criteria and reports that abnormal bowel movements are usually constipation (i.e., types 1 or 2 on BSS).

IBS-D (Predominant Diarrhea)

More than one-fourth (>25%) of bowel movements with BSS types 6 or 7 and less than one-fourth (<25%) of bowel movements with BSS types 1 or 2. Alternative for clinical practice: Patient meets IBS criteria and reports that abnormal bowel movements are usually diarrhea (i.e., types 6 or 7 on BSS).

IBS-M (Mixed Stool Pattern)

More than one-fourth (>25%) of bowel movements with BSS types 1 or 2 **and more than** one-fourth (>25%) of bowel movements with BSS types 6 or 7. Alternative for clinical practice: Patient meets IBS criteria and reports that abnormal bowel movements are both constipation and diarrhea (at least 25% constipation and at least 25% diarrhea).

IBS-U (Unclassified)

Patients who meet the criteria for IBS but whose bowel habits cannot be accurately categorized into one of the three groups above. This category is not common, but often results if patients continually alter their diets or cannot fully stop medications to be evaluated properly.

Physical Exam and Exclusion of Other Conditions

It is important when dealing with the potential diagnosis of IBS (or any other FGID) that the clinician rule out other conditions that may cause lower abdominal pain or alter bowel habits for more than a few weeks. Abdominal swelling, hepatosplenomegaly or an abdominal mass should be investigated. According to Rome IV, an anorectal examination is mandatory to identify anorectal causes of bleeding, evaluate anorectal tone and squeeze pressure, and identify dyssynergic defecation (anismus).[3]

Laboratory Diagnostics

There is no definitive biomarker for IBS or any of its subtypes.[6,7] However, several laboratory tests can be performed (in addition to standard tests like a CBC) to help the clinician rule out conditions with similar symptoms, or help uncover an underlying root cause contributing to the dysfunction and symptoms. The

clinician should be aware that many patients with IBS have become frustrated with years of testing by other clinicians with limited interpretive benefit and may be financially and emotionally reluctant to submit to a broad range of tests (especially since none are definitive for the diagnosis). Therefore, clinicians should choose to do tests intended to rule out more serious organic diseases, or those that are more likely to change their therapeutic recommendations.

· **Inflammatory Markers**
  C-reactive protein (CRP) is a non-specific inflammatory marker that can be used with fecal calprotectin to rule out patients with inflammatory bowel diseases (see page 169 for IBD and page 173 for fecal calprotectin). According to a recent meta-analysis, CRP levels of ≤0.5 mg/dl or calprotectin levels of ≤40 μg/g, essentially excludes IBD in patients

meeting the criteria for IBS.[8] As we mention below, these markers may be higher in IBS patients than in healthy controls, and therefore these markers have been used to detect chronic low levels of inflammation in IBS patients. It is also important to note that some subjects meet the diagnostic criteria for both IBS and IBD, so this can only rule out IBD, not IBS.

· **Food Allergy and Sensitivity Testing**
Since a variety of food allergies, sensitivities and intolerances can trigger IBS-like symptoms (e.g., lactose intolerance), clinicians should ensure a comprehensive diet history (preferably a diet diary used with a stool diary) is used to help understand the relationship between intake of particular foods and the timing of IBS-like symptoms. Testing for food allergies and/or sensitivities is often helpful when investigating root-cause issues in anyone with a functional gastrointestinal disorder, especially wheat, yeast, dairy (lactose intolerance and protein allergens), soy and nickel.

· **Stool Analysis for Pathogens**
Stool analysis for specific bacteria or parasite pathogens may be a helpful tool, especially when diarrhea is the predominant symptom and the patient lives in, or has recently traveled to, an area where they may have encountered a new GI organism.[9]

· **Celiac Testing**
While a gluten-free diet may be an empirical way to test for gluten sensitivity or celiac disease, clinicians may want to test a patient for gluten reactivity/celiac disease using traditional test methods. See page 147 for tests for celiac disease and gluten sensitivity.

· **Emerging Biomarker Panels/Algorithms**
A group from the Netherlands has published a biomarker panel reported to discriminate IBS patients from healthy controls (non-symptomatic subjects) with high sensitivity (88.1%) and specificity (86.5%).[10] The eight biomarkers of this panel, selected from 15 candidates using univariate analysis, are the serum markers IL-1β, IL-6, IL-12p70, TNF-α; and the fecal markers CgA (chromogranin A), HBD2 (human β-defensin),

calprotectin, and caproate (a short-chain fatty acid). These biomarkers appear to combine activities of the immune system, endothelial protection and microbial community. While this biomarker panel has yet to be validated beyond this group and is not known to be currently available in any commercial lab, such panels may be available in the future to help confirm a case of IBS.

Also, a test that measures two serum antibodies has been proposed by Pimentel et al. as a way to distinguish IBS-D from other conditions that include chronic diarrhea (i.e., IBD).[11] The two antibodies, anti-cytolethal distending toxin B and anti-vinculin are remnants of an intestinal infection by one of several common bacteria that cause food poisoning. This test may be commercially available under the name IBSchek™ (see also "Is Food Poisoning a Key Trigger for IBS?" sidebar on page 198).

Other Tests
Because the potential root cause(s) may be any number of dysfunctions within the five basic functions of the GI tract (digestion, elimination, barrier function, microbial ecosystem and neuroendocrine), a number of other tests will be discussed in the context of these root causes below. Such tests might include comprehensive stool test (i.e., CDSA™), breath test for SIBO or *H. pylori*, test for intestinal permeability, tests for digestive function (stomach acid/ pancreatic function), or metagenomics test of the gut microbiota.

Colonoscopy
Most guidelines suggest a screening colonoscopy in patients 50 or older, independent of a suspicion of IBS or another dysfunction. When evaluating a patient who meets the criteria for IBS, colonoscopy is indicated when there are alarm features such as a positive family history of colorectal cancer, rectal bleeding in the absence of a documented hemorrhoid or anal fissure, or unintentional weight loss. Microscopic colitis can be ruled out using biopsy, though fecal calprotectin levels may also differentiate this condition from IBS.[12] Colorectal cancer incidence the first year after diagnosis of IBS is ~1% higher than the general population, though it is the same as the general population after the first year.[13]

Assessing and Treating Predisposing Factors and Root Causes of IBS

Since IBS is defined by the lack of specific organic disease on the one hand and the presence of dysfunctions leading to symptoms that persist on the other hand, defining a cause for IBS is obviously difficult. As Figure 37 illustrates, IBS is considered to be the convergence of numerous physiological and psychological disturbances mediated through pathways that are generally referred to as "Gut/Brain Signaling". Therapies designed to address these underlying dysfunctions will have more long-term success than those designed to limit the symptoms of diarrhea or constipation alone.

Genetics

Large national surveys of IBS patients and their relatives indicate a genetic component related to this dysfunction. However, compared to other gastrointestinal conditions, and most other chronic diseases, there is limited evidence linking specific genetic loci with the increased risk for IBS.[14] More than 60 candidate genes have been studied, many involved with serotonin synthesis, mucosal immunity,

neuropeptide signaling (including CRH; see below in HPA axis), pain signaling, bile acid synthesis and a variety of intestinal secretions. While many of these have helped researchers investigate the complex pathophysiology related to IBS (or a rare loss-of-function mutation), there is currently no specific gene (allele or polymorphism) that, if identified, is likely to help a clinician diagnose or manage a patient who fits the diagnostic criteria for IBS.[15]

Psychological Factors

It does not take a trained scientist to realize there is a connection between the functions of the GI tract (especially motility) and the feelings of anxiety, fear and stress. There is a strong interaction between the way we perceive the world around us and the function of the gastrointestinal tract, mediated by what is often called the gut-brain axis. IBS specifically, and the majority of other functional gastrointestinal disorders according to Rome IV, are now referred to as "Disorders of Gut-Brain Interaction."[16]

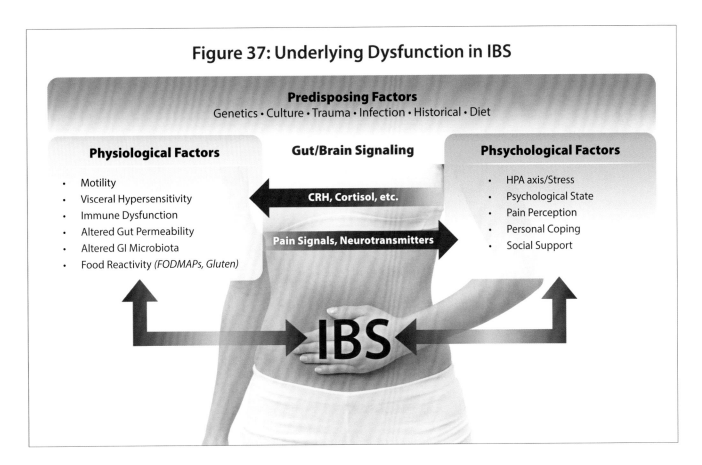

Figure 37: Underlying Dysfunction in IBS

Predisposing Factors
Genetics • Culture • Trauma • Infection • Historical • Diet

Physiological Factors
- Motility
- Visceral Hypersensitivity
- Immune Dysfunction
- Altered Gut Permeability
- Altered GI Microbiota
- Food Reactivity *(FODMAPs, Gluten)*

Gut/Brain Signaling
CRH, Cortisol, etc.
Pain Signals, Neurotransmitters

Phsychological Factors
- HPA axis/Stress
- Psychological State
- Pain Perception
- Personal Coping
- Social Support

IBS

Using various Rome criteria for diagnosis, 54 to 94% of those seeking treatment for IBS also meet the diagnostic criteria for a psychiatric disorder.[17,18] However, since most subjects meeting the diagnostic criteria for IBS do not seek medical treatment, these numbers may represent more severe cases of IBS or subjects more likely to be under medical care for other conditions also highly prevalent in IBS patients (fibromyalgia, chronic fatigue, TMJ, pelvic pain). Psychological conditions most linked with IBS are panic disorder/agoraphobia,[19] generalized anxiety disorder,[20,21] PTSD,[22] and major depression.[23] It is important that a clinician get a complete health history of each patient with IBS to discover sources of stress and traumatic events. Clinicians should treat (or refer) appropriately to help the patient manage the psychiatric disorder as the treatment of such disorders is beyond the scope of this handbook. The use and efficacy of psychological therapies, antidepressants, anxiolytics and other CNS-acting drugs for IBS have recently been reviewed.[24,25,26,27]

The HPA Axis and Stress

We have extensively covered the mechanisms and HPA axis-driven dysfunctions related to various stressors in our previous book, *The Role of Stress and the HPA Axis in Chronic Disease Management* (Point Institute, 2015). Here, we will briefly discuss the links between the HPA axis and IBS pathophysiology.

There has been quite a bit of investigation into how the stress responses of both the sympatho-adreno-medulary system (catecholamines) and the hypothalamic pituitary adrenal axis (CRH-ACTH-cortisol) influence GI function. In particular, because chronic stress has a predictable response on the HPA axis and is related to many of the same conditions known to be associated with IBS, clinical research has attempted to link particular HPA axis dysfunctions with IBS or other functional gastrointestinal disorders.

In general, they have discovered HPA axis dysfunction (upregulation, downregulation, stress hyper-responsiveness) is quite common in IBS subjects,

but distinct patterns of dysfunction are difficult to categorize. While this may be partly due to the heterogeneity of the clinical studies performed, this may also be inherent within the progressive and adaptive nature of the HPA axis to chronic stress and the signaling of the gut-brain axis itself. There are numerous mechanisms linking the HPA axis with alterations in GI function including direct corticotropin-releasing factor (CRF) and related urocortin signaling in the gut, mast cell-induced alterations in intestinal permeability, changes in the gut microbiota, altered immune-reactivity, changes in gastric (slower) and gut (faster) motility and increased pain sensitivity.

CRH is released in the hypothalamus as a consolidation of its assessment of internal and external stressors, modulated by the feedback inhibition of cortisol already in circulation (see Figures 38 and 39). In the classic understanding of the stress response, CRH then makes its way from the hypothalamus to receptors within the anterior pituitary where it triggers the release

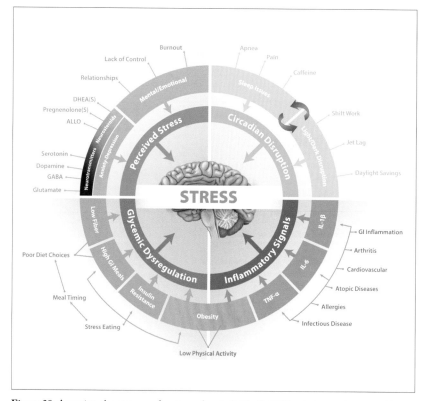

Figure 38: Assessing the status or function of an individual's HPA axis is not the same thing as identifying those unique stressor(s) that have contributed to that status or function. Thankfully, while there are hundreds of internal and external signals that affect the HPA axis, most of them can be collected into just a few simple categories. In most subjects with chronic HPA axis dysfunction, creating strategies to modify the stress-signals coming from one or more of these categories will result in great improvement within the stress response system and, ultimately, overall chronic disease progression.

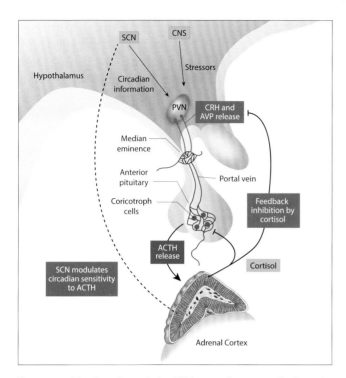

Figure 39: The Signaling of the HPA axis. Stress signals from the CNS and circadian signals from the suprachiasmatic nucleus (SCN) are coordinated by the paraventricular nucleus (PVN) of the hypothalamus. CRH and AVP are released from the PVN into the anterior pituitary where ACTH is produced and released. ACTH triggers cortisol production from the adrenal cortex. Cortisol travels to target tissues, including cells within the hypothalamus, pituitary and CNS where cortisol acts to inhibit the signals of the HPA axis. The SCN also modulates the ACTH sensitivity of cortisol-producing adrenal cortex cells to enhance the circadian function of the HPA axis.

of ACTH, which in turn causes the release of cortisol from within the adrenal cortex. However, CRH is actually one of several corticotropic releasing factors called urocortins, which have been shown to be produced and have receptor-mediated activities in other parts of the brain and periphery, including the gut.[28]

For many years it has been known that CRH and related peptides are produced in the gut (either by immune cells or enteric neurons) and, combined with signals coming from the CNS, can stimulate gut activities through CRH-receptors on gut enterocytes leading to changes in gut motility, permeability, cell secretions and inflammation.[29,30,31,32] In addition, several gene variants and polymorphisms related to CRH/urocortins or CRH-receptor genes have been linked to increased incidence of functional bowel disorders, especially IBS.[33,34] Interestingly, healthy

volunteers given CRH-injections had small bowel constriction and water transfer from the small bowel to the colon in a manner than mimicked the symptoms of IBS-D.[35] There is also significant research showing that the expression pattern and circadian modulation mediated through the glucocorticoid receptor (i.e., cortisol receptor) has a strong influence on the gut-brain axis.[36]

While the mechanistic links between the HPA axis and IBS pathophysiology is becoming clearer, the clinical picture linking stress and the HPA axis with IBS symptoms in patients is still a bit foggy. The best, and easiest in our estimation, tool for assessing a patient's HPA axis is measuring diurnal and waking levels of cortisol in the saliva (we discuss the nuances of salivary cortisol testing and the cortisol awakening response in our book, *The Role of Stress and the HPA Axis in Chronic Disease Management*). Again, since IBS can be associated with both hyper and hypo-activity of the HPA axis (high and low unstimulated cortisol), clinicians must assess each patient's HPA axis to understand the level of cortisol and DHEA(S) output and the stressors most likely contributing to the clinical picture.[37] We should note that while measures of salivary cortisol in IBS patients are somewhat heterogeneous, most studies show a robust diurnal pattern, similar to healthy subjects.[38] One study of 57 women with IBS (compared to 20 controls) showed that those with IBS-D had a higher waking level of cortisol (first sample upon waking), but a blunted cortisol awakening response (CAR change over the next 45 minutes).[39] This is somewhat consistent with the notion that IBS-D subjects appear to have a high anticipation of stress, perhaps suggesting that the HPA axis (ACTH/Cortisol) is already elevated upon awakening; though another small study (n=41) showed blunted early morning ACTH secretion in women with IBS, compared to controls.[40] Since some of these subjects also have a blunted response to a stimulated psychological stressor (Trier social stress test), this reduced CAR could indicate a reduced plasticity (adaptive downregulation) within the HPA axis itself.

It is very important to assess any patient with a functional gastrointestinal disorder, especially IBS, for HPA axis dysfunction (e.g., cortisol and DHEA(S)), *and* to assess the root stressors of the HPA axis that are likely driving these dysfunctions (i.e., perceived stress, circadian disruption, glycemic dysregulation and inflammatory signaling;

see Figure 38). We encourage clinicians to address the root causes of HPA axis dysfunction using diet and lifestyle intervention directly, while concurrently helping to relieve the patient's immediate GI-related symptoms (i.e., diarrhea, constipation). While moderate exercise is known to improve both HPA axis stress and IBS symptoms, strenuous exercise is known to exacerbate both and should be limited until both issues are managed appropriately.[41]

Intestinal Permeability

We have previously discussed the importance and mechanisms related to the barrier functions of the gut (see pages 141-163). Maintaining an appropriate barrier between the gut lumen and the mucosal layers of the GI tract is critically important; disruption of which is known to lead to a number of GI, immune and systemic-related consequences. Not surprisingly, intestinal permeability (i.e., leaky gut) is commonly described as part of the IBS pathophysiology.[42,43] In fact, one of the key mediators of the stress and immune-related triggers leading to IBS symptoms is thought to occur through mast cells residing within the gut mucosa. These mast cells are easily triggered by neuronal signals, CRH (stress response), and immune signals (esp. immunoglobulins) that lead to changes in intestinal permeability and mucosal secretions.[44] Furthermore, mast cell degranulation (from any trigger) increases excitability of vagal, splanchnic, and mesenteric afferent nerves, leading to increased pain signaling.[45,46,47]

This discovery has led to the idea that mast cells may be a potential therapeutic target for treating IBS. Though small and limited studies have shown beneficial symptomatic relief in IBS patients given synthetic mast cell stabilizing agents (e.g., sodium cromelyn), no studies looking at the more powerful natural mast cell stabilizers (e.g., quercetin, fisetin, etc.)[48] have been published. We should note, however, that some evidence suggests that quercetin and related flavonoids may directly improve tight junction integrity, leading to improved barrier function in cell culture experiments where mast cells are excluded.[49,50,51]

In most cases, studies investigating the intestinal permeability within IBS patients show a greater permeability compared to healthy controls, especially in IBS-D subjects (though some have shown no statistical difference).[52,53,54] Therefore, clinicians may choose to perform a standard test for intestinal

permeability (e.g., lactulose/mannitol permeability test; see page 150) if they believe having this additional information will alter their therapeutic strategy. The initiation of a therapeutic strategy using the 4R approach (see page 22) and incorporating specific nutrients that reduce the mediators of intestinal permeability or directly strengthen enterocyte tight junction integrity should be considered (see page 153 for specific strategies to improve gut integrity).

Inflammation and Immune Dysregulation

Ironically, while IBS is often distinguished from inflammatory bowel diseases by the fact that the latter is characterized by elevated serum or fecal inflammatory markers, low-grade chronic inflammation is still considered a key part of IBS pathophysiology.[55] For instance, while the use of fecal calprotectin levels is often used to distinguish IBD from IBS; depending on the cut-off point used (e.g., 40 or 50 µg/g), these levels may still lead to false positives (for IBD) in many IBS subjects (and unnecessary referral for colonoscopy) due to underlying chronic inflammation.[56]

Evaluation of immune cytokines and cells in subjects meeting the diagnostic criteria for IBS shows a number of immune-related differences, compared to healthy controls.[43,57,58] As mentioned above, mast cells appear to be more active and numerous in IBS patients, and have been shown to mediate many of the known pathophysiological changes related to the symptoms of IBS. It is difficult, however, to determine whether these immune-system functional changes are a precursor to IBS pathophysiology, or whether they are an adaptive response to changes in the lumen due to food triggers, altered microbiota or stress-induced changes mediated through CRH, cortisol, or direct innervation.

Therefore, we remind clinicians that even after having "ruled-out" IBD in any given patient with IBS, this does not mean that immune-related or even inflammatory-mediated phenomena are absent from the clinical picture. Therapies designed to reduce inflammation may, in fact, be helpful in some subjects with IBS, though perhaps not directly altering IBS symptoms or outcomes (though the drug mesalazine, often used for the treatment of IBD, appears to have no benefit in IBS subjects).[59,60]

Microbiota and IBS

We have already covered the many different general

functions and imbalances that occur related to the gut microbiota (see pages 103); as well as the relationship between bowel transit time and the relative abundance of species within the microbiota when measured by fecal stool analysis (see pages 100). The fact that IBS is, by definition, characterized by altered stool frequency and bowel transit; as well a host of other immune and secretory alterations that are known to be associated with changes to the microbiota, it should come as no surprise that subjects with IBS (and other FGIDs) have various patterns of dysbiosis within their gut microbiome.[61,62] However, due to the complex interplay between the microbiota within the lumen and the GI mucosa, gut-associated lymphoid tissues (GALT) and the CNS, the cause and effect relationship between IBS and various measures of dysbiosis are cyclical in nature and can differ based on IBS-subtype, chronicity of the condition and even the dietary and therapeutic changes used to manage the symptoms.

Characterizing the typical microbiota of a typical IBS patient is extremely difficult since there are few "typical" IBS patients and the definition of a "typical microbiota" in the healthy general population is still in dispute. Nonetheless, the IBS-related microbiota is generally characterized as being less diverse, less stable and more vulnerable to perturbations.[63,64] In some studies, specific phyla, family or genera of bacteria are similarly altered in IBS subjects compared to controls, while some studies even suggest there is a microbiota signature associated with specific subtypes of IBS.[65,66,67,68] However, while some of these features are similar across different populations of IBS patients (e.g., reduced *Lactobacilli*, reduced *Bifidobacterium*, and increased *Firmicutes*, etc.), these features are absent or non-statistical in other populations.[69] Therefore, while we highly recommend that clinicians test the fecal metagenomics of IBS patients (or those with a suspected FGID), we cannot yet suggest any specific metagenomic diagnostic criteria linking these results to different therapeutic strategies.

One particular animal experiment suggests that, indeed, an "IBS-prone" microbiota may be highly influential in driving IBS pathology. Researchers transferred fecal microbiota from IBS patients, noted for hypersensitive colorectal distention, into the GI tract of germ-free mice and subsequently transferred both the dysbiosis and the increased colon hypersensitivity to these mice, when compared to germ-free mice given fecal microbiota from healthy controls.[70] This experiment suggests that two things might be possible: 1) that unknown "functional" disorders may be inadvertently passed from one person to another during a fecal microbiota transfer (FMT), or 2) that FMTs may have the potential to treat IBS, when using healthy donor feces. Since neither of these possibilities have been investigated in any systematic way, and limited reports of FMT use for IBS outcomes exists, we will need to wait for more research to make any recommendations or precautions.[71]

Post-Infectious IBS

IBS is commonly triggered by an infectious disturbance of the microbiota, a condition commonly called post-infectious IBS (PI-IBS).[72] In fact, reports suggest that 10 to 17% of IBS patients say their symptoms commenced after an episode of infectious diarrhea.[63,73] There are many different types of enteric infections linked with PI-IBS, including norovirus,[74] *Camplylobacter*,[75] *Salmonella*,[76] *Shigella*,[77] *C. difficile*,[78] and unidentified traveler's diarrhea.[79] Likely any major disturbance leading to significant diarrhea, including the use of antibiotics for these infections or other reasons can cause or exacerbate PI-IBS.[80] Clinicians should be sure to ask patients about any significant incidence of infectious diarrhea over the previous three to five years (along with the therapies used at the time), as this can be a helpful record of the progressive history of the microbiota or the presence of an altered "IBS-prone" microbiome (see also sidebar "Is Food Poisoning a Key Trigger for IBS?" on page 198).

IBS and Small Intestinal Bowel Overgrowth

There is ample evidence that IBS subjects have an increased incidence of small intestinal bacteria overgrowth (SIBO), though there is considerable debate about the diagnostic relationship between these two conditions (see page 231 for more comprehensive discussion of SIBO).[81] This is partly due to the low sensitivity of the tests used to diagnose SIBO (culturing or breath tests), and the overlapping symptoms related to these two conditions.[82] Subjects with IBS-D appear to have a higher incidence of SIBO

Is Food Poisoning a Key Trigger for IBS?

Food poisoning is a leading cause of gastroenteritis; which in turn, is a common precursor for IBS (e.g., post-infectious IBS). This connection normally links food poisoning gastroenteritis to the dysbiosis caused by diarrhea or the antibiotics used to treat the infection. While specific dysbiotic profiles do link food-borne pathogens and IBS, several lines of research are now investigating the role of bacterial toxins, especially cytolethal distending toxin (CDT), that are produced by several gram-negative bacteria that cause food poisoning (e.g., *Shigella*, *E. coli*, *Campylobacter*, *Salmonella*) with the pathophysiology of IBS (and SIBO).[1]

Using animal models, Pimental et al. have shown that CDT from *Camplobacter jejuni* infections can lead to specific changes in intestinal physiology that may linger even after the organism is eliminated. Such changes include alterations in intestinal permeability, immune system signaling, and neuroanatomy.[2,3] While some of these outcomes are a direct result of the toxin itself, they have discovered that an autoimmune cross-reactivity (molecular mimicry) against the vinculin protein is also partly responsible for the intestinal permeability and motility changes.[4] Vinculin is an important protein in the cytoskeleton of gastrointestinal cells, particularly interstitial cells of Cajal (ICC), which are neuron-like cells that interface between the enteric nervous system and smooth muscles in the GI tract. These cells are important in maintaining proper rhythmic smooth muscle contraction in the small intestines. In animal models, GI exposure to CDT (from *Camplobacter* infection) causes an increase in antibodies against the toxin, as well as vinculin, and reduces the number of ICC.[5] These changes in gut motility are thought to help promote small intestinal bacteria overgrowth (SIBO) leading to related IBS symptoms such as gas, bloating, diarrhea, and intestinal pain.

This animal model has led to the proposed use of both anti-CDT and anti-vinculin antibody testing as a means to distinguish IBS-D patients from subjects with other non-IBS chronic diarrhea conditions (IBD or celiac disease). Circulating anti-CDT (CdtB specifically) and anti-vinculin antibodies were measured in 2375 subjects meeting the Rome III criteria for IBS-D and in subjects with IBD (n=142), celiac disease (n=121) and healthy controls (n=43). Both antibody titers were significantly higher in IBS-D subjects compared to the other groups tested. These antibodies are now used in a commercially-available test (e.g., IBSchek™) which clinicians may use as a biomarker to identify IBS-D subjects.[6]

This line of research is very intriguing, and also very controversial. It suggests that at least one major subtype of IBS is not a functional bowel disorder after all, but a post-infectious pathophysiological alteration of the cells that manage the immune, permeability and motility functions of the small intestines, with further consequences to the commensal organisms in the small bowel. Currently, while there are ways to directly treat the SIBO consequences (see page 233), there are no proposed strategies to eliminate the residual effects of these food-borne toxins or the auto-immune cross reactivity to vinculin. Further studies are needed to assess ways to reduce autoimmune signaling as a means to affect IBS outcomes.

References

1. Sung J, Morales W, Kim G, et al. Effect of repeated Campylobacter jejuni infection on gut flora and mucosal defense in a rat model of post infectious functional and microbial bowel changes. *Neurogastroenterol Motil.* 2013 Jun;25(6):529-37.
2. Morales W, Pimentel M, Hwang L, et al. Acute and chronic histological changes of the small bowel secondary to C. jejuni infection in a rat model for post-infectious IBS. *Dig Dis Sci.* 2011 Sep;56(9):2575-84.
3. Pokkunuri V, Pimentel M, Morales W, et al. Role of Cytolethal Distending Toxin in Altered Stool Form and Bowel Phenotypes in a Rat Model of Post-infectious Irritable Bowel Syndrome. *J Neurogastroenterol Motil.* 2012 Oct;18(4):434-42.
4. Pimentel M, Morales W, Pokkunuri V, et al. Autoimmunity Links Vinculin to the Pathophysiology of Chronic Functional Bowel Changes Following Campylobacter jejuni Infection in a Rat Model. *Dig Dis Sci.* 2015 May;60(5):1195-205.
5. Jee SR, Morales W, Low K, et al. ICC density predicts bacterial overgrowth in a rat model of post-infectious IBS. *World J Gastroenterol.* 2010 Aug 7;16(29):3680-6.
6. Pimentel M, Morales W, Rezaie A, et al. Development and validation of a biomarker for diarrhea-predominant irritable bowel syndrome in human subjects. *PLoS One.* 2015 May 13;10(5):e0126438.

(by either measure), and this condition is often linked with more abdominal bloating and gas.[81,83] In addition, treatments designed to treat SIBO (e.g., rifaxamin) are associated with significant relief of IBS symptoms, especially in subjects *without* constipation (see below for role of antibiotics for IBS).

Clinicians should become familiar with the signs and symptoms of SIBO, along with the tests that may be helpful to confirm this condition in patients with IBS (see page 191). Since many of the treatments for IBS and SIBO are similar, a diagnosis of SIBO may help the clinician prioritize those treatments that are known to be beneficial for both conditions.

The Role of Antibiotics for IBS Therapy

The use of antibiotic therapy for IBS is controversial. Since most antibiotics are absorbed systemically, and virtually all are known to influence the antibiotic resistance of certain microbes and/or lead to negative changes in the gut microbiota, these agents can potentially destabilize an already vulnerable GI micro-environment. For this reason, nearly all antibiotics are discouraged as part of the treatment for IBS (though some may be necessary for non-IBS infections in an individual with IBS).

The exception to this rule has been rifaximin, a semi-synthetic rifamycin-derivative that has virtually no systemic absorption.[84,85] Rifaximin is now FDA-approved for IBS-D (since 2015) at a dose of 550 mg, TID for 14 days (it is also approved for traveler's diarrhea and hepatic encephalopathy at different dosing). It should be noted that while rifaximin therapy has been shown to be statistically superior to placebo in most cases of IBS without constipation; in many of these clinical trials rifaximin treatment was ineffective in more than 50% of subjects and may be more effective when subjects have SIBO.[86]

Antimicrobial herbs have been compared to rifaxamin for their ability to kill bacteria and/or modulate symptoms in IBS subjects. While some of these reports have been positive, they are either cell-culture studies or the products used are very heterogeneous (using up to 10 ingredients), making specific recommendations difficult.[87,88] Promising ingredients include thyme (extracts or oil), oregano (oil), berberine or berberine-containing plant extracts, lemon balm extracts, tea tree oil, coriander seed, peppermint and spearmint. Except for peppermint oil (see page 201), none of these agents have been studied in prospective clinical trials for IBS outcomes.

Probiotics and IBS

The use of probiotics to improve the microbiome and reduce symptoms in subjects with IBS is a fairly common practice around the world.[89] In fact, so common is the practice that well over 50 clinical trials, using most of the commercially-available *Lactobacilli* and/or *Bifidobacterium* strains, have been performed and published over the past few decades; and at least 10 systematic reviews and meta-analysis have been performed on various subsets of these trials.[90] One might assume that with this much data, there would be a clear understanding of the role of probiotics in IBS subjects. However, since these studies were performed by dozens of different groups around the world, using different strains (single strain products or mixed strain products), doses, length of treatments and delivery mechanisms; along with the complex diagnostic and subtyping issues inherent with IBS, the picture is all but clear.

Therefore, depending on which subset of published trials are collected for the given meta-analysis, a different recommendation (or no specific recommendation) is made.[91,92,93] What we can say at this time by combining the published literature on this topic and discussion of the use of probiotics for IBS with healthcare providers is this: 1) probiotic therapy is safe in subjects with IBS, adverse effects are very limited and cease when probiotic is stopped, 2) the same strains or combinations of strains will not work in all subjects with IBS or even in every subtype of IBS, 3) symptom improvement using a particular probiotic may diminish (or improve) over time, especially in subjects with IBS-M, 4) positive benefits have been seen at relatively low doses (<10 billion CFU/day) as well as very high doses (450 to 900 billion CFU/day); clinicians should be willing to start low and consider high doses (see page 130).

Dietary Components and IBS (Triggers and Treatments)[94,95]

The link between certain foods and the triggering of gastrointestinal symptoms is extremely common, especially in subjects with recurrent functional gastrointestinal disorders.[96] Surveys of IBS patients suggest that meals or specific foods are common triggers for symptoms. In one survey of 197 IBS subjects living in Sweden, the most common foods associated with symptoms were fried and fatty foods (52%), dairy products (49%), beans/lentils (36%), apple (28%), flour (24%), and plum (23%). Also, 58% of these subjects reported experiencing GI symptoms from foods rich in biogenic amines, such as wine/beer (31%), salami (22%), and cheese (20%); and histamine-releasing foods, such as milk (43%), wine/beer (31%), and pork (21%).[97] To gain any benefit from a diet and lifestyle approach for IBS, clinicians must ask patients about known food triggers or whether they are already on a self-prescribed elimination diet. If possible, clinicians should direct patients to work closely with a trusted nutritionist/dietitian that can help them make diet-symptom connections through diet diary or diet recall. In many cases, IBS patients will have dramatic symptom improvements when specific foods or food categories are eliminated from the diet.

Gluten

It is now well-documented that gluten can trigger a number of symptoms in non-celiac subjects, many of which mirror the symptoms experienced by IBS patients. In addition, reports show subjects who meet the Rome III criteria for IBS have a higher likelihood of a positive antibody reaction to gluten or biopsy confirmation of celiac disease, compared to healthy controls.[98] A meta-analysis of 14 studies evaluating the role of gluten-reactivity/celiac disease in IBS subjects estimates that biopsy-positive celiac is four-fold higher in IBS subjects than healthy controls, and up to one-third of IBS patients may exhibit some form of gluten or wheat-protein sensitivity.[99,100] Therefore, it is strongly recommended that clinicians determine the gluten-reactivity of each patient that meets the criteria for IBS or other FGIDs (see page 148 for algorithm); or at a minimum, use a gluten-free diet and re-challenge to empirically assess the role of gluten in IBS patients.

A limited number of studies suggest that gluten-free diets improve IBS symptoms, especially those with subtype IBS-D. Researchers at the Mayo Clinic randomized 45 non-celiac, IBS-D patients either to a gluten-containing or a gluten-free diet for four weeks and followed patients for bowel function, colonic transit, intestinal permeability, immune system activation and even specific GI transcripts of tight junction protein genes.[101] They found that when IBS-D subjects consumed gluten, they had more bowel movements and higher small intestinal permeability; both of which were exaggerated in subjects with genetic predisposition for celiac disease (i.e., HLA DQ2 or DQ8 positive). IBS-D subjects also had significantly lower bowel expression of important tight junction proteins (zonula occludens-1, claudin-1 and occludin); again affected to a greater extent in genetically vulnerable subjects. Other small clinical trials or case studies confirm the potential benefit of a gluten-free diet in subjects with IBS.[102,103]

Fiber and FODMAPs

There has been great debate in past years about the role of dietary fiber intake (soluble and insoluble), fermentable fiber intake (prebiotics), or the intake of various carbohydrates that fit the definition of FODMAPs and the IBS patient.[62] Since all of these substrates have the potential to alter the microbiota and/or bowel transit time, and many other GI-related functions mediated by these two factors, they may be considered helpful or harmful. In general, it appears that soluble fibers that are only modest substrates for bacterial fermentation appear to be helpful for patients with IBS-C, while the limited intake of fermentable fibers and carbohydrates (i.e., FODMAPs) may be beneficial for a range of IBS patients (For more information on fiber/constipation, see page 56; for prebiotics, see page 108; and for FODMAP diet specifics, see page 236).

Clinical research on the use of fibers in IBS patients is plagued with the same heterogeneity as most other dietary intervention in IBS patients. Dozens of clinical trials have been performed, though many were of poor quality using different doses of different types of fibers in ill-defined subjects.[104] The best evidence is for the use of soluble fiber, mostly psyllium/isphagula, in subjects with unspecified IBS or IBS-C. The best trials testing insoluble fiber were mostly performed using wheat fiber, a substance that may have inadvertently triggered symptoms due to unmeasured gluten or wheat protein reactivity, thereby neutralizing any benefits realized by the fiber. In general, when a fiber supplement improves the symptoms of constipation, it is likely to help relieve symptoms in IBS-C subjects.

Unlike with fiber, there is now a growing consensus as to the usefulness of the low FODMAP diet in patients with IBS. Essentially this diet limits the intake of a range of foods and supplements that contain fermentable oligo-, di-, and monosaccharides and polyols (see list on page 237), essentially limiting excessive fermentation within the gut. While fermentation of several of these carbohydrates have been shown to be helpful in the general population (e.g., prebiotic stimulation of *Bifidobacterium*), and IBS subjects are even noted to have low amounts of *Bifidobacterium*, this diet has been highly successful in reducing IBS-related symptoms in a large number of subjects across a wide range of clinical trials.[105,106,107] Notably, the British Dietetic Association recently (2016) updated their evidence-based guidelines for the dietary management of IBS in adults and included a recommendation for the low FODMAP diet in these patients; additionally, national guidelines from Japan and the UK recommend the low FODMAP diet in IBS management.[108,109,110]

Patients meeting the criteria for IBS should be given instructions to attempt a FODMAP-restricted diet for at least four to six weeks, followed by a re-challenge of FODMAP-containing foods (though symptom improvement may occur within only a few days). Since the list of FODMAP containing foods is broad and includes many that are beneficial for GI health, we do not recommend that a patient maintain a strict FODMAP-restricted diet indefinitely. Certain foods should be added back one-by-one to allow for as many fermentable carbohydrates as the patient can tolerate based on symptoms (more details on the low FODMAP diet can be found on page 236).

Peppermint Oil and Other Herbal Remedies

A large number of herbal remedies, botanical extracts and concentrated phytochemicals have been used to manage symptoms in patients with IBS or related FGIDs, some of which have quality published research. Recent reviews and clinical trials have been published on many herbal remedies from Eastern medical traditions, including those used within Traditional Chinese Medicine (TCM), Ayurvedic, Tibetan and Kampo medicine; though they use different quite different diagnostic criteria for "IBS."[111,112,113,114]

The use of herbs and botanical extracts within Western medical traditions using Rome criteria for IBS is common, though few have been systematically studied. Numerous single-herb or multi-herb formulas with antimicrobial, antispasmodic, carminative,

choleretic, laxative, or mucilaginous properties have been recommended.[115,116,117] However, the herbal therapy most studied is peppermint oil, usually delivered as an enteric-coated soft gel capsule.

Over 25 published clinical studies have used some form of peppermint oil in subjects with IBS (mostly defined by Rome criteria). While many of these studies were poorly designed and/or controlled, the most stringent of systematic reviews and meta-analysis conclude these preparations are both safe and effective for relieving symptoms in IBS patients.[118] Most of these studies used capsules containing between 0.1 to 0.2 mL (or describes as 50 to 225 mg) of peppermint oil, using various doses (one or two capsules consumed two to three times daily). In the analysis of the five best studies reporting global improvement of IBS symptoms, 69% of patients receiving peppermint oil had improved symptoms compared to only 31% of subjects consuming placebo (RR 2.23).

IBS Summary

- Teach patient to use Bristol Stool Form Scale for proper category diagnosis

- Rule out organic or other factors with overlapping symptoms

- Investigate with diet and stool diary for food triggers

- Evaluate patient for HPA axis dysfunction (treat accordingly)

- Consider soluble fiber for IBS-C

- Recommend FODMAP-limited diet (avoid prebiotics initially)

- Consider the need for gluten-free diet

- Recommend probiotic (dose and strains variable, see what works)

- Consider peppermint oil soft gel capsule (two to six capsules per day, in divided doses)

- Consider the need for rifaximin

References

1.   Drossman DA. Functional Gastrointestinal Disorders: History, Pathophysiology, Clinical Features and Rome IV. *Gastroenterology*. 2016 Feb 19. pii: S0016-5085(16)00223-7.
2.   Thompson WG, Dotevall G, Drossman DA, et al. Irritable bowel syndrome: guidelines for the diagnosis. *Gastroenterol Int*. 1989;2:92-95.
3.   Mearin F, Lacy BE, Chang L, Chey WD, et al. Bowel Disorders. *Gastroenterology*. 2016 Feb 18; 150:1393-1407.
4.   Canavan C, West J, Card T. The epidemiology of irritable bowel syndrome. *Clin Epidemiol*. 2014 Feb 4;6:71-80.
5.   Hungin AP, Chang L, Locke GR, et al. Irritable bowel syndrome in the United States: prevalence, symptom patterns and impact. *Aliment Pharmacol Ther*. 2005 Jun 1;21(11):1365-75.
6.   Chira A, Dumitrascu DL. Serum biomarkers for irritable bowel syndrome. *Clujul Med*. 2015;88(3):258-64.
7.   Corsetti M, Van Oudenhove L, Tack J. The quest for biomarkers in IBS-where should it lead us? *Neurogastroenterol Motil*. 2014 Dec;26(12):1669-76.
8.   Menees SB, Powell C, Kurlander J, Goel A, Chey WD. A meta-analysis of the utility of C-reactive protein, erythrocyte sedimentation rate, fecal calprotectin, and fecal lactoferrin to exclude inflammatory bowel disease in adults with IBS. *Am J Gastroenterol*. 2015 Mar;110(3):444-54.
9.   Vasquez-Rios G, Machicado JD, Terashima A, Marcos LA. Irritable bowel syndrome and intestinal parasites: a view from South America. *Rev Gastroenterol Peru*. 2016 Apr-Jun;36(2):153-158.
10. Mujagic Z, Tigchelaar EF, Zhernakova A, et al. A novel biomarker panel for irritable bowel syndrome and the application in the general population. *Sci Rep*. 2016 Jun 6;6:26420.
11. Pimentel M, Morales W, Rezaie A, et al. Development and validation of a biomarker for diarrhea-predominant irritable bowel syndrome in human subjects. *PLoS One*. 2015 May 13;10(5):e0126438.
12. von Arnim U, Wex T, Ganzert C, Schulz C, Malfertheiner P. Fecal calprotectin: a marker for clinical differentiation of microscopic colitis and irritable bowel syndrome. *Clin Exp Gastroenterol*. 2016 Apr 21;9:97-103.
13. García Rodríguez LA, Ruigómez A, Wallander MA, et al. Detection of colorectal tumor and inflammatory bowel disease during follow-up of patients with initial diagnosis of irritable bowel syndrome. *Scand J Gastroenterol*. 2000 Mar;35(3):306-11.
14. Henström M, D'Amato M. Genetics of irritable bowel syndrome. *Mol Cell Pediatr*. 2016 Dec;3(1):7.
15. Makker J, Chilimuri S, Bella JN. Genetic epidemiology of irritable bowel syndrome. *World J Gastroenterol*. 2015 Oct 28;21(40):11353-61.
16. Drossman DA, Hasler WL. Rome IV-Functional GI Disorders: Disorders of Gut-Brain Interaction. *Gastroenterology*. 2016 May;150(6):1257-61.
17. Fadgyas-Stanculete M, Buga AM, Popa-Wagner A, Dumitrascu DL. The relationship between irritable bowel syndrome and psychiatric disorders: from molecular changes to clinical manifestations. *J Mol Psychiatry*. 2014 Jun 27;2(1):4.
18. Whitehead WE, Palsson O, Jones KR. Systematic review of the comorbidity of irritable bowel syndrome with other disorders: what are the causes and implications? *Gastroenterology*. 2002 Apr;122(4):1140-56.
19. Sugaya N, Yoshida E, Yasuda S, et al. Irritable bowel syndrome, its cognition, anxiety sensitivity, and anticipatory anxiety in panic disorder patients. *Psychiatry Clin Neurosci*. 2013 Sep;67(6):397-404.
20. Popa SL, Dumitrascu DL. Anxiety and IBS revisited: ten years later. *Clujul Med*. 2015;88(3):253-7.
21. Gros DF, Antony MM, McCabe RE, Swinson RP. Frequency and severity of the symptoms of irritable bowel syndrome across the anxiety disorders and depression. *J Anxiety Disord*. 2009 Mar;23(2):290-6.
22. White DL, Savas LS, Daci K, et al. Trauma history and risk of the irritable bowel syndrome in women veterans. *Aliment Pharmacol Ther*. 2010 Aug;32(4):551-61.
23. Fond G, Loundou A, Hamdani N, et al. Anxiety and depression comorbidities in irritable bowel syndrome (IBS): a systematic review and meta-analysis. *Eur Arch Psychiatry Clin Neurosci*. 2014 Dec;264(8):651-60.
24. Laird KT, Tanner-Smith EE, Russell AC, Hollon SD, Walker LS. Short-term and Long-term Efficacy of Psychological Therapies for Irritable Bowel Syndrome: A Systematic Review and Meta-analysis. *Clin Gastroenterol Hepatol*. 2016 Jul;14(7):937-947.e4.
25. Ford AC, Quigley EM, Lacy BE, et al. Effect of antidepressants and psychological therapies, including hypnotherapy, in irritable bowel syndrome: systematic review and meta-analysis. *Am J Gastroenterol*. 2014 Sep;109(9):1350-65.
26. Bundeff AW, Woodis CB. Selective serotonin reuptake inhibitors for the treatment of irritable bowel syndrome. *Ann Pharmacother*. 2014 Jun;48(6):777-84.
27. Canavan JB, Bennett K, Feely J, O'Moráin CA, O'Connor HJ. Significant psychological morbidity occurs in irritable bowel syndrome: a case-control study using a pharmacy reimbursement database. *Aliment Pharmacol Ther*. 2009 Feb 15;29(4):440-9.
28. Taché Y, Brunnhuber S. From Hans Selye's discovery of biological stress to the identification of corticotropin-releasing factor signaling pathways: implication in stress-related functional bowel diseases. *Ann N Y Acad Sci*. 2008 Dec;1148:29-41.
29. Fukudo S. Role of corticotropin-releasing hormone in irritable bowel syndrome and intestinal inflammation. *J Gastroenterol*. 2007 Jan;42 Suppl 17:48-51.
30. Chang YM, El-Zaatari M, Kao JY. Does stress induce bowel dysfunction? *Expert Rev Gastroenterol Hepatol*. 2014 Aug;8(6):583-5.
31. Bunnett NW. The stressed gut: contributions of intestinal stress peptides to inflammation and motility. *Proc Natl Acad Sci U S A*. 2005 May 24;102(21):7409-10.
32. Larauche M, Kiank C, Tache Y. Corticotropin releasing factor signaling in colon and ileum: regulation by stress and pathophysiological implications. *J Physiol Pharmacol*. 2009 Dec;60 Suppl 7:33-46.
33. Komuro H, Sato N, Sasaki A, et al. Corticotropin-Releasing Hormone Receptor 2 Gene Variants in Irritable Bowel Syndrome. *PLoS One*. 2016 Jan 25;11(1):e0147817.
34. Sasaki A, Sato N, Suzuki N, et al. Associations between Single-Nucleotide Polymorphisms in Corticotropin-Releasing Hormone-Related Genes and Irritable Bowel Syndrome. *PLoS One*. 2016 Feb 16;11(2):e0149322.
35. Pritchard SE, Garsed KC, Hoad CL, et al. Effect of experimental stress on the small bowel and colon in healthy humans. *Neurogastroenterol Motil*. 2015 Apr;27(4):542-9.
36. Wiley JW, Higgins GA, Athey BD. Stress and glucocorticoid receptor transcriptional programming in time and space: Implications for the brain-gut axis. *Neurogastroenterol Motil*. 2016 Jan;28(1):12-25.
37. Ehlert U, Nater UM, Böhmelt A. High and low unstimulated salivary cortisol levels correspond to different symptoms of functional gastrointestinal disorders. *J Psychosom Res*. 2005 Jul;59(1):7-10.
38. Patacchioli FR, Angelucci L, Dellerba G, Monnazzi P, Leri O. Actual stress, psychopathology and salivary cortisol levels in the irritable bowel syndrome (IBS). *J Endocrinol Invest*. 2001 Mar;24(3):173-7.
39. Suárez-Hitz KA, Otto B, Bidlingmaier M, et al. Altered psychobiological responsiveness in women with irritable bowel syndrome. *Psychosom Med*. 2012 Feb-Mar;74(2):221-31.
40. Chang L, Sundaresh S, Elliott J, et al. Dysregulation of the hypothalamic-pituitary-adrenal (HPA) axis in irritable bowel syndrome. *Neurogastroenterol Motil*. 2009 Feb;21(2):149-59.
41. Johannesson E, Ringström G, Abrahamsson H, Sadik R. Intervention to increase physical activity in irritable bowel syndrome shows long-term positive effects. *World J Gastroenterol*. 2015 Jan 14;21(2):600-8.
42. González-Castro AM, Martínez C, Salvo-Romero E, et al. Mucosal pathobiology and molecular signature of epithelial barrier dysfunction in the small intestine in Irritable Bowel Syndrome. *J Gastroenterol Hepatol*. 2016 Apr 18. doi: 10.1111/jgh.13417. [Epub ahead of print]
43. Matricon J, Meleine M, Gelot A, et al. Review article: Associations between immune activation, intestinal permeability and the irritable bowel syndrome. *Aliment Pharmacol Ther*. 2012 Dec;36(11-12):1009-31.
44. Overman EL, Rivier JE, Moeser AJ. CRF induces intestinal epithelial barrier injury via the release of mast cell proteases and TNF-α. *PLoS One*. 2012;7(6):e39935.
45. Zhang L, Song J, Hou X. Mast Cells and Irritable Bowel Syndrome: From the Bench to the Bedside. *J Neurogastroenterol Motil*. 2016 Apr 30;22(2):181-92.
46. Lee H, Park JH, Park DI, et al. Mucosal mast cell count is associated with intestinal permeability in patients with diarrhea predominant irritable bowel syndrome. *J Neurogastroenterol Motil*. 2013 Apr;19(2):244-50.
47. Vanuytsel T, van Wanrooy S, Vanheel H, et al. Psychological stress and corticotropin-releasing hormone increase intestinal permeability in humans by a mast cell-dependent mechanism. *Gut*. 2014 Aug;63(8):1293-9.

48. Weng Z, Zhang B, Asadi S, et al. Quercetin is more effective than cromolyn in blocking human mast cell cytokine release and inhibits contact dermatitis and photosensitivity in humans. *PLoS One.* 2012;7(3):e33805.

49. Suzuki T, Hara H. Quercetin enhances intestinal barrier function through the assembly of zonula [corrected] occludens-2, occludin, and claudin-1 and the expression of claudin-4 in Caco-2 cells. *J Nutr.* 2009 May;139(5):965-74.

50. Amasheh M, Schlichter S, Amasheh S, et al. Quercetin enhances epithelial barrier function and increases claudin-4 expression in Caco-2 cells. *J Nutr.* 2008 Jun;138(6):1067-73.

51. Chuenkitiyanon S, Pengsuparp T, Jianmongkol S. Protective effect of quercetin on hydrogen peroxide-induced tight junction disruption. *Int J Toxicol.* 2010 Jul;29(4):418-24.

52. Gecse K, Róka R, Séra T, et al. Leaky gut in patients with diarrhea-predominant irritable bowel syndrome and inactive ulcerative colitis. *Digestion.* 2012;85(1):40-6.

53. Dunlop SP, Hebden J, Campbell E, et al. Abnormal intestinal permeability in subgroups of diarrhea-predominant irritable bowel syndromes. *Am J Gastroenterol.* 2006 Jun;101(6):1288-94.

54. Del Valle-Pinero AY, Van Deventer HE, et al. Gastrointestinal permeability in patients with irritable bowel syndrome assessed using a four probe permeability solution. *Clin Chim Acta.* 2013 Mar 15;418:97-101.

55. Sinagra E, Pompei G, Tomasello G, et al. Inflammation in irritable bowel syndrome: Myth or new treatment target? *World J Gastroenterol.* 2016 Feb 21;22(7):2242-55.

56. Waugh N, Cummins E, Royle P et al. Faecal calprotectin testing for differentiating amongst inflammatory and non-inflammatory bowel diseases: systematic review and economic evaluation. *Health Technol Assess.* 2013 Nov;17(55):xv-xix, 1-211.

57. O'Malley D. Immunomodulation of enteric neural function in irritable bowel syndrome. *World J Gastroenterol.* 2015 Jun 28;21(24):7362-6.

58. Bashashati M, Rezaei N, Shafieyoun A, et al. Cytokine imbalance in irritable bowel syndrome: a systematic review and meta-analysis. *Neurogastroenterol Motil.* 2014 Jul;26(7):1036-48.

59. Barbara G, Cremon C, Annese V, et al. Randomised controlled trial of mesalazine in IBS. *Gut.* 2016 Jan;65(1):82-90.

60. Lam C, Tan W, Leighton M, et al. A mechanistic multicentre, parallel group, randomised placebo-controlled trial of mesalazine for the treatment of IBS with diarrhoea (IBS-D). *Gut.* 2016 Jan;65(1):91-9.

61. Simrén M, Barbara G, Flint HJ, et al. Intestinal microbiota in functional bowel disorders: a Rome foundation report. *Gut.* 2013 Jan;62(1):159-76.

62. Staudacher HM, Whelan K. Altered gastrointestinal microbiota in irritable bowel syndrome and its modification by diet: probiotics, prebiotics and the low FODMAP diet. *Proc Nutr Soc.* 2016 Feb 24:1-13.

63. Distrutti E, Monaldi L, Ricci P, Fiorucci S. Gut microbiota role in irritable bowel syndrome: New therapeutic strategies. *World J Gastroenterol.* 2016 Feb 21;22(7):2219-41.

64. Durbán A, Abellán JJ, Jiménez-Hernández N, et al. Instability of the faecal microbiota in diarrhoea-predominant irritable bowel syndrome. *FEMS Microbiol Ecol.* 2013 Dec;86(3):581-9.

65. Chassard C, Dapoigny M, Scott KP, et al. Functional dysbiosis within the gut microbiota of patients with constipated-irritable bowel syndrome. *Aliment Pharmacol Ther.* 2012 Apr;35(7):828-38.

66. Ringel-Kulka T, Benson AK, Carroll IM, et al. Molecular characterization of the intestinal microbiota in patients with and without abdominal bloating. *Am J Physiol Gastrointest Liver Physiol.* 2016 Mar 15;310(6):G417-26.

67. Chung CS, Chang PF, Liao CH, et al. Differences of microbiota in small bowel and faeces between irritable bowel syndrome patients and healthy subjects. *Scand J Gastroenterol.* 2016;51(4):410-9.

68. Liu Y, Zhang L, Wang X, et al. Similar Fecal Microbiota Signatures in Patients With Diarrhea-predominant Irritable Bowel Syndrome and Patients With Depression. *Clin Gastroenterol Hepatol.* 2016 Jun 3. pii: S1542-3565(16)30268-3.

69. Zhuang X, Xiong L, Li L, Li M, Chen MH. Alterations of gut microbiota in patients with irritable bowel syndrome: A systematic review and meta-analysis. *J Gastroenterol Hepatol.* 2016 Jun 14. doi: 10.1111/jgh.13471. [Epub ahead of print]

70. Crouzet L, Gaultier E, Del'Homme C, et al. The hypersensitivity to colonic distension of IBS patients can be transferred to rats through their fecal microbiota. *Neurogastroenterol Motil.* 2013 Apr;25(4):e272-82.

71. Pinn DM, Aroniadis OC, Brandt LJ. Is fecal microbiota transplantation (FMT) an effective treatment for patients with functional gastrointestinal disorders (FGID)? *Neurogastroenterol Motil.* 2015 Jan;27(1):19-29.

72. Beatty JK, Bhargava A, Buret AG. Post-infectious irritable bowel syndrome: mechanistic insights into chronic disturbances following enteric infection. *World J Gastroenterol.* 2014 Apr 14;20(14):3976-85.

73. Kanazawa M, Fukudo S. Relationship between infectious gastroenteritis and irritable bowel syndrome. *Clin J Gastroenterol.* 2014 Feb;7(1):14-8.

74. Zanini B, Ricci C, Bandera F, at al. Incidence of post-infectious irritable bowel syndrome and functional intestinal disorders following a water-borne viral gastroenteritis outbreak. *Am J Gastroenterol.* 2012 Jun;107(6):891-9.

75. Nielsen HL, Engberg J, Ejlertsen T, Nielsen H. Psychometric scores and persistence of irritable bowel after Campylobacter concisus infection. *Scand J Gastroenterol.* 2014 May;49(5):545-51.

76. Schwille-Kiuntke J, Enck P, Zendler C, Postinfectious irritable bowel syndrome: follow-up of a patient cohort of confirmed cases of bacterial infection with Salmonella or Campylobacter. *Neurogastroenterol Motil.* 2011 Nov;23(11):e479-88.

77. Youn YH, Kim HC, Lim HC, et al. Long-term Clinical Course of Post-infectious Irritable Bowel Syndrome After Shigellosis: A 10-year Follow-up Study. *J Neurogastroenterol Motil.* 2016 Jul 30;22(3):490-6.

78. Wadhwa A, Al Nahhas MF, Dierkhising RA, et al. High risk of post-infectious irritable bowel syndrome in patients with Clostridium difficile infection. *Aliment Pharmacol Ther.* 2016 Jul 22. doi: 10.1111/apt.13737. [Epub ahead of print]

79. Schwille-Kiuntke J, Mazurak N, Enck P. Systematic review with meta-analysis: post-infectious irritable bowel syndrome after travellers' diarrhoea. *Aliment Pharmacol Ther.* 2015 Jun;41(11):1029-37.

80. Paula H, Grover M, Halder SL, et al. Non-enteric infections, antibiotic use, and risk of development of functional gastrointestinal disorders. *Neurogastroenterol Motil.* 2015 Nov;27(11):1580-6.

81. Ghoshal UC, Srivastava D. Irritable bowel syndrome and small intestinal bacterial overgrowth: meaningful association or unnecessary hype. *World J Gastroenterol.* 2014 Mar 14;20(10):2482-91.

82. Ghoshal UC, Srivastava D, Ghoshal U, Misra A. Breath tests in the diagnosis of small intestinal bacterial overgrowth in patients with irritable bowel syndrome in comparison with quantitative upper gut aspirate culture. *Eur J Gastroenterol Hepatol.* 2014 Jul;26(7):753-60.

83. Ghoshal UC, Kumar S, Mehrotra M, Lakshmi C, Misra A. Frequency of small intestinal bacterial overgrowth in patients with irritable bowel syndrome and chronic non-specific diarrhea. *J Neurogastroenterol Motil.* 2010 Jan;16(1):40-6.

84. Schey R, Rao SS. The role of rifaximin therapy in patients with irritable bowel syndrome without constipation. *Expert Rev Gastroenterol Hepatol.* 2011 Aug;5(4):461-4.

85. Acosta A, Camilleri M, Shin A, et al. Effects of Rifaximin on Transit, Permeability, Fecal Microbiome, and Organic Acid Excretion in Irritable Bowel Syndrome. *Clin Transl Gastroenterol.* 2016 May 26;7:e173.

86. Pimentel M. Review article: potential mechanisms of action of rifaximin in the management of irritable bowel syndrome with diarrhoea. *Aliment Pharmacol Ther.* 2016 Jan;43 Suppl 1:37-49.

87. Thompson A, Meah D, Ahmed N, et al. Comparison of the antibacterial activity of essential oils and extracts of medicinal and culinary herbs to investigate potential new treatments for irritable bowel syndrome. *BMC Complement Altern Med.* 2013 Nov 28;13:338.

88. Chedid V, Dhalla S, Clarke JO, et al. Herbal therapy is equivalent to rifaximin for the treatment of small intestinal bacterial overgrowth. *Glob Adv Health Med.* 2014 May;3(3):16-24.

89. Quigley EM. Probiotics in Irritable Bowel Syndrome: The Science and the Evidence. *J Clin Gastroenterol.* 2015 Nov-Dec;49 Suppl 1:S60-4.

90. Mazurak N, Broelz E, Storr M, Enck P. Probiotic Therapy of the Irritable Bowel Syndrome: Why Is the Evidence Still Poor and What Can Be Done About It? *J Neurogastroenterol Motil.* 2015 Oct 1;21(4):471-85.

91. Zhang Y, Li L, Guo C, et al. Effects of probiotic type, dose and treatment duration on irritable bowel syndrome diagnosed by Rome III criteria: a meta-analysis. *BMC Gastroenterol.* 2016 Jun 13;16(1):62.

92. McKenzie YA, Thompson J, Gulia P, et al. British Dietetic Association systematic review of systematic reviews and evidence-based practice guidelines for the use of probiotics in the management of irritable bowel syndrome in adults (2016 update). *J Hum Nutr Diet.* 2016 Jun 6. doi: 10.1111/jhn.12386. [Epub ahead of print]

93. Didari T, Mozaffari S, Nikfar S, Abdollahi M. Effectiveness of probiotics in irritable bowel syndrome: Updated systematic review with meta-analysis. *World J Gastroenterol.* 2015 Mar 14;21(10):3072-84.

94. Shah SL, Lacy BE. Dietary Interventions and Irritable Bowel Syndrome: A Review of the Evidence. *Curr Gastroenterol Rep.* 2016 Aug;18(8):41.

95. Chey WD. Food: The Main Course to Wellness and Illness in Patients with Irritable Bowel Syndrome. *Am J Gastroenterol.* 2016 Mar;111(3):366-71.

96. Gibson PR, Varney J, Malakar S, Muir JG. Food components and irritable bowel syndrome. *Gastroenterology.* 2015 May;148(6):1158-74.e4.

97. Böhn L, Störsrud S, Törnblom H, et al. Self-reported food-related gastrointestinal symptoms in IBS are common and associated with more severe symptoms and reduced quality of life. *Am J Gastroenterol.* 2013 May;108(5):634-41.

98. Sánchez-Vargas LA, Thomas-Dupont P, Torres-Aguilera M, et al. Prevalence of celiac disease and related antibodies in patients diagnosed with irritable bowel syndrome according to the Rome III criteria. A case-control study. *Neurogastroenterol Motil.* 2016 Jul;28(7):994-1000.

99. Ford AC, Chey WD, Talley NJ, Malhotra A, Spiegel BM, Moayyedi P. Yield of diagnostic tests for celiac disease in individuals with symptoms suggestive of irritable bowel syndrome: systematic review and meta-analysis. *Arch Intern Med.* 2009 Apr 13;169(7):651-8.

100. De Giorgio R, Volta U, Gibson PR. Sensitivity to wheat, gluten and FODMAPs in IBS: facts or fiction? *Gut.* 2016 Jan;65(1):169-78.

101. Vazquez-Roque MI, Camilleri M, Smyrk T, et al. A controlled trial of gluten-free diet in patients with irritable bowel syndrome-diarrhea: effects on bowel frequency and intestinal function. *Gastroenterology.* 2013 May;144(5):903-911.e3.

102. Aziz I, Trott N, Briggs R, North JR, Hadjivassiliou M, Sanders DS. Efficacy of a Gluten-Free Diet in Subjects With Irritable Bowel Syndrome-Diarrhea Unaware of Their HLA-DQ2/8 Genotype. *Clin Gastroenterol Hepatol.* 2016 May;14(5):696-703.e1.

103. Rodrigo L, Blanco I, Bobes J, de Serres FJ. Effect of one year of a gluten-free diet on the clinical evolution of irritable bowel syndrome plus fibromyalgia in patients with associated lymphocytic enteritis: a case-control study. *Arthritis Res Ther.* 2014 Aug 27;16(4):421.

104. Nagarajan N, Morden A, Bischof D, et al. The role of fiber supplementation in the treatment of irritable bowel syndrome: a systematic review and meta-analysis. *Eur J Gastroenterol Hepatol.* 2015 Sep;27(9):1002-10.

105. Nanayakkara WS, Skidmore PM, et al. Efficacy of the low FODMAP diet for treating irritable bowel syndrome: the evidence to date. *Clin Exp Gastroenterol.* 2016 Jun 17;9:131-42.

106. Mansueto P, Seidita A, D'Alcamo A, Carroccio A. Role of FODMAPs in Patients With Irritable Bowel Syndrome. *Nutr Clin Pract.* 2015 Oct;30(5):665-82.

107. Khan MA, Nusrat S, Khan MI, Nawras A, Bielefeldt K. Low-FODMAP Diet for Irritable Bowel Syndrome: Is It Ready for Prime Time? *Dig Dis Sci.* 2015 May;60(5):1169-77.

108. McKenzie YA, Bowyer RK, Leach H, et al. British Dietetic Association systematic review and evidence-based practice guidelines for the dietary management of irritable bowel syndrome in adults (2016 update). *J Hum Nutr Diet.* 2016 Jun 8. doi: 10.1111/jhn.12385. [Epub ahead of print]

109. National Institute for Health and Clinical Excellence (2015) Irritable bowel syndrome in adults. Diagnosis and management of irritable bowel syndrome in primary care. Clinical Guideline 61 Update 2015. Available at: http://www.nice.org.uk/Guidance/CG61.

110. Fukudo S, Kaneko H, Akiho H, et al. Evidence-based clinical practice guidelines for irritable bowel syndrome. *J Gastroenterol.* 2015 Jan;50(1):11-30.

111. Liu JP, Yang M, Liu YX, Wei M, Grimsgaard S. Herbal medicines for treatment of irritable bowel syndrome. *Cochrane Database Syst Rev.* 2006 Jan 25;(1):CD004116.

112. Xiao HT, Zhong L, Tsang SW, Lin ZS, Bian ZX. Traditional Chinese medicine formulas for irritable bowel syndrome: from ancient wisdoms to scientific understandings. *Am J Chin Med.* 2015;43(1):1-23.

113. Oka T, Okumi H, Nishida S, et al. Effects of Kampo on functional gastrointestinal disorders. *Biopsychosoc Med.* 2014 Jan 21;8(1):5.

114. Sahib AS. Treatment of irritable bowel syndrome using a selected herbal combination of Iraqi folk medicines. *J Ethnopharmacol.* 2013 Jul 30;148(3):1008-12.

115. Bone K, Mills S. Principles and Practice of Phytotherapy, 2nd Ed. London, England: Churchill Livingstone, 2013, pp199-210.

116. Ottillinger B, Storr M, Malfertheiner P, Allescher HD. STW 5 (Iberogast®)--a safe and effective standard in the treatment of functional gastrointestinal disorders. *Wien Med Wochenschr.* 2013 Feb;163(3-4):65-72.

117. Sallon S, Ben-Arye E, Davidson R, et al. A novel treatment for constipation-predominant irritable bowel syndrome using Padma Lax, a Tibetan herbal formula. *Digestion.* 2002;65(3):161-71.

118. Khanna R, MacDonald JK, Levesque BG. Peppermint oil for the treatment of irritable bowel syndrome: a systematic review and meta-analysis. *J Clin Gastroenterol.* 2014 Jul;48(6):505-12.

Understanding and Treating *H. pylori* Infections

Helicobacter pylori are motile, gram-negative spiral-shaped bacteria that take up residence in the stomach upon ingestion.[1,2] There is a debate about whether they should be deemed commensals or pathogens; we prefer to classify them as pathobionts.[3] Therefore, the use of the term "infection" could be rendered "colonization," though we will use the former term in this chapter as it is the most common term found in the literature.

Infection with *H. pylori* is linked to gastritis, hypochlorhydria or hyperchlorhydria (depending on location of colonization), peptic ulcer, duodenal ulcer, MALT lymphomas and gastric adenocarcinoma.[4] The bacterium grows optimally at a pH of 6.0 to 7.0, and has several characteristics allowing colonization within the stomach (luminal pH 1.0 to 2.0) that will be outlined below. *H. pylori* was discovered by Marshall and Warren in 1984; the pair was awarded the Nobel Prize in Physiology or Medicine in 2005.[5] The World Health Organization has since classified *H. pylori* as a class 1 carcinogen because of its connection to gastric cancer, making it the only bacterium to be classified as such.[6] Epidemiological studies suggest the prevalence of *H. pylori* infection in humans is decreasing; however, treatment is becoming increasingly difficult as antibiotic resistance rates increase in parts of the world.[7]

Epidemiology of *H. pylori*

Prevalence

Although about 50% of the world's population is estimated to be infected with *H. pylori*, the prevalence of infection is not proportionally distributed within or between countries.[8] Generally between countries, the prevalence of infection is greater in the developing world compared to the developed world (prevalence estimates range from 22 to 95% in developing countries and 1 to 58% in developed countries).[9] Prevalence of *H. pylori* in the United States has been reported as 17.1%; in Japan, prevalence is also relatively low (39.6%). Latin American countries have relatively higher prevalence of *H. pylori* (79.4%), China has been reported at 83.4%, and in the Italian village of Calabria, prevalence is 71.6%.[10,11] Within countries, prevalence has been shown to correlate with socioeconomic status, with those of low socioeconomic status having greater prevalence of infection. The prevalence of various *H. pylori* virulence factors also varies considerably by region, and Eastern Asia is associated with the highest prevalence of one of the most well-characterized virulence factors, CagA. These virulence factors will be discussed further below.[12] In the United States, infection with *H. pylori* has been shown to be greater in African-Americans or Hispanics compared to non-Hispanic whites.[13] Thus, although *H. pylori* infection is less prevalent in the Western world compared to the developing world, there may be sub-populations within the Western world with high prevalence.

Incidence and prevalence of *H. pylori* vary considerably by age, mostly because of the mode of transmission and the persistence of the infection. Generally, transmission of *H. pylori* occurs during childhood and, consequently, incidence of infection is higher in children compared to adults. However, a birth-cohort effect has been observed in developed countries, whereby the incidence of childhood infection of *H. pylori* in successive birth cohorts is decreasing.[14,15,16] Generally, *H. pylori* infection persists throughout life unless eradicated by treatment measures; therefore, prevalence of *H. pylori* infection is generally higher in older birth cohorts because the incidence of infection was more frequent when they were children, and the infection has persisted (even if asymptomatic) with the individual throughout life.[8] Transient infection with *H. pylori* may occur in infants and toddlers.[17]

Transmission

As previously stated, transmission most frequently occurs during childhood, but the major modes for *H. pylori* transmission are not fully understood. The majority of current evidence suggests humans are the only known reservoir for *H. pylori*, and, as such, transmission generally occurs via the human-to-human route. It is unknown if the route is through contact with infected digestive tract secretions via the fecal-oral, oral-oral, or gastric-oral routes. Vertical transmission from mother to child may be an important route.[8,18] It is unclear whether other environmental reservoirs may contribute to human infection. Several studies have suggested that the oral cavity may be an important reservoir for *H. pylori*, and oral infection may be implicated in gastric re-infection with *H. pylori*.[19,20] A Cochrane review has evaluated the effect of adjunctive periodontal treatment plus eradication therapy versus eradication therapy alone; the group found periodontal treatment was associated with better *H. pylori* eradication outcomes.[21] However, the included studies were all performed in developing countries and may have poor generalizability for the developed world.

The estimated incidence of *H. pylori* infection in children living in Western countries is higher than in adults, particularly in early childhood. In some studies, *H. pylori* incidence rates peak between the ages of two and three, and decline thereafter. A recent systematic review and meta-analysis by Carreira et al. found breastfeeding may contribute a protective effect against *H. pylori* infection in economically less-developed regions.[22]

Risk Factors

The greatest risk factor for infection with *H. pylori* is low socioeconomic conditions, especially in childhood. Many studies found an inverse association between risk of *H. pylori* infection and factors related to socioeconomic status including educational level and income.[14] Other risk factors include contaminated drinking water source and the presence of *H. pylori* infection in siblings or caregivers (for children), hygiene factors, and a high density of people in the household.[23,24] Moderate increases in risk for *H. pylori* infection have been observed in daycare settings for children.[25] Incidence rates are higher for adult travelers to high prevalence areas. Immigrant and migrant populations moving from a high prevalence country tend to have higher prevalence of *H. pylori* infection in Western countries, and the same is true of their children.[14]

Recurrence of Infection

Zhang et al. studied the worldwide "true" re-infection rate of *H. pylori* after successful eradication, and found re-infection to be relatively uncommon in adults (less than 1%) in many developed and developing countries.[26] Some developing countries (e.g., Mexico, Iran and Korea) had re-infection rates greater than 10%. The authors note many studies exploring the recurrence rates of *H. pylori* generally are influenced by "recrudescence," or the incomplete eradication of *H. pylori*, and this is why they chose to study strict criteria for "true" re-infection (defined as the complete eradication of one's original *H. pylori* strain and the subsequent re-infection by either a genetically distant strain, or a second exposure to the original *H. pylori* strain). In other studies, recurrence of *H. pylori* has been associated with the reappearance of gastritis and relapse of peptic ulcer disease.[26] Interfamilial transmission, particularly mother to child, is believed to be a major cause of re-infection.[26]

Colonization and Virulence of *H. pylori*

The factors underlying the pathogenesis and virulence of *H. pylori* are complicated, and depend on both bacterial factors and host factors.[27,28] Colonization, persistence and pathology of *H. pylori* depend on four important factors: 1) survival under acidic conditions, 2) movement toward epithelial cells through flagella-mediated motility, 3) attachment to host receptors by adhesins, and 4) release of tissue-damaging toxins.[29] Without eradication treatment, these unique mechanisms allow lifelong colonization with *H. pylori*, a reason some consider *H. pylori* to be the most successful bacterial pathogen.[30] These mechanisms will be briefly explained below.

1. **Surviving the Acidic Stomach**

   Generally, the stomach is viewed as an inhospitable niche for bacterial colonization and proliferation; however, *H. pylori* have many unique features affording it the ability to thrive within the stomach. It has a urease enzyme that converts host derived urea into ammonia and carbon dioxide, which buffers the microenvironment surrounding the bacterium as it finds its way to its preferred niche within the more neutral gastric mucosa.[29,30] The enzyme urease has greatest activity at low pH, a proton-gated channel UreI permits urea entry only under acidic conditions; the UreI channel is fully open at pH of 5.0 or below and closed at a pH of 7.0 to avoid lethal alkalization in an alkaline environment.[29] By altering the pH immediately surrounding the cell, the bacterium is able to change the viscosity of the mucosal layer making it more fluid-like, which aids in colonization.[27] This neutral zone allows for *H. pylori* to survive short exposures to acid. Urease has also been proposed to disrupt the epithelial tight junctions.[30]

2. Flagella-mediated Motility

Chemotaxis allows *H. pylori* to use physiochemical signals (e.g., pH, urea, amino acids, metals, bicarbonate, etc.) to move via its sheathed flagella from the lumen of the stomach to an optimal location within the more neutral mucosal layer.[27,29] *H. pylori* also uses quorum sensing in addition to chemotaxis in its search for an optimal niche to colonize.[27] The helical shape allows for a rotational corkscrew motility pattern, which aids in colonization by allowing for efficient movement through the vicious mucus layer.[27] In animal models knocking out the motility gene, *H. pylori* has reduced ability to colonize.[31] Once the organism reaches the mucosal layer, *H. pylori* can thrive fairly well, thereby allowing for prolonged colonization, as the rate of chemical diffusion is low and the pH is generally more neutral.[27]

3. Host Receptor Attachment

The next step to successful colonization relies on the adhesion of *H. pylori* to host receptors by outer membrane proteins or adhesins. Examples of these adhesins include blood-antigen binding adhesin (BabA), sialic acid-binding adhesin (SabA), neutrophil activating protein A, heat shock protein 60, adherence associated lipoprotein A and B (AlpA/B), and outer inflammatory protein A (OipA).[29,30] Of the adhesin molecules, BabA and SabA are the most widely studied thus far. These adhesins are important for bacterial attachment to host cells, and increase the fitness of the bacteria by: 1) protecting *H. pylori* from displacement caused by peristalsis and gastric emptying, 2) allowing the bacteria

to use host nutrients and metabolic substrates for growth, and 3) providing proximity to host cells to maximize effective toxin concentration. Polymorphisms have been found in many of these adhesin molecules, which may be important to virulence.[27]

4. Toxin Release

Cytotoxin-associated gene A (CagA) and vacuolating cytotoxin A (VacA) are two well-studied toxins released by *H. pylori* that are important to its virulence. CagA is a component of and a marker for the *cag* pathogenicity island (PAI), which is a group of genes that encodes a type IV secretion system (T4SS). The T4SS is a needle-like structure used to inject bacterial effectors into the host cell, and CagA is an effector injected into the cytoplasm of cells.[27,32,33] Once in the host cell, CagA has been shown to affect phosphorylation-mediated proliferation, cytoskeletal changes, signal transduction cascades, gene expression, inflammatory changes, cell elongation and disruption of tight junctions in the host cell.[27,29,32] The effects of CagA on the host cell depend on whether it is phosphorylated or not.[33]

The second well-studied toxin, VacA, is polymorphic due to its mosaic gene structure, and is considered a multifunctional toxin because of its diverse actions on the cell.[30] VacA is internalized, forms pores in the cell membrane and releases bicarbonate and organic acids into the host cytoplasm.[29] VacA is also associated with cellular apoptosis with release of pro-inflammatory proteins in a mitochondria mediated fashion, the inhibition of T cell functions, and cellular vacuolation, and may be involved in disruption of the polarized epithelial barrier.[27,30] VacA can also induce acute inflammatory responses through inducing host cell release of IL-8.[29]

H. pylori may be able to invade the epithelial cells and multiply via double-layered vesicles either in the plasma membrane or in the cytoplasm.[29] It has also been reported that *H. pylori* forms biofilms within the stomach. Both the multiplication of *H. pylori* and its ability to form biofilms may have considerable impact on its resistance to antibacterial therapy.

Pathophysiology of *H. pylori* Infection

The pathogenicity of *H. pylori* is highly variable amongst individuals and likely depends on many factors, including host factors (e.g., genetics, lifestyle factors, etc.), bacterial factors (e.g., genetics, virulence factors), environmental factors, and the interaction between the three. *H. pylori* is genetically highly variable, and this variation affects its virulence factors, which may affect the pathogenicity of some strains.[33] In all cases, *H. pylori* infection induces gastritis, but only a minority (10 to 15%) of those infected present clinical symptoms related to gastritis.[30] Therefore, in most cases (about 80%), *H. pylori* infection remains clinically silent. However, in a smaller proportion of cases, *H. pylori* infection is an etiological factor for peptic ulcer disease (about 10% of those infected), gastric cancer (in about 1 to 3% of those infected) and mucosa-associated lymphoid tissue (MALT) lymphoma (in about 0.1% of those infected).[8,57]

Both CagA and VacA are polymorphic, and epidemiological and animal studies have shown certain polymorphisms for VacA (i.e., s1/i1/m1) and seropostivity for CagA may be associated with increased degrees of chronic inflammation, neurophilic activity, epithelial damage in the gastric mucosa, increased risk of gastric atrophy and gastric cancer. The details of these associations are beyond the scope of this review; readers are referred to a recent review on this topic.[33] Epidemiologically, the prevalence of CagA positive strains in Western countries is estimated at 60-70%, while in Asian countries estimates are near 90%. Furthermore, studies in transgenic mice suggest the East Asian-type CagA is more carcinogenic than the Western-type CagA. Epidemiologically, CagA positive strains are important, as several studies indicate these strains are directly associated with acute gastritis, gastric ulcer and gastric cancer development. Further, CagA strains can be divided into the Western type CagA and the East Asian type CagA; the latter is associated with more cytoskeletal changes and is more likely to be associated with gastric cancer.

The location of *H. pylori* colonization within the stomach may be important to the resultant effect on host health. *H. pylori* generally colonizes in an antral-predominant or a corpus-predominant manner; if *H. pylori* colonization is distributed evenly throughout all gastric areas, it is defined as pangastritis. Colonization of the body of the stomach has been associated with hypochlorhydria and greater risk for gastric cancer compared to antrum-predominant gastritis, which is associated with hyperchlorhydria and duodenal ulcer disease.[34] A prospective study involving 1,526 Japanese patients (1,246 had *H. pylori* infection, 280 were uninfected) found patients with corpus-predominant gastritis had a high risk of gastric cancer (RR: 34.5; 95% CI: 7.1-166.7).[35] This phenomenon seems most important for those on chronic proton pump inhibitor drugs, as chronic use of these drugs has been associated with a location shift from antrum-predominant *H. pylori* colonization to the corpus region colonization.[36,37] A systematic review and meta-analysis found *H. pylori*-positive patients on long-term treatment with PPIs were at a significantly higher risk for developing corpus gastritis than *H. pylori*-negative patients (OR: 11.45, p < 0.00001).[38] The Maastricht IV/Florence consensus report recommends *H. pylori* be eradicated prior to long-term PPI treatment.[54] Long-term PPI use has also been shown to decrease the abundance of *H. pylori*, and *H. pylori* infection has been shown to increase the acid-suppressive effect of PPIs.[34,36]

Additionally, *H. pylori* infection can increase the risk of ulceration and bleeding in patients taking NSAIDs, and is responsible for symptoms in a subset of patients with functional dyspepsia.[8] *H. pylori* eradication has been associated with improved platelet counts in children and adults with idiopathic thrombocytopenic pupura.[39,40] Iron deficiency anemia is also associated with *H. pylori* colonization; systematic reviews and meta-analysis have shown *H. pylori* eradication with iron administration was more effective than iron administration alone in those with iron deficiency anemia.[41,42] A meta-analysis has shown *H. pylori* colonization is associated with decreased ascorbic acid and decreased cobalamin levels; levels of both ascorbic acid and cobalamin may be improved after *H. pylori* eradication.[43] Other micronutrients were investigated in this meta-analysis (e.g., folate, beta-carotene, alpha-tocopherol, calcium, magnesium, phosphorus, selenium, and zinc), however, the evidence was insufficient to draw conclusions. Despite the potential for harm in those infected, many individuals infected with *H. pylori* remain asymptomatic throughout life and some research has suggested *H. pylori* infection may have some protective benefit (see below). This has led to a debate about whether asymptomatic infections (i.e., colonization) should be treated at all.

Should *H. Pylori* be Eradicated in All Who Are Infected?

Many argue that *H. pylori* should be considered a commensal organism that merely creates negative host consequences in certain situations.[44] They will point, for instance, to archeological evidence that *H. pylori* has been discovered to have colonized the stomach of humans from prehistoric time. Furthermore, there have been reports that eradiation of *H. pylori* increases the incidence or complication of GERD; though more recent reviews and meta-analysis suggest this link is weak or non-existent.[45,46] Inverse relationships have also been reported between *H. pylori* infection and asthma and even childhood obesity, though these associations have been challenged by other investigators.[47,48,49]

The other main objection for the need to eradicate *H.pylori* in asymptomatic individuals is the eradication therapy itself (discussed further below). The use of antibiotics, the core of the therapy, is well-known to negatively affect the rest of the microbiome, and increase the likelihood of increasing antibiotic resistance (of *H.pylori* and other species in the gut). In fact, some antibiotics for the treatment of *H. pylori* cannot be used in some regions of the world due to the prevalence of antibiotic resistant strains in those areas. Therefore, there is great interest in developing new alternatives for eradication therapy and in investigating whether complete eradication of the infection is necessary, or if reducing the level and/or virulence of the colonization will result in a reduced risk of disease or disease severity.[50]

We should note that arguments for eradication, even in asymptomatic subjects, are still quite common. Though research shows that eradication of *H. pylori* leads to better outcomes in those who are symptomatic and successful treatment of *H. pylori* is associated with ulcer healing rates greater than 90%, eradication has also been shown to prevent gastric cancer and leads to eventual regression of acute and chronic inflammation.[51,52]

Diagnostic Tools[53]

Generally, invasive tests are more reliable than non-invasive tests for diagnosing infection.

Invasive tests
- **Histopathology staining**
- **Visual observation via endoscopy**
  Expensive, unpleasant, requires highly specialized operator to perform test
- **Bacterial culture**
  "Gold standard"
- **Biopsy sample**
  Rapid urease test
- **PCR**

Non-invasive tests
- **Urea Breath Test (UBT)**
  Preferred non-invasive test, "gold standard," for *in vivo* detection, effective means to evaluate whether therapy has successfully eradicated the organism, may be less reliable for children because they produce less CO_2 compared to adults.

  Sensitivity is 88 to 95% and specificity is 95 to 100%.[54]

- **Fecal antigen test**
  Highly sensitive and precise, good for children who are unable to perform breath test, false-negative results may be due to PPI.

  May be less acceptable in some cultures, but equally as valid as the UBT with a sensitivity of 94% and a specificity of 92%.[55]

- **Serological methods (ELISA, Western blotting)**
  Antibody specific to *H. pylori* in serum, whole blood, saliva, and stool.

  Antibodies against *H. pylori* and especially against its most specific antigen CagA remain elevated despite transient decreases of the bacterial load and even for long periods of time (months and even years) after disappearance of *H. pylori* from the stomach[56]

  May be used frequently on an epidemiological scale.

According to the Maastricht IV consensus report, in patients treated with PPIs: if possible, PPIs should be stopped for two weeks prior to testing by culture, histology, rapid urease test, UBT or stool test.[54]

STANDARD REGIMENS FOR *H. PYLORI* ERADICATION	
Standard triple therapy (7-14 d)	PPI - standard dose, *bid* Clarithromycin - 500 mg, *bid* Amoxicillin - 1 g, *bid*
Bismuth quadruple therapy (10-14 d)	PPI - standard dose, *bid* Bismuth - standard dose, *qid* Tetracycline - 500 mg, *qid* Metronidazole - 500 mg, *tid*
Sequential therapy (5 d dual therapy followed by a 5 d triple therapy)	Dual therapy; PPI - standard dose, *bid* Amoxicillin - 1 g, *bid* Triple therapy; PPI - standard dose, *bid* Clarithromycin - 500 mg, *bid* Metronidazole - 500 mg, *bid*
Concomitant therapy (7-10 d)	PPI - standard dose, *bid* Clarithromycin - 500 mg, *bid* Amoxicillin - 1 g, *bid* Metronidazole - 500 mg, *bid*
Hybrid therapy (7 d dual therapy followed by a 7 d quadruple therapy)	Dual therapy; PPI - standard dose, *bid* Amoxicillin - 1 g, *bid* Triple therapy; PPI - standard dose, *bid* Amoxicillin - 1 g, *bid* Clarithromycin - 500 mg, *bid* Metronidazole - 500 mg, *bid*
Levofloxacin-based triple therapy (10 d)	PPI - standard dose, *bid* Levofloxacin - 500 mg, *qd* Amoxicillin - 1 g, *bid*
Rifabutin-based triple therapy (7-14 d)	PPI - standard dose, *bid* Amoxicillin - 1 g, *bid* Rifabutin - 150 mg, *qd*
Culture-guided therapy (10 d)	PPI - standard dose, *bid* Bismuth - standard dose, *qid* Two antibiotics selected by antimicrobial sensitivity tests

Table 8: From: Ermis F, Senocak Tasci E. Current Helicobacter pylori treatment in 2014. *World J Methodol.* 2015 Jun 26;5(2):101-7. Licensed under a Creative Commons Attribution 4.0 License. qd: once daily; bid: twice daily; tid: three times daily; qid: four times daily.

Standard Eradication of *H. pylori*

The first eradication strategy for *H. pylori*, triple therapy, was proposed in 1987 by Thomas Borody for the treatment of duodenal ulcers. Standard triple therapy generally consists of a PPI and two antibiotics taken for seven to fourteen days, the most common triple therapy for *H. pylori* eradication historically has consisted of a PPI, clarithromycin, and metronidazole or amoxicillin. However, this treatment regime is falling out of favor due to increasing antibiotic resistance to clarithromycin around the world, and consequent declining treatment success rates to lower than the acceptable level of 80% in many parts of the world.[57] Other factors affecting eradication success rates include, patient compliance and host and bacterial factors. Consequently, the eradication of *H. pylori* is not straightforward, and many regimes (e.g., dual therapy, sequential therapy, concomitant therapy, hybrid therapy, reverse hybrid therapy, etc) and combinations of a PPI, antibiotics, and non-antibiotics (i.e., bismuth) have been proposed (see Table 7). After failed eradication therapy, antimicrobial sensitivity testing is recommended to guide further treatment protocols. Smoking has been shown to increase the treatment failure of *H. pylori* eradication efforts.[58] The details of all these regimes are beyond the scope of this text, and helpful reviews have been published.[59,60]

Why Are Proton Pump Inhibitors Used for *H. Pylori* Eradication?

The biological rationale behind the use of proton pump inhibitors in *H. pylori* eradication regimes is that of creating a favorable environment for the action of some antibiotics. The mechanism of action behind some antibiotics (e.g., amoxicillin, clarithromycin, tetracycline, etc.) requires an actively replicating bacterium for maximal efficacy. At the physiological pH of the stomach, *H. pylori* is generally quiescent and embedded with the mucus layer because of the acidic conditions associated with the lumen. With the use of proton pump inhibitors, the intragastric pH of the lumen is increased, allowing for conditions favorable for *H. pylori* growth. Despite the biological rationale behind this theory, it has been proposed that the median intragastric pH achieved by PPIs is about 4.0, which is still low enough for many *H. pylori* organisms to remain non-replicating and associated with the mucosal layer.[57]

Non-Pharmacological Agents

Since *H. pylori* infections are a global concern, there have been ongoing investigations to find alternatives for the use of pharmacological antibiotics or adjuncts to improve eradication rates (or to limit the side effects of the antibiotics). Many other agents have been tested for their ability to affect the growth and colonization of *H. pylori* in cell culture, animal and human clinical studies. These include natural antimicrobial agents and compounds that destabilize the mucosal biofilm, alter stomach pH or those that affect the gastrointestinal microbiota. Here, we overview some of the more promising agents that have been reported in clinical trials.

N-acetyl Cysteine

It has been suggested that *H. pylori* treatment failure may be due to the ability of *H. pylori* to form biofilms, which may undermine the current antimicrobial treatment protocols.[61] Carron et al. were the first to study the presence of *H. pylori* biofilms *in vivo* through the use of scanning electron microscopy of endoscopically directed gastric biopsies; the group found mature biofilms were present and attached to cell surfaces on *H. pylori* positive specimens (determined by rapid urease testing), though biofilms were not present in the urease-negative specimens.[62] Due to the general lack of success of standard *H. pylori* treatment protocols, use of biofilm inhibitors or biofilm-destabilizing agents have been proposed as a means to increase successful eradication. N-acetyl cysteine, known for its ability to cleave disulfide bonds that cross-link glycoproteins, such as those involved in mucosal biofilm matrixes, has been studied in a number of experimental models and clinical trials.[63,64]

In an open label, randomized clinical trial involving 40 patients in Italy with at least four *H. pylori* eradication failures, Cammarota et al. (2010) found a one-week pretreatment course with 600 mg NAC/day before a culture-guided, one-week treatment regime (two antibiotics plus one proton pump inhibitor) was superior (p<0.01) than the same treatment regime without pretreatment with NAC on *H. pylori* eradication rates as assessed by urea breath testing.[65] At the start of the study, all patients were evaluated for *H. pylori* biofilm formation via scanning electron microscopy; after treatment 60% of patients elected to perform repeat endoscopic examination to determine *H. pylori* biofilm status; all subjects in which *H. pylori* had been eradicated showed disappearance of *H. pylori* biofilms upon scanning electron microscopy. This same study featured an *in vitro* study, prior to the clinical trial, which illustrated the ability of NAC to disrupt cultured *H. pylori* biofilms.

A recent RCT (n=79) by Hamidian et al. (2015) showed a 14-day triple therapy eradication regime with amoxicillin/clarithromycin/omeprazole plus NAC (600 mg bid) was superior when compared to the triple therapy regime without NAC (72.9% and 60.9%, respectively, p = 0.005); *H. pylori* eradication was measured via urea breath test four weeks after treatment.[66] Another early Turkish study compared dual antibiotic therapy with lansoprazole (30 mg bid) and clarithromycin (500 mg bid) for 10 days plus NAC liquid (400 mg tid) or dual therapy without NAC for ten days.[67] After one month, treatment with dual therapy plus NAC was associated with a 50% eradication rate (14 of 28 patients), while the control group achieved an eradication rate of 23.3% (7 of 30 patients, p = 0.034); eradication was evaluated by gastric biopsy for histopathological study and rapid urease test.

A few studies have failed to achieve a statistical improvement when using NAC. A prospective, randomized open-label clinical trial by Emami et al. (2014) found the addition of NAC (600 mg tablet bid) to standard quadruple therapy (500 mg amoxicillin, four times/day), bismuth citrate (120 mg qid), omeprazole (20 mg bid), and clarithromycin (500 mg bid) compared to standard quadruple therapy alone did not affect eradication rates of *H. pylori* as assessed by stool antigen test (p = 0.96, by intention-to-treat analysis [ITT]).[68] Eradication rates in the group receiving quadruple therapy alone had an eradication rate of 49/60 (81.7%, 95% CI: 71.6-91.8) and the group receiving NAC in addition to quadruple therapy had an eradication rate of 50/61 (82%, 95% CI: 72-91.9%) by ITT. A South Korean study by Yoon et al. (2016) studied the effect of sequential therapy with and without NAC on *H. pylori* eradication.[69] Sequential therapy was as follows: rabeprazole (20 mg bid) and amoxicillin (1 g bid) for the first five days, followed by rabeprazole (20 mg bid), clarithromycin (500 mg bid), and metronidazole (500 mg bid) for the remaining five days. Subjects were randomized to sequential therapy plus NAC (400 mg bid, only for the first five days of sequential therapy) or sequential therapy alone. The ITT eradication rates for sequential therapy alone were 58% (95% CI: 43.8-72.2) and the sequential therapy plus NAC rates were 67.3% (95% CI: 53.7-81.0). Although sequential therapy plus NAC showed numerically higher eradication rates, the difference between groups was not significant (p= 0.336). None of these trials reported serious adverse events related to adjunct treatment with NAC for *H. pylori* eradication, and other reviews have confirmed the safety of oral NAC.[70]

We believe these data suggest that NAC may be a safe and potentially beneficial adjunct therapy during *H. pylori* eradication. Doses of 600 mg/day appear to be effective, and should be started one week prior to the eradication protocol and for the duration of the eradication protocol.

Bismuth Citrate

There are a number of bismuth salts used throughout the world, but three in particular have been studied for their anti-*H. pylori* action: bismuth subsalicylate, colloidal bismuth subcitrate, and ranitidine bismuth citrate.[72] The first bismuth salts to be tested *in vitro* for anti-*H. pylori* activity were bismuth subsalicylate (OTC as Pepto Bismol®) and bismuth subcitrate (available as a dietary supplement). Bismuth salts have been used historically for gastrointestinal indications dating back as far as the 19th century.[71] Eventually, bismuth was replaced with antacids, histamine-2 receptor antagonists, and proton pump inhibitors for the treatment of dyspepsia and peptic ulcer disease. Bismuth reappeared in the 1980s when many clinical trials were attempting to eradicate *H. pylori* infections proved to be ineffective; Tom Borody found successful eradication rates (94/100) with a regime of bismuth subcitrate (120 mg qid), and tetracycline (500 mg qid) for 28 days and metronidazole (200 mg qid) for 14 days. Later, metronidazole resistance reduced the effectiveness of this regime, and bismuth containing quadruple therapies were developed which included a PPI, bismuth, and two antibiotics. The different dosages, duration of therapy and use of different PPIs/antibiotics in studies complicate the understanding of the optimal regime.

Ingested bismuth compounds form salts in the stomach where their solubility is influenced by gastric pH and the unique chemistry of the compound.[72] Due to poor water solubility, most bismuth salts are weakly absorbed, and therefore exert local effect in the GI tract.[73] Bismuth levels have been measured greater than the minimum inhibitory concentration for the eradication of *H. pylori* within the gastric mucosa; bismuth levels fall quickly over three hours with mucus turnover. Although the mechanism of action of bismuth salts against *H. pylori* is unclear, some proposed mechanisms include the ability of bismuth to form complexes with the bacterial cell wall or periplasmic space, inhibition of important bacterial enzymes (i.e., urease, catalase, lipase, phospholipase), inhibition of ATP synthesis, and inhibition of *H. pylori* adherence to the surface of epithelial cells.[72]

Dark stools may present as a transient side effect during the use of bismuth compounds. It has been proposed that the dark stools may be a result of colonic anaerobic bacterial production of hydrogen sulfide from non-absorbed bismuth salts.[74]

Mastic Gum *(Pistacia lentiscus)*

Mastic gum is a resin from the *Pistacia lentiscus* tree grown in the southern region of Chios Island, Greece.[75] Many *in vitro* studies have shown mastic gum and its essential oil contain a variety of biological compounds with antibacterial activity against clinical isolates of *H. pylori*, even some isolates with antibiotic resistance against clarithromycin and metronidazole.[76,77,78] Mastic gum-extracted arabinogalactan proteins have been shown to reduce neutrophil activation induced from a virulence factor of *H. pylori* (*H.pylori* neutrophil-activating protein), an effect that may reduce gastric mucosal inflammation.[79,80]

A recent randomized trial evaluated the effects of mastic gum on *H. pylori* eradication in 52 *H. pylori*-positive human subjects.[81] The investigators randomized subjects to four treatment groups: 1) low dose mastic gum monotherapy (350 mg tid) for 14 days, 2) high dose mastic gum monotherapy (1.05 g tid) for 14 days, 3) dual regime of mastic gum (350 mg tid) and pantoprazole (20 mg bid) for 14 days, or 4) standard triple therapy consisting of pantoprazole (20 mg bid), amoxicillin (1 g bid) and clarithromycin (500 mg bid) for 10 days. Mastic gum was dispensed in capsules containing 350 mg. Urea breath testing was performed before randomization and again five weeks after treatment termination to assess *H. pylori* eradication. Upon testing UBT post treatment, standard triple therapy achieved the highest eradication rate (76.9%); those in the low-dose mastic gum monotherapy group had an eradication rate of 30.8%, and those in the high-dose mastic gum monotherapy group had an eradication rate of 38.5%. Interestingly, no one assigned to the combination treatment with pantoprazole and mastic gum achieved *H. pylori* eradication. Upon comparing pretreatment UBT measures to post-treatment UBT measures, only triple therapy achieved statistical significance (p=0.01), both the low and high dose mastic gum monotherapy groups approached significance (p=0.08 and p=0.064, respectively). The mastic gum was well tolerated by subjects, and it was concluded that mastic gum has antibacterial activity against *H. pylori in vivo*. Although mastic gum was not able to reach acceptable eradication rates, it was able to eradicate *H. pylori* in some individuals and may be an alternative *H. pylori* eradication regime.

Despite the positive results discussed above, an early small scale human clinical trial found treatment with mastic gum did not have any effect on *H. pylori* eradication.[82] In this study, eight *H. pylori* positive subjects were given 1 g mastic gum in capsule form four times per day for 14 days. After treatment, all subjects remained *H. pylori* positive as assessed by UBT. An animal study also showed monotherapy with mastic gum (2 g/day) had no effect on *H. pylori* eradication.[83]

Zinc

There is a small amount of data published using zinc L-carnosine (polaprezinc) for *H. pylori*-related outcomes. While only one clinical trial is published, most of the published *in vitro* and animal studies suggest zinc L-carnosine may exert its protective effect via anti-inflammatory mechanisms at the gastric mucosa. Ishihara et al. studied the effect of polaprezinc on *H. pylori*-associated gastritis in a Mongolian gerbil model of *H. pylori* infection.[84] Treatment with 0.02%

polaprezinc (given in chow pellets *ad libitum*) for 12 weeks did not have an effect on *H. pylori* density in the pyloric and fundic mucosa; however, zinc L-carnosine was shown to reduce *H. pylori*-induced inflammation. Zinc L-carnosine administration significantly reduced the development of polymorphonuclear neutrophil activity, mononuclear infiltration and surface epithelial erosion in the pyloric and fundic regions compared to control animals. An *in vitro* experiment within the trial showed the reduction in inflammation may be mediated through the scavenging of monochloramine by zinc L-carnosine. Another study evaluating polaprezinc in Mongolian gerbils with a higher dose (0.06%, 100 mg/kg, 10 times the usual clinical dose) found similar results; the treatment had no effect on the eradication of *H. pylori*, though it attenuated gastric mucosal inflammation and measures of oxidative stress.[85] *In vitro* studies have also found anti-inflammatory effects of polaprezinc on the gastric mucosa.[86]

A clinical trial randomized 66 patients (28 with peptic ulcers, and 38 with non-ulcer dyspepsia) to two groups: 1) "LAC" regime consisting of lansoprazole (30 mg bd), amoxicillin (500 mg bid) and clarithromycin (400 mg bd), or 2) the LAC regime plus polaprezinc (zinc L-carnosine, 150 mg bid).[87] Each group was treated for seven days. Subjects were evaluated for *H. pylori* before and four weeks after treatment via rapid urease test, histology and culture. Upon intention-to-treat analysis, the eradication rate in the LAC group was 77% (95% CI: 62-93%), and in the group treated with LAC plus zinc L-carnosine, the eradication rate was 94% (95% CI: 86-100%). Adverse events were minor and similar amongst the two groups; the most frequent adverse event was diarrhea. One subject in the LAC group and two subjects in the group receiving LAC/ zinc L-carnosine discontinued treatment due to severe diarrhea. Overall, it was concluded that the *H. pylori* eradication rate was significantly improved (p<0.05) with the addition of zinc L-carnosine to the triple therapy regime.

Probiotics and *H. pylori*

Many *in vitro* and animal studies have been performed suggesting probiotics may inhibit *H. pylori* by a number of different mechanisms, including the modification of host immune responses, the secretion of antibacterial substances (i.e., lactic acid, short chain fatty acids, hydrogen peroxide, bacteriocins, autolysins, etc.), increase of mucin production, and direct competition with *H. pylori* for mucosal adhesion sites.[88,89] Human clinical trials have also been performed using probiotics as adjunctive therapy or even as a monotherapy for the eradication of *H. pylori*.

Probiotics as an Adjunctive Therapy for *H. pylori* Eradication:

Numerous systematic reviews and meta-analyses have been published to evaluate the benefit of adjunctive probiotic use for improving *H. pylori* eradication rates with mostly, though not universally, positive outcomes.[90,91,92,93,94,95] Further, the Maastricht IV/Florence Consensus Report guidelines note that certain prebiotics and probiotics may be promising as an adjuvant treatment for *H. pylori* eradication simply by reducing side effects of antibiotic use.[54]

Unfortunately many of the studies evaluating probiotics for *H. pylori* outcomes have been small, of low methodological quality (e.g., absence of blinding, no placebo groups, etc.), and have been heterogeneous in terms of the probiotic agent tested (e.g., multi-strain or single strain, dose, duration of treatment, strain/species of probiotic tested, etc.) or heterogeneous in terms of the *H. pylori* eradication treatment used (e.g., concomitant therapy, bismuth quadruple therapy, standard triple therapy) and duration of treatment. Another variable affecting the inconsistency in the overall association between probiotics and *H. pylori* eradication treatment is the choice of antibiotics and the location of the study, as antibiotic resistance patterns vary by geography. In their meta-analysis, Dang et al. suggest that the ability of probiotics to improve *H. pylori* eradication rates may depend on the overall efficacy of the *H. pylori* eradication strategy chosen, with probiotics showing greater improvements when the *H. pylori* eradication regime effectiveness is low.[90] Thus, given the available evidence base, it is difficult to determine the optimal strain and dose of probiotics for improving *H. pylori* eradiation rates though a few species/strains have been studied more than others and associations may be drawn.

Saccharomyces boulardii

In a randomized, open study evaluating 182 children from a low-income socioeconomic district in Santiago, Chile, Gotteland et al. studied the effect of three treatments on the eradication of *H. pylori*: 1) antibiotic treatment with lansoprazole (1 mg/kg, bid), amoxicillin (50 mg/kg, tid), and clarithromycin (15 mg/kg bid) for eight days; 2) *Lactobacillus acidophilus* LB, heat-killed and lyophilized in a capsule (10^9 CFU bid) for eight weeks; and 3) *Saccharomyces boulardii* plus inulin (250 mg *S. boulardii*, 5 g inulin in a sachet, bid) for eight weeks.[96] *H. pylori* levels were measured by urea breath test before and after treatment. Sixty-six percent (30/45) of the children randomized to antibiotics had successful eradiation of *H. pylori* after treatment; lower rates of eradication were found in the probiotic groups. In the heat-killed *L. acidophilus* group, 6.5% (3/46) of subjects were successfully eradicated, and in the *S. boulardii* plus inulin group 12% (6/51) were successfully eradicated from *H. pylori*. An additional 81 children were tested as *H. pylori*-positive and followed for the eight weeks without treatment; in this group, spontaneous eradication was not found.

A recent meta-analysis of *S. boulardii* as an adjuvant therapy to triple therapy shows moderate evidence for improved eradication (RR: 1.11, 95% CI: 1.06-1.17) and for reduction in adverse effects (RR: 0.44, 95% CI: 0.31-0.64).[97] High-quality evidence was specifically shown for reduction in diarrhea in those supplemented with *S. boulardii* (RR: 0.51, 95% CI: 0.42-0.62). Although *S. boulardii* was able to improve *H. pylori* eradication rates, the rate was still below the desired level of success and the authors suggest other, possibly more effective eradication measures may be more useful to study (e.g., concomitant therapy, bismuth quadruple therapy) in conjunction with *S. boulardii* adjuvant treatment. In this study, the daily dose of *S. boulardii* ranged from 500 mg to 1,000 mg, and the duration of treatment ranged from one to four weeks.

Lactobacillus reuteri

A small-scale human study (10 healthy volunteers and nine with ileostomy) has shown *L. reuteri* ATCC 55730 (4 x 10^8 CFU, for 28 days) is able to colonize the gastric mucosa.[98] Human clinical trials studying *L. reuteri* as monotherapy for *H. pylori* eradication suggest supplementation with *L. reuteri* may reduce total *H.*

pylori bacterial counts, but alone may not fully eradicate *H. pylori*.[99] Francavilla et al. randomized 40 *H. pylori*-positive subjects to supplementation with a chewable tablet of *L. reuteri* ATCC 55730 (10^8 CFU, taken once per day, two hours before meals) or to placebo for 28 days.[100] After treatment, subjects randomized to *L. reuteri* had significantly reduced bacterial loads of *H. pylori* compared to baseline (p<0.05), and significantly improved rating on the Gastrointestinal Symptom Rating Scale compared to pretreatment value (p<0.05); no change was seen in the placebo group for either parameter. After treatment with either *L. reuteri* or placebo, both groups were given a 10-day sequential *H. pylori* eradication treatment; eradication rates following sequential therapy were similar in both groups (initially given *L. reuteri*: 88% vs. initially given placebo: 82%, p= 0.8).

Emara et al. studied the addition of *L. reuteri* to standard triple therapy in a randomized clinical trial.[101] Seventy treatment naïve subjects were randomized into two groups: 1) triple therapy plus *L. reuteri* (mixture of *L. reuteri* DSM 17938 and *L. reuteri* ATCC PTA 6475 in a chewable tablet, 2×10^8 CFU/day) for two weeks followed by *L. reuteri* tablet alone for an additional two weeks, or 2) triple therapy plus placebo for two weeks followed by placebo alone for an additional two weeks. In both groups, triple therapy consisted of omeprazole (20 mg bid), amoxicillin (1,000 mg bid), and clarithromycin (500 mg bid). After treatment, the eradication rate for the *L. reuteri* group was 74.3% (26/35), and for the placebo group, 65.7% (23/35), though the difference between groups was not statistically significant (p=0.603). After treatment, Gastrointestinal Symptom Rating Scale scores were lower in the *L. reuteri* group (4.77 ± 2.446) compared to the placebo group (9.06 ± 5.291) (p<0.001), indicating better symptom scores in the *L. reuteri* group. Additionally, the *L. reuteri* treatment improved histological features of the *H. pylori* infection. No serious adverse events were noted in either group studied. A similar study by Francavilla et al. (n=100) found treatment with *L. reuteri* (2×10^8 CFU, DSM 17938 and ATCC PTA 6475) in monotherapy had an inhibitory effect on *H. pylori* growth (^{13}C urea breath test value decreased by 13% in the *L. reuteri* group compared to 4% in the placebo group); and when given in addition to eradication therapy, *L. reuteri* significantly reduced antibiotic-associated side effects.[102]

Lactobacillus rhamnosus GG
L. rhamnosus GG (LGG) has been noted in a few studies investigating its effect as an adjunctive agent for *H. pylori* eradication. One study in adult patients found LGG administration (6×10^9 CFU) reduced eradication therapy related side effects and improved treatment tolerability, but did not affect success of eradication rate.[103] A study in 83 children found LGG supplementation (10^9 CFU bid) given alongside a triple therapy eradication regime did not improve eradication rates, nor improve side effects compared to placebo.[104]

Probiotics as a Standalone Therapy for *H. pylori* Eradication
A few experimental and low-quality human trials have evaluated probiotics as monotherapy against *H. pylori*.[105] Most of these human trials have tested a variety of strains and dosages of probiotics, and generally find that although probiotics are not able to consistently eradicate *H. pylori*, probiotics can reduce the density of *H. pylori* usually measured by urea breath testing. These studies have published eradication rates ranging from 6.5 to 14.9%. Some researchers have suggested probiotics delivered via fermented milk products (FMP) may have advantages over other types of probiotic formulations (e.g., capsules, sachets, etc.). These advantages, the authors suggest, may be due to additional components found in FMP preparations such as bovine lactoferrin, alpha-lactalbumin, glycomacropeptide, and lactic acid.[106,107] Of these components, bovine lactoferrin seems to have the most evidence related to *H. pylori* eradication.

Many proposed mechanisms have been suggested for the potential role of bovine lactoferrin in the eradication of *H. pylori*: 1) bovine lactoferrin has iron binding affinity and may limit iron utilization by bacteria, 2) it has antioxidant activity, 3) it may limit *H. pylori* attachment to the stomach, 4) it may influence structural changes in the microbial cell wall, amongst others.[107,108] A meta-analysis of nine trials has shown lactoferrin as an adjunctive agent to *H. pylori* eradication regimes may increase eradication rates and may reduce side-effects (especially nausea) of anti-*H. pylori* therapy.[109] Another meta-analysis of five studies, published in the same year, notes lactoferrin given as an adjunctive agent to *H. pylori* eradication regimes is potentially more beneficial than lactoferrin given alone for the eradication of *H. pylori*; however, the authors note more research is needed as the included studies point in the direction of benefit for bovine lactoferrin improving *H.pylori* eradication rates, but the majority of these studies are of low methodological quality (only one double-blind RCT).[110] The included studies of both meta-analyses used lactoferrin at a dose of 200 mg bid. Based on this evidence, it seems the use of bovine lactoferrin appear promising as adjunctive agents to *H. pylori* eradication; however, more research is needed in this area to better understand the potential advantage of lactoferrin (or FMP) in the context of *H. pylori* eradication.

Conclusion of Probiotics and *H. pylori*

Since the majority of *H. pylori* eradication regimes rely heavily on the use of antibiotics, concomitant probiotic use should be advised to avoid antibiotic therapy associated side effects such as AAD and CDAD (see AAD/CDAD section on page 164). In fact, many of the same meta-analyses cited above reported benefits for probiotics in reducing the side effects of *H. pylori*

eradication therapy such as diarrhea, nausea, epigastric pain, taste disturbance and vomiting.[91,92,93] Because patient compliance is necessary for both eradication success and for avoiding increasing antibiotic resistant bacteria, incorporating probiotics into *H. pylori* eradication therapy may be helpful for therapeutic success.

Overall, probiotics mechanistically may help create an unfavorable milieu for *H. pylori*. However, when given as a monotherapy, probiotics show limited ability to eradicate *H. pylori* on their own, though they may reduce *H. pylori* density. Furthermore, meta-analyses report a benefit of probiotics on increased *H. pylori* eradication rates when given as an adjuvant therapy, and perhaps a stronger benefit when eradication by standard treatment regimes is low. In any event, we suggest probiotics should be given anytime antibiotics are prescribed (see page 134), independent of their ability to increase eradication rates.

References

1.   Carroll KC, Hobden JA, Miller S, et al. Vibrio, Campylobacter, and Helicobacter. In: Carroll KC, Hobden JA, Miller S, Morse SA, Mietzner TA, Detrick B, Mitchell TG, McKerrow JH, Sakanari JA. eds. Jawetz, Melnick, & Adelberg's Medical Microbiology, 27e. New York, NY: McGraw-Hill; 2015.
2.   Levinson W. Brief Summaries of Medically Important Organisms. In: Levinson W. eds. Review of Medical Microbiology and Immunology, 13e. New York, NY: McGraw-Hill; 2014.
3.   Whalen MB1, Massidda O. Helicobacter pylori: enemy, commensal or, sometimes, friend? *J Infect Dev Ctries*. 2015 Jul 4;9(6):674-8.
4.   Kao CY, Sheu BS, Wu JJ. Helicobacter pylori infection: An overview of bacterial virulence factors and pathogenesis. *Biomed J*. 2016 Feb;39(1):14-23.
5.   Marshall BJ, Warren JR. Unidentified curved bacilli in the stomach of patients with gastritis and peptic ulceration. *Lancet*. 1984 Jun 16;1(8390):1311-5.
6.   Schistosomes, liver flukes and Helicobacter pylori. IARC Working Group on the Evaluation of Carcinogenic Risks to Humans. Lyon, 7-14 June 1994. IARC Monogr Eval Carcinog Risks Hum. 1994;61:1-241.
7.   Cui R, Zhou L. Helicobacter pylori infection: an overview in 2013, focus on therapy. *Chin Med J (Engl)*. 2014;127(3):568-73.
8.   Mitchell H, Katelaris P. Epidemiology, clinical impacts and current clinical management of Helicobacter pylori infection. *Med J Aust*. 2016 Jun 6;204(10):376-80.
9.   Sierra MS, Hastings EV, Fagan-Garcia K, Colquhoun A, Goodman KJ. Epidemiology, Transmission and Public Health Implications of Helicobacter pylori Infection in Western Countries. *Helicobacter Pylori: A Worldwide Perspective*. 2014, 25-79.
10. Calvet X, Ramírez Lázaro MJ, Lehours P, Mégraud F. Diagnosis and epidemiology of Helicobacter pylori infection. *Helicobacter*. 2013 Sep;18 Suppl 1:5-11.
11. Mentis A, Lehours P, Mégraud F. Epidemiology and Diagnosis of Helicobacter pylori infection. *Helicobacter*. 2015 Sep;20 Suppl 1:1-7.
12. Laird-Fick HS, Saini S, Hillard JR. Gastric adenocarcinoma: the role of Helicobacter pylori in pathogenesis and prevention efforts. *Postgrad Med J*. 2016 Aug;92(1090):471-7.
13. Nguyen T, Ramsey D, Graham D, et al. The Prevalence of Helicobacter pylori Remains High in African American and Hispanic Veterans. *Helicobacter*. 2015 Aug;20(4):305-15.
14. Eusebi LH, Zagari RM, Bazzoli F. Epidemiology of Helicobacter pylori infection. *Helicobacter*. 2014 Sep;19 Suppl 1:1-5.
15. IARC Working Group. Helicobacter Pylori. 2012. Retrieved from: http://monographs.iarc.fr/ENG/Monographs/vol100B/mono100B-15.pdf
16. The EUROGAST Study Group. Epidemiology of, and risk factors for, Helicobacter pylori infection among 3194 asymptomatic subjects in 17 populations. The EUROGAST Study Group. *Gut*. 1993 Dec;34(12):1672-6.
17. Sustmann A, Okuda M, Koletzko S. Helicobacter pylori in children. *Helicobacter*. 2016 Sep;21 Suppl 1:49-54.
18. Osaki T, Konno M, Yonezawa H, et al. Analysis of intra-familial transmission of Helicobacter pylori in Japanese families. *J Med Microbiol*. 2015 Jan;64(Pt 1):67-73.
19. Payão SL, Rasmussen LT. Helicobacter pylori and its reservoirs: A correlation with the gastric infection. *World J Gastrointest Pharmacol Ther*. 2016 Feb 6;7(1):126-32.
20. Yee JK. Helicobacter pylori colonization of the oral cavity: A milestone discovery. *World J Gastroenterol*. 2016 Jan 14;22(2):641-8.
21. Ren Q, Yan X, Zhou Y, Li WX. Periodontal therapy as adjunctive treatment for gastric Helicobacter pylori infection. *Cochrane Database Syst Rev*. 2016 Feb 7;2:CD009477.
22. Carreira H, Bastos A, Peleteiro B, Lunet N. Breast-feeding and Helicobacter pylori infection: systematic review and meta-analysis. *Public Health Nutr*. 2015 Feb;18(3):500-20.
23. Yucel O. Prevention of Helicobacter pylori infection in childhood. *World J Gastroenterol*. 2014 Aug 14;20(30):10348-54.
24. Iwańczak B, Francavailla R. Helicobacter pylori infection in pediatrics. *Helicobacter*. 2014 Sep;19 Suppl 1:46-51.
25. Bastos J, Carreira H, La Vecchia C, Lunet N. Childcare attendance and Helicobacter pylori infection: systematic review and meta-analysis. *Eur J Cancer Prev*. 2013 Jul;22(4):311-9.
26. Zhang YY, Xia HH, Zhuang ZH, Zhong J. Review article: 'true' re-infection of Helicobacter pylori after successful eradication--worldwide annual rates, risk factors and clinical implications. *Aliment Pharmacol Ther*. 2009 Jan;29(2):145-60.
27. Keilberg D, Ottemann KM. How Helicobacter pylori senses, targets and interacts with the gastric epithelium. *Environ Microbiol*. 2016 Mar;18(3):791-806.
28. Sgouras DN, Trang TT, Yamaoka Y. Pathogenesis of Helicobacter pylori Infection. *Helicobacter*. 2015 Sep;20 Suppl 1:8-16.
29. Kao CY, Sheu BS, Wu JJ. Helicobacter pylori infection: An overview of bacterial virulence factors and pathogenesis. *Biomed J*. 2016 Feb;39(1):14-23.
30. Posselt G, Backert S, Wessler S. The functional interplay of Helicobacter pylori factors with gastric epithelial cells induces a multi-step process in pathogenesis. *Cell Commun Signal*. 2013 Oct 7;11:77.
31. Ottemann KM, Lowenthal AC. Helicobacter pylori uses motility for initial colonization and to attain robust infection. *Infect Immun*. 2002 Apr;70(4):1984-90.
32. Atherton JC, Blaser MJ. Helicobacter pylori Infections. In: Kasper D, Fauci A, Hauser S, Longo D, Jameson J, Loscalzo J. eds. Harrison's Principles of Internal Medicine, 19e. New York, NY: McGraw-Hill; 2015.

33. Ferreira RM, Machado JC, Figueiredo C. Clinical relevance of Helicobacter pylori vacA and cagA genotypes in gastric carcinoma. *Best Pract Res Clin Gastroenterol*. 2014 Dec;28(6):1003-15.

34. Malfertheiner P. The intriguing relationship of Helicobacter pylori infection and acid secretion in peptic ulcer disease and gastric cancer. *Dig Dis*. 2011;29(5):459-64.

35. Uemura N, Okamoto S, Yamamoto S, et al. Helicobacter pylori infection and the development of gastric cancer. *N Engl J Med*. 2001 Sep 13;345(11):784-9.

36. Freedberg DE, Lebwohl B, Abrams JA. The impact of proton pump inhibitors on the human gastrointestinal microbiome. *Clin Lab Med*. 2014 Dec;34(4):771-85.

37. Moayyedi P, Wason C, Peacock R, et al. Changing patterns of Helicobacter pylori gastritis in long-standing acid suppression. *Helicobacter*. 2000 Dec;5(4):206-14.

38. Lundell L, Vieth M, Gibson F, Nagy P, Kahrilas PJ. Systematic review: the effects of long-term proton pump inhibitor use on serum gastrin levels and gastric histology. *Aliment Pharmacol Ther*. 2015 Sep;42(6):649-63.

39. Kodama M, Kitadai Y, Ito M. et al. Immune response to CagA protein is associated with improved platelet count after Helicobacter pylori eradication in patients with idiopathic thrombocytopenic purpura. *Helicobacter*. 2007 Feb;12(1):36-42.

40. Ferrara M, Capozzi L, Russo R. Effect of Helicobacter pylori eradication on platelet count in children with chronic idiopathic thrombocytopenic purpura. *Hematology*. 2009 Oct;14(5):282-5.

41. Hudak L, Jaraisy A, Haj S, Muhsen K. An updated systematic review and meta-analysis on the association between Helicobacter pylori infection and iron deficiency anemia. *Helicobacter*. 2016 Jul 13. doi: 10.1111/hel.12330.

42. Huang X, Qu X, Yan W, et al. Iron deficiency anaemia can be improved after eradication of Helicobacter pylori. *Postgrad Med J*. 2010 May;86(1015):272-8.

43. Lahner E, Persechino S, Annibale B. Micronutrients (Other than iron) and Helicobacter pylori infection: a systematic review. *Helicobacter*. 2012 Feb;17(1):1-15.

44. Otero LL, Ruiz VE, Perez Perez GI. Helicobacter pylori: the balance between a role as colonizer and pathogen. *Best Pract Res Clin Gastroenterol*. 2014 Dec;28(6):1017-29.

45. Xie T1, Cui X, Zheng H, et al. Meta-analysis: eradication of Helicobacter pylori infection is associated with the development of endoscopic gastroesophageal reflux disease. *Eur J Gastroenterol Hepatol*. 2013 Oct;25(10):1195-205.

46. Tan J, Wang Y, Sun X, et al. The effect of Helicobacter pylori eradication therapy on the development of gastroesophageal reflux disease. *Am J Med Sci*. 2015 Apr;349(4):364-71.

47. Zhou X, Wu J, Zhang G. Association between Helicobacter pylori and asthma: a meta-analysis. *Eur J Gastroenterol Hepatol*. 2013 Apr;25(4):460-8.

48. Wang Q, Yu C, Sun Y. The association between asthma and Helicobacter pylori: a meta-analysis. *Helicobacter*. 2013 Feb;18(1):41-53.

49. Wang Y, Bi Y, Zhang L, Wang C. Is Helicobacter pylori infection associated with asthma risk? A meta-analysis based on 770 cases and 785 controls. *Int J Med Sci*. 2012;9(7):603-10.

50. Kim SY, Choi DJ, Chung JW Antibiotic treatment for Helicobacter pylori: Is the end coming? *World J Gastrointest Pharmacol Ther*. 2015 Nov 6;6(4):183-98.

51. Doorakkers E, Lagergren J, Engstrand L, Brusselaers N. Eradication of Helicobacter pylori and Gastric Cancer: A Systematic Review and Meta-analysis of Cohort Studies. *J Natl Cancer Inst*. 2016 Jul 14;108(9).

52. Lee YC, Chiang TH, Chou CK, et al. Association Between Helicobacter pylori Eradication and Gastric Cancer Incidence: A Systematic Review and Meta-analysis. *Gastroenterology*. 2016 May;150(5):1113-1124.e5.

53. Khalilpour A, Kazemzadeh-Narbat M, Tamayol A, et al. Biomarkers and diagnostic tools for detection of Helicobacter pylori. *Appl Microbiol Biotechnol*. 2016 Jun;100(11):4723-34.

54. Malfertheiner P, Megraud F, O'Morain CA, et al. Management of Helicobacter pylori infection--the Maastricht IV/ Florence Consensus Report. *Gut*. 2012 May;61(5):646-64.

55. Vaira D, Malfertheiner P, Mégraud F, et al. Diagnosis of Helicobacter pylori infection with a new non-invasive antigen-based assay. HpSA European study group. *Lancet*. 1999 Jul 3;354(9172):30 3.

56. Ekström AM, Held M, Hansson LE, et al. Helicobacter pylori in gastric cancer established by CagA immunoblot as a marker of past infection. *Gastroenterology*. 2001 Oct;121(4):784-91.

57. Sachs G, Scott DR. Helicobacter pylori: Eradication or Preservation. *F1000 Med Rep*. 2012;4:7.

58. Suzuki T, Matsuo K, Ito H, et al. Smoking increases the treatment failure for Helicobacter pylori eradication. *Am J Med*. 2006 Mar;119(3):217-24.

59. Marcus EA, Sachs G, Scott DR. Eradication of Helicobacter pylori Infection. *Curr Gastroenterol Rep*. 2016 Jul;18(7):33.

60. Liou JM, Wu MS, Lin JT. Treatment of Helicobacter pylori Infection- Where are we now? *J Gastroenterol Hepatol*. 2016 Apr 18.

61. García A, Salas-Jara MJ, Herrera C, González C. Biofilm and Helicobacter pylori: from environment to human host. *World J Gastroenterol*. 2014 May 21;20(19):5632-8.

62. Carron MA, Tran VR, Sugawa C, Coticchia JM. Identification of Helicobacter pylori biofilms in human gastric mucosa. *J Gastrointest Surg*. 2006 May;10(5):712-7.

63. Makipour K, Friedenberg FK. The potential role of N-acetylcysteine for the treatment of Helicobacter pylori. *J Clin Gastroenterol*. 2011 Nov-Dec;45(10):841-3.

64. Samuni Y, Goldstein S, Dean OM, Berk M. The chemistry and biological activities of N-acetylcysteine. *Biochim Biophys Acta*. 2013 Aug;1830(8):4117-29.

65. Cammarota G, Branca G, Ardito F, et al. Biofilm demolition and antibiotic treatment to eradicate resistant Helicobacter pylori: a clinical trial. *Clin Gastroenterol Hepatol*. 2010 Sep;8(9):817-820.e3.

66. Hamidian SM, Aletaha NS, Taslimi R, Montazeri M. An Additive Effect of Oral N-Acetyl Cysteine on Eradication of Helicobacter pylori. *J Pathog*. 2015;2015:540271.

67. Gurbuz AK, Ozel AM, Ozturk R, et al. Effect of N-acetyl cysteine on Helicobacter pylori. *South Med J*. 2005 Nov;98(11):1095-7.

68. Emami MH, Zobeiri M, Rahimi H, et al. N-acetyl cysteine as an adjunct to standard anti-Helicobacter pylori eradication regimen in patients with dyspepsia: A prospective randomized, open-label trial. *Adv Biomed Res*. 2014 Sep 8;3:189.

69. Yoon H, Lee DH, Jang ES, et al. Effects of N-acetylcysteine on First-Line Sequential Therapy for Helicobacter pylori Infection: A Randomized Controlled Pilot Trial. *Gut Liver*. 2016 Jul 15;10(4):520-5.

70. Atkuri KR, Mantovani JJ, Herzenberg LA, Herzenberg LA. N-Acetylcysteine--a safe antidote for cysteine/glutathione deficiency. *Curr Opin Pharmacol*. 2007 Aug;7(4):355-9.

71. Graham DY, Lee SY. How to Effectively Use Bismuth Quadruple Therapy: The Good, the Bad, and the Ugly. *Gastroenterol Clin North Am*. 2015 Sep;44(3):537-63.

72. Lambert JR, Midolo P. The actions of bismuth in the treatment of Helicobacter pylori infection. *Aliment Pharmacol Ther*. 1997 Apr;11 Suppl 1:27-33.

73. Yang JC, Lu CW, Lin CJ. Treatment of Helicobacter pylori infection: current status and future concepts. *World J Gastroenterol*. 2014 May 14;20(18):5283-93.

74. Bierer DW. Bismuth subsalicylate: history, chemistry, and safety. *Rev Infect Dis*. 1990 Jan-Feb;12 Suppl 1:S3-8.

75. Dimas KS, Pantazis P, Ramanujam R. Review: Chios mastic gum: a plant-produced resin exhibiting numerous diverse pharmaceutical and biomedical properties. *In Vivo*. 2012 Sep-Oct;26(5):777-85.

76. Marone P, Bono L, Leone E, Bona S, Carretto E, Perversi L. Bactericidal activity of Pistacia lentiscus mastic gum against Helicobacter pylori. *J Chemother*. 2001 Dec;13(6):611-4.

77. Miyamoto T, Okimoto T, Kuwano M. Chemical Composition of the Essential Oil of Mastic Gum and their Antibacterial Activity Against Drug-Resistant Helicobacter pylori. *Nat Prod Bioprospect*. 2014 Aug;4(4):227-31.

78. Sharifi MS, Hazell SL. Isolation, analysis and antimicrobial activity of the acidic fractions of Mastic, Kurdica, Mutica and Cabolica gums from genus Pistacia. *Glob J Health Sci*. 2011 Dec 29;4(1):217-28.

79. Kottakis F, Kouzi-Koliakou K, Pendas S, et al. Effects of mastic gum Pistacia lentiscus var. Chia on innate cellular immune effectors. *Eur J Gastroenterol Hepatol*. 2009 Feb;21(2):143-9.

80. Choli-Papadopoulou T, Kottakis F, Papadopoulos G, Pendas S. Helicobacter pylori neutrophil activating protein as target for new drugs against H. pylori inflammation. *World J Gastroenterol*. 2011 Jun 7;17(21):2585-91.

81. Dabos KJ, Sfika E, Vlatta LJ, Giannikopoulos G. The effect of mastic gum on Helicobacter pylori: a randomized pilot study. *Phytomedicine*. 2010 Mar;17(3-4):296-9.

82. Bebb JR, Bailey-Flitter N, Ala'Aldeen D, Atherton JC. Mastic gum has no effect on Helicobacter pylori load in vivo. *J Antimicrob Chemother*. 2003 Sep;52(3):522-3.

83. Loughlin MF, Ala'Aldeen DA, Jenks PJ. Monotherapy with mastic does not eradicate Helicobacter pylori infection from mice. *J Antimicrob Chemother*. 2003 Feb;51(2):367-71.

84. Ishihara R, Iishi H, Sakai N, et al. Polaprezinc attenuates Helicobacter pylori-associated gastritis in Mongolian gerbils. *Helicobacter*. 2002 Dec;7(6):384-9.

85. Suzuki H, Mori M, Seto K, et al. Polaprezinc attenuates the Helicobacter pylori-induced gastric mucosal leucocyte activation in Mongolian gerbils--a study using intravital videomicroscopy. *Aliment Pharmacol Ther*. 2001 May;15(5):715-25.

86. Shimada T, Watanabe N, Ohtsuka Y, et al. Polaprezinc down-regulates proinflammatory cytokine-induced nuclear factor-kappaB activiation and interleukin-8 expression in gastric epithelial cells. *J Pharmacol Exp Ther*. 1999 Oct;291(1):345-52.

87. Kashimura H, Suzuki K, Hassan M, et al. Polaprezinc, a mucosal protective agent, in combination with lansoprazole, amoxycillin and clarithromycin increases the cure rate of Helicobacter pylori infection. *Aliment Pharmacol Ther*. 1999 Apr;13(4):483-7.

88. Homan M, Orel R. Are probiotics useful in Helicobacter pylori eradication? *World J Gastroenterol*. 2015 Oct 7;21(37):10644-53.

89. Dore MP, Goni E, Di Mario F. Is There a Role for Probiotics in Helicobacter pylori Therapy? *Gastroenterol Clin North Am*. 2015 Sep;44(3):565-75.

90. Dang Y, Reinhardt JD, Zhou X, Zhang G. The effect of probiotics supplementation on Helicobacter pylori eradication rates and side effects during eradication therapy: a meta-analysis. *PLoS One*. 2014 Nov 3;9(11):e111030.

91. Gong Y, Li Y, Sun Q. Probiotics improve efficacy and tolerability of triple therapy to eradicate Helicobacter pylori: a meta-analysis of randomized controlled trials. *Int J Clin Exp Med*. 2015 Apr 15;8(4):6530-43.

92. Zhang MM, Qian W, Qin YY, He J, Zhou YH. Probiotics in Helicobacter pylori eradication therapy: a systematic review and meta-analysis. *World J Gastroenterol*. 2015 Apr 14;21(14):4345-57.

93. Wang ZH, Gao QY, Fang JY. Meta-analysis of the efficacy and safety of Lactobacillus-containing and Bifidobacterium-containing probiotic compound preparation in Helicobacter pylori eradication therapy. *J Clin Gastroenterol*. 2013 Jan;47(1):25-32.

94. McFarland LV, Huang Y, Wang L, Malfertheiner P. Systematic review and meta-analysis: Multi-strain probiotics as adjunct therapy for Helicobacter pylori eradication and prevention of adverse events. *United European Gastroenterol J*. 2016 Aug;4(4):546-61.

95. Lu C, Sang J, He H, et al. Probiotic supplementation does not improve eradication rate of Helicobacter pylori infection compared to placebo based on standard therapy: a meta-analysis. *Sci Rep*. 2016 Mar 21;6:23522.

96. Gotteland M, Poliak L, Cruchet S, Brunser O. Effect of regular ingestion of Saccharomyces boulardii plus inulin or Lactobacillus acidophilus LB in children colonized by Helicobacter pylori. *Acta Paediatr*. 2005 Dec;94(12):1747-51.

97. Szajewska H, Horvath A. Systematic review with meta-analysis: Saccharomyces boulardii supplementation and eradication of Helicobacter pylori infection. *Aliment Pharmacol Ther*. 2015 Jun;41(12):1237-45.

98. Mukai T, Asasaka T, Sato E, et al. Inhibition of binding of Helicobacter pylori to the glycolipid receptors by probiotic Lactobacillus reuteri. *FEMS Immunol Med Microbiol*. 2002 Jan 14;32(2):105-10.

99. Imase K, Tanaka A, Tokunaga K, et al. Lactobacillus reuteri tablets suppress Helicobacter pylori infection--a double-blind randomised placebo-controlled cross-over clinical study. *Kansenshogaku Zasshi*. 2007 Jul;81(4):387-93.

100. Francavilla R, Lionetti E, Castellaneta SP, et al. Inhibition of Helicobacter pylori infection in humans by Lactobacillus reuteri ATCC 55730 and effect on eradication therapy: a pilot study. *Helicobacter*. 2008 Apr;13(2):127-34.

101. Emara MH, Mohamed SY, Abdel-Aziz HR. Lactobacillus reuteri in management of Helicobacter pylori infection in dyspeptic patients: a double-blind placebo-controlled randomized clinical trial. *Therap Adv Gastroenterol*. 2014 Jan;7(1):4-13.

102. Francavilla R, Polimeno L, Demichina A, et al. Lactobacillus reuteri strain combination in Helicobacter pylori infection: a randomized, double-blind, placebo-controlled study. *J Clin Gastroenterol*. 2014 May-Jun;48(5):407-13.

103. Armuzzi A, Cremonini F, Bartolozzi F, et al. The effect of oral administration of Lactobacillus GG on antibiotic-associated gastrointestinal side-effects during Helicobacter pylori eradication therapy. *Aliment Pharmacol Ther*. 2001 Feb;15(2):163-9.

104. Szajewska H, Albrecht P, Topczewska-Cabanek A. Randomized, double-blind, placebo-controlled trial: effect of lactobacillus GG supplementation on Helicobacter pylori eradication rates and side effects during treatment in children. *J Pediatr Gastroenterol Nutr*. 2009 Apr;48(4):431-6.

105. Boltin D. Probiotics in Helicobacter pylori-induced peptic ulcer disease. *Best Pract Res Clin Gastroenterol*. 2016 Feb;30(1):99-109.

106. Sachdeva A, Nagpal J. Effect of fermented milk-based probiotic preparations on Helicobacter pylori eradication: a systematic review and meta-analysis of randomized-controlled trials. *Eur J Gastroenterol Hepatol*. 2009 Jan;21(1):45-53.

107. Sachdeva A, Rawat S, Nagpal J. Efficacy of fermented milk and whey proteins in Helicobacter pylori eradication: a review. *World J Gastroenterol*. 2014 Jan 21;20(3):724-37.

108. Wada T, Aiba Y, Shimizu K, et al. The therapeutic effect of bovine lactoferrin in the host infected with Helicobacter pylori. *Scand J Gastroenterol*. 1999 Mar;34(3):238-43.

109. Zou J, Dong J, Yu XF. Meta-analysis: the effect of supplementation with lactoferrin on eradication rates and adverse events during Helicobacter pylori eradication therapy. *Helicobacter*. 2009 Apr;14(2):119-27.

110. Sachdeva A, Nagpal J. Meta-analysis: efficacy of bovine lactoferrin in Helicobacter pylori eradication. *Aliment Pharmacol Ther*. 2009 Apr 1;29(7):720-30.

Clinical Consequences of Proton Pump Inhibitor Overuse

The rampant use of proton pump inhibitors (PPIs include omeprazole/Prilosec®, lansoprazole/Prevacid®, rabeprazole/Aciphex, esomeprazole/Nexium®) is a concern to many clinicians, even those who believe them to be a useful tool in certain patients. The control of HCl production is tightly managed by a series of overlapping signaling mechanisms (see page 29), which PPIs completely obliterate. The hypochlorhydria/achlorhydria induced by PPI use has been shown to have many negative consequences[1,2,3,4,5] Most of the evidence supporting these associations is based on epidemiological data, often making causality difficult to determine, and hence many of these associations are controversial.

Microbiome Changes

- Changes within the microbiome of PPI-users versus non-users in all areas of the GI tract from the esophagus to the colonic microbiome have been reported.[6] A significant decrease in diversity and over-representation of oral bacteria was reported in the fecal microbiome of PPI-users.[7]

- *C. difficile*-Associated Diarrhea (CDAD): Although most studies are of low quality and heterogeneous, it appears that PPI users have a higher risk for CDAD.[8,9,10] A recent systematic review and meta-analysis has found the evidence supporting this association to be of low quality, though the FDA released a safety announcement in 2015 regarding the association between CDAD and PPI use.[11,12]

- SIBO: A recent systematic review and meta-analysis found an increased risk of SIBO in PPI users, but only when the presence of SIBO was tested via duodenal or jejunal aspirate culture (OR: 7.587, 95% CI: 1.805-31.894) versus glucose hydrogen breath test (OR: 1.93, 95% CI: 0.69-5.42).[13] Based on the wide confidence intervals of this study and the heterogeneity amongst included trials, more research should be done in this area to help determine causality. For more discussion of SIBO, see page 231.

Micronutrient Malabsorption

The reduced acidity associated with PPI use has been proposed as a mechanism behind the malabsorption of several micronutrients; effects that may be more pronounced in special populations such as the elderly and the malnourished. A comprehensive review has been published on this topic.[14] Some details will be expanded upon below.

- **Magnesium**
  - Most data for hypomagnesemia has been published in case reports.[14]
  - A cross-sectional study has shown an association between standard and high-dose PPI treatment and risk of hypomagnesemia (adjusted OR: 2.50; 95% CI: 1.43-4.36).[15] The authors conclude long-term PPI use may be associated with sub-clinical magnesium insufficiency or deficiency status.
  - In 2011, the FDA released a safety announcement regarding the long-term use (defined as > 1 year) of PPIs and the risk for low serum magnesium levels. Further, in about a quarter of the cases examined, magnesium supplementation did not improve serum magnesium levels and PPI use had to be stopped.[16]
  - The FDA safety statement also recommended that physicians take baseline serum magnesium levels on patients for which they anticipate long-term PPI therapy and to periodically measure levels during treatment.
  - According to the FDA, after discontinuing the PPI, the median time required for magnesium to normalize is one week.

- **Calcium**
  Acid suppression with PPI may interfere with the ionization of insoluble calcium salts.[17] There are limited data on the effect of PPI on calcium absorption; however, O'Connell et al. showed omeprazole decreased calcium carbonate absorption efficiency in elderly (>65 years) fasted women by an average of 41% compared to placebo.[18]

- **Vitamin B12**

  Adequate stomach acid is required to separate vitamin B12 from protein in food sources, and elevated pH due to PPI therapy may interfere with this separation.[19] A cross-sectional study (n=659 adults) showed prolonged PPI use was associated with low serum B12 levels (p<0.00005), but not with prolonged use of H2 blockers (p=0.1036).[20] Co-therapy with oral B12 supplementation based on the RDA slowed but did not prevent the decline in B12 status (p=0.0125).[21]

- **Iron**

  Based on molecular studies, dietary iron is absorbed in the ferrous (II) form; in order to reduce dietary ferric (III) iron to the ferrous form, an adequate proton gradient by gastric acid is reported to be necessary. Omeprazole has been shown to decrease the absorption of oral iron supplements (ferrous sulfate) in iron deficient subjects; though this effect on iron absorption was not seen in iron-replete healthy subjects (n=9) on a normal diet when supplemented with 650 mg ferrous sulfate (130 mg elemental iron).[22,23,24] A retrospective cohort study including subjects who received PPI therapy for at least one year, compared to matched controls, found PPI therapy significantly decreased hematologic indices from baseline compared to controls.[25] After adjusting for confounders, long-term PPI therapy was associated with an OR of 5.03 (95% CI: 1.71-14.78, p<0.01) for decreasing hemoglobin by 1g/dL and an OR of 5.46 (95% CI: 1.67-17.85, p<0.01) for decreasing hematocrit by 3%.

- **Vitamin C**

  The use of PPIs may decrease vitamin C bioavailability by reducing its concentration in gastric fluid and by reducing the amount of the active form of ascorbic acid These effects have been mostly, sometimes exclusively, limited to individuals infected with *H. pylori*.[26,27]

Fracture:

- Several epidemiological studies have been published linking PPI use to increased risk of osteoporotic fractures; however, not all studies have confirmed this effect.[28] Calcium malabsorption is thought to be a mechanism underlying this effect.

Adverse Drug Reactions:

- The drug interactions of omeprazole have been published, and are quite numerous because of its moderate inhibition of CYP2C19 and CYP3A4.[22] Generally the most cited drug interaction is between omeprazole and the antiplatelet agent clopidogrel. Because of its effect on CYP2C19, omeprazole is suggested to attenuate the antiplatelet activity of clopidogrel.[29] Ironically, PPI therapy is often used alongside clopidogrel therapy to reduce the risk of GI bleeding due to the use of clopidogrel.

Pneumonia:

- A systematic review of 26 other systematic reviews and meta-analyses has recently been published.[30] This report confirms that PPI therapy has been associated with an increased risk of community acquired pneumonia (CAP). This report additionally suggests that CAP risk is greatest during early treatment periods with PPI therapy (30 days after initiation of PPI) compared to long-term PPI use. Another meta-analysis suggested that high-dose PPI treatment is also associated with a higher risk of CAP, while treatment >180 days with PPI is not associated with CAP.[31]

Rebound Acid Hypersecretion (RAHS):

- RAHS, or the increased HCl secretion above pretreatment levels following acid suppression treatment, has been shown to occur in human clinical trials following PPI treatment.[32] RAHS is clinically relevant because it has been associated with acid-related rebound symptoms such as dyspepsia, heartburn and acid regurgitation—symptoms that may lead patients to reinitiate acid suppression via PPI use.[33] Therefore, understanding the nature of RAHS may help inform PPI cessation protocols.

- Generally, the RAHS effect is usually temporary with the time-course, perhaps dependent on duration of PPI therapy.[33] Following short-term therapy (< 2 months) RAHS has been shown to be present for about eight weeks, whereas long-term therapy (> 1 year) has been associated with RAHS for eight to 26 weeks.[33,34]

- An underlying mechanism for RAHS has been proposed to be related to hypergastrinemia caused from prolonged elevations in gastric pH due to PPI therapy, and secondary ECL cell hyperplasia.[35]

Protocol for PPI Withdrawal:

- A systematic review evaluating six clinical studies for the discontinuation of proton pump inhibitors has been published.[36] Although the studies evaluated varied in design, discontinuation of PPI was reported across all studies ranging from 14% to 64%. Gradually reducing or tapering treatment seemed to have better success compared to abrupt cessation; an approach that may allow for an adaptation within the cells controlling HCl production. The authors further suggest giving an alginate or antacid to manage possible acid-related symptoms during the cessation period.

- The best outcomes, associated with a 64% discontinuation rate after three months, utilized patient education as a key intervention.[37] The subjects in this trial attended a nurse-led dyspepsia clinic, where they were screened for *H. pylori* infection and treated appropriately, if positive. The nurse helped subjects create an individual action plan to reduce or stop PPI administration; subjects were also offered a prescription for an alginate for rebound symptoms. At 12 months, 34% of subjects remained off PPIs and 50% reduced their dosage.

- Therefore, incorporating patient education may be a necessary factor for successful discontinuation of PPI use; it is especially important to educate patients about the potential for acid rebound symptoms and to give them an estimation of the duration of symptoms. The patient should be made aware of and understand that the symptoms of rebound will eventually subside without reverting back to PPI use.

References

1. Mössner J. The Indications, Applications, and Risks of Proton Pump Inhibitors. *Dtsch Arztebl Int.* 2016 Jul 11;113(27-28):477-83.
2. Coté GA, Howden CW. Potential adverse effects of proton pump inhibitors. *Curr Gastroenterol Rep.* 2008 Jun;10(3):208-14.
3. Chapman DB, Rees CJ, Lippert D Adverse effects of long-term proton pump inhibitor use: a review for the otolaryngologist. *J Voice.* 2011 Mar;25(2):236-40.
4. McCarthy DM. Adverse effects of proton pump inhibitor drugs: clues and conclusions. *Curr Opin Gastroenterol.* 2010 Nov;26(6):624-31.
5. Reimer C. Safety of long-term PPI therapy. *Best Pract Res Clin Gastroenterol.* 2013 Jun;27(3):443-54.
6. Freedberg DE, Lebwohl B, Abrams JA. The impact of proton pump inhibitors on the human gastrointestinal microbiome. *Clin Lab Med.* 2014 Dec;34(4):771-85.
7. Imhann F, Bonder MJ, Vich Vila A, et al. Proton pump inhibitors affect the gut microbiome. *Gut.* 2016 May;65(5):740-8.
8. McCarthy DM. Adverse effects of proton pump inhibitor drugs: clues and conclusions. *Curr Opin Gastroenterol.* 2010 Nov;26(6):624-31.
9. Janarthanan S, Ditah I, Adler DG, Ehrinpreis MN. Clostridium difficile-associated diarrhea and proton pump inhibitor therapy: a meta-analysis. *Am J Gastroenterol.* 2012 Jul;107(7):1001-10.
10. Kwok CS, Arthur AK, Anibueze CI, et al. Risk of Clostridium difficile infection with acid suppressing drugs and antibiotics: meta-analysis. *Am J Gastroenterol.* 2012 Jul;107(7):1011-9.
11. Tleyjeh IM, Bin Abdulhak AA, Riaz M, et al. Association between proton pump inhibitor therapy and clostridium difficile infection: a contemporary systematic review and meta-analysis. *PLoS One.* 2012;7(12):e50836.
12. http://www.fda.gov/Drugs/DrugSafety/ucm290510.htm
13. Lo WK, Chan WW. Proton pump inhibitor use and the risk of small intestinal bacterial overgrowth: a meta-analysis. *Clin Gastroenterol Hepatol.* 2013 May;11(5):483-90.
14. Heidelbaugh JJ. Proton pump inhibitors and risk of vitamin and mineral deficiency: evidence and clinical implications. *Ther Adv Drug Saf.* 2013 Jun;4(3):125-33.
15. Gau JT, Yang YX, Chen R, Kao TC. Uses of proton pump inhibitors and hypomagnesemia. *Pharmacoepidemiol Drug Saf.* 2012 May;21(5):553-9.
16. http://www.fda.gov/Drugs/DrugSafety/ucm245011.htm
17. Yang YX. Chronic proton pump inihibitor therapy and calcium metabolism. *Curr Gastroenterol Rep.* 2012 Dec;14(6):473-9.
18. O'Connell MB, Madden DM, Murray AM, et al. Effects of proton pump inhibitors on calcium carbonate absorption in women: a randomized crossover trial. *Am J Med.* 2005 Jul;118(7):778-81.
19. Linder L, Tamboue C, Clements JN. Drug-Induced Vitamin B12 Deficiency: A Focus on Proton Pump Inhibitors and Histamine-2 Antagonists. *J Pharm Pract.* 2016 Aug 12. pii: 0897190016663092.
20. Dharmarajan TS, Kanagala MR, Murakonda P, et al. Do acid-lowering agents affect vitamin B12 status in older adults? *J Am Med Dir Assoc.* 2008 Mar;9(3):162-7.
21. Lam JR, Schneider JL, Zhao W, Corley DA. Proton pump inhibitor and histamine 2 receptor antagonist use and vitamin B12 deficiency. *JAMA.* 2013 Dec 11;310(22):2435-42.
22. Li W, Zeng S, Yu LS, Zhou Q. Pharmacokinetic drug interaction profile of omeprazole with adverse consequences and clinical risk management. *Ther Clin Risk Manag.* 2013;9:259-71.
23. Ajmera AV, Shastri GS, Gajera MJ, Judge TA. Suboptimal response to ferrous sulfate in iron-deficient patients taking omeprazole. *Am J Ther.* 2012 May;19(3):185-9.
24. Tempel M, Chawla A, Messina C, Celiker MY. Effects of omeprazole on iron absorption: preliminary study. *Turk J Haematol.* 2013 Sep;30(3):307-10.
25. Sarzynski E, Puttarajappa C, Xie Y, et al. Association between proton pump inhibitor use and anemia: a retrospective cohort study. *Dig Dis Sci.* 2011 Aug;56(8):2349-53.
26. McColl KE. Effect of proton pump inhibitors on vitamins and iron. *Am J Gastroenterol.* 2009 Mar;104 Suppl 2:S5-9.
27. Henry EB, Carswell A, Wirz A, et al. Proton pump inhibitors reduce the bioavailability of dietary vitamin C. *Aliment Pharmacol Ther.* 2005 Sep 15;22(6):539-45.

28. Lau AN, Tomizza M, Wong-Pack M, Papaioannou A, Adachi JD. The relationship between long-term proton pump inhibitor therapy and skeletal frailty. *Endocrine*. 2015 Aug;49(3):606-10.

29. Bouziana SD, Tziomalos K. Clinical relevance of clopidogrel-proton pump inhibitors interaction. *World J Gastrointest Pharmacol Ther*. 2015 May 6;6(2):17-21.

30. Abramowitz J, Thakkar P, Isa A, et al. Adverse Event Reporting for Proton Pump Inhibitor Therapy: An Overview of Systematic Reviews. *Otolaryngol Head Neck Surg*. 2016 May 17. pii: 0194599816648298.

31. Giuliano C, Wilhelm SM, Kale-Pradhan PB. Are proton pump inhibitors associated with the development of community-acquired pneumonia? A meta-analysis. *Expert Rev Clin Pharmacol*. 2012 May;5(3):337-44.

32. Dacha S, Razvi M, Massaad J, Cai Q, Wehbi M. Hypergastrinemia. *Gastroenterol Rep (Oxf)*. 2015 Aug;3(3):201-8.

33. Książdzyna D, Szeląg A, Paradowski L. Overuse of proton pump inhibitors. *Pol Arch Med Wewn*. 2015;125(4):289-98.

34. Fossmark R, Johnsen G, Johanessen E, Waldum HL. Rebound acid hypersecretion after long-term inhibition of gastric acid secretion. *Aliment Pharmacol Ther*. 2005 Jan 15;21(2):149-54.

35. Lerotić I, Baršić N, Stojsavljević S, Duvnjak M. Acid inhibition and the acid rebound effect. *Dig Dis*. 2011;29(5):482-6.

36. Haastrup P, Paulsen MS, Begtrup LM, et al. Strategies for discontinuation of proton pump inhibitors: a systematic review. *Fam Pract*. 2014 Dec;31(6):625-30.

37. Murie J, Allen J, Simmonds R, de Wet C. Glad you brought it up: a patient-centred programme to reduce proton-pump inhibitor prescribing in general medical practice. *Qual Prim Care*. 2012;20(2):141-8.

GERD: A Lifestyle and Nutrient Approach

Gastroesophageal reflux disease (GERD) is a common diagnosis in Western societies that negatively affects the quality of life of those afflicted.[1] Characterized by reflux of gastric contents into the esophagus, the refluxate itself may contain heterogeneous components including acid, pepsin, gas or even contents of the duodenum, including bile acid and pancreatic enzymes.[2,3] Symptoms of GERD are often described as typical, atypical or extra-esophageal.[4] Typical symptoms of GERD include heartburn and/or regurgitation; atypical symptoms include epigastric discomfort, non-cardiac chest pain, nausea, satiety, dysphagia, globus, eructation, and hematemesis. Extra-esophageal symptoms include chronic cough, wheezing, sore throat, hoarseness, and dental erosions. GERD may present as erosive or non-erosive reflux disease (NERD) depending on the appearance of the esophageal mucosa upon endoscopy. NERD is actually the more common phenotype (about 70% of cases) compared to erosive reflux disease (about 30% of cases).[5]

While the most sensitive test for diagnosis of GERD is 24-hour ambulatory pH monitoring, it is most often "diagnosed" by empiric symptom relief using acid suppressing drugs. Endoscopy is suggested in subjects with reflux symptoms refractory to anti-secretory therapy; in those with alarm symptoms, such as dysphagia, weight loss, or gastrointestinal bleeding; and in those with recurrent dyspepsia after treatment that is not clearly due to reflux on clinical grounds alone. Endoscopy should be considered in patients with long-standing (≥10 years) GERD, as they have a six-fold increased risk of Barrett's esophagus compared to a patient with <1 year of reflux symptoms.[6]

Risk Factors for GERD[2]

The prevalence of GERD varies in different populations around the world and is generally higher in Western countries: 18 to 28% in North America, 9 to 26% in Europe, 2 to 8% in East Asia, 9 to 33% in the Middle East, 12% in Australia and 23% in South America.[7] Since 1995, prevalence for GERD has increased, particularly in North America and East Asia. The following list represents the most common and statistically significant risk factors associated with GERD:

- **Dietary factors:** See pages 225-227
- **Obesity:** GERD diagnosis rates have been reported to be higher in those who are overweight and obese, and the prevalence of GERD appears to increase with higher BMI.[8,9] Abdominal obesity may increase the pressure over the gastroesophageal junction through gastric distension, thus facilitating transient esophageal sphincter relaxations and reflux.

- **Smoking:** In an epidemiological study by Nisson et al., cigarette smoking was shown to increase the risk of GERD in a dose-dependent manner.[10] Smoking daily for more than 20 years was associated with an OR of 1.7 (95% CI: 1.5-1.9) compared to non-smokers. Other studies have confirmed this relationship.[11]

- **Physical activity:** Although the association between physical activity and GERD is controversial, Festi et al. conclude in their review that moderate physical activity and a diet high in dietary fiber and low in fat likely are beneficial for the prevention of GERD.[12]

- **Psychological stress:** In an epidemiological study carried out in Japan, strong psychological stress was significantly associated with NERD (OR: 1.77, 95% CI: 1.18-2.62) compared to a control group.[13] Psychological stress has been linked to a heighted perception of pain related to GERD.[14]

- **Genetic predisposition:** Twin studies have suggested a genetic component to GERD, and more recently a genome-wide association study identified potential genes related to GERD.[15,16,17] More research is needed to discover the clinical relevance for patient genetic testing and GERD.

- **Pregnancy:** A prospective longitudinal study found GERD prevalence to increase during the first, second and third trimesters (16.9%, 25.3%, and 51.2%, respectively).[18]

- **Medications decreasing LES pressure:** These include nitrates, calcium channel blockers, NSAIDs, theophylline, morphine, meperidone, diazepam, barbiturates, and sildenafil.[2]

- **Sleep disturbance:** A bidirectional relationship between sleep disturbance and GERD has been studied; see melatonin section below.

Pathophysiology of GERD

Although the complete pathophysiological mechanism of GERD is not fully understood, many technological advances in the past several years have provided more insight into understanding the many mechanisms underlying GERD.[19] The pathophysiological factors underlying GERD include sliding hiatal hernia, low pressure at the lower esophageal sphincter (LES), transient LES relaxations (TLESRs), the acid pocket, increased intra-abdominal distension (obesity), prolonged acid clearance, impaired saliva flow, esophageal hypersensitivity, and delayed gastric emptying.[20,21,22] In infants and children, food allergy (especially to bovine milk proteins) has been associated with GERD.[23,24,25] Ironically, measures of stomach pH are similar in subjects with symptoms of GERD compared to healthy control subjects, suggesting that excess stomach acid production is unrelated to reflux and not a root cause of GERD symptoms.[26] Furthermore, while some evidence suggests low stomach acid production (hypochlorhydria) may be a contributor of GERD in some subjects (due to delayed stomach emptying or supine position),[24,27] there is limited evidence to suggest hypochlorhydria is common in subjects with GERD (see page 30 for discussion of hypochlorhydria/achlorhydria).

Barrett's esophagus (BE) is a premalignant condition of the esophagus wherein the normal stratified squamous epithelium of the distal esophagus is replaced by columnar mucosal cells.[28] In the general population, it is estimated that the prevalence of BE is about 0.5 to 2%, whereas in those with GERD the BE prevalence estimates generally range from 5 to 15%.[29] Spechler and Souza note "patients with long-segment BE typically have severe GERD with erosive esophagitis, whereas short-segment BE is not associated with GERD symptoms or endoscopic signs of reflux esophagitis."[30] BE is detected upon endoscopy and is a major risk factor for esophageal adenocarcinoma. Ironically, BE and the associated risk for esophageal adenocarcinoma has increased, rather than decreased, since the advent of the use of PPIs.[31]

Treatments for GERD

Conventional
Conventional pharmaceutical treatment of GERD is highly dependent upon the use of proton pump inhibitors (PPIs), histamine H_2-receptor antagonists (H2RAs), and prokinetic medications.[19] PPIs are by far the most commonly used treatment because of their potent suppression of symptoms for the patient; however, their use is not without long-term health risks. Anti-secretory therapies such as PPIs and H2RAs simply mask the symptoms of GERD but do not address the most common root cause of the dysfunction leading to GERD symptoms: an incompetent lower esophageal sphincter. In fact, reflux will rarely resolve when taking a PPI, but the drug is effective at raising the pH of the refluxate so the sensation of burning in the esophagus diminishes.[32] Rebound acidity in addition to a number of long-term side effects including increased fracture risk, impaired absorption of vitamins and minerals, and bacterial overgrowth are associated with long-term PPI use (see page 219 for more on PPI-related consequences). Furthermore, PPI therapy is unsuccessful for symptomatic relief in some patients with erosive GERD and, especially, NERD.[33]

Histamine H_2-receptor antagonists provide temporary symptomatic relief (about six hours), and their onset is slower in duration than antacids (because they require systemic absorption). Their long-term use is not recommended because the body can build up a tolerance within one to two weeks and they are not as effective against erosive esophagitis.[34,64] Prokinetic drugs are used to increase esophageal clearance in GERD subjects, but their onset is slow and of short duration (four to eight hours).[34] Also, their side effect profile is unfavorable: tremors, tardive dyskinesia, fatigue, and increased risk for cardiac events.[34]

Because conventional treatments carry inherent short-term and long-term risks, and because the causes of GERD are multifactorial, a comprehensive treatment approach to GERD would include temporary symptom suppression with agents offering less risk and the evaluation of lifestyle behaviors that may contribute to GERD.[4] Once lifestyle behaviors are identified, it is important to educate the patient on adopting lifestyle modifications aimed at addressing the root cause of their symptoms. For some, this may include losing weight, smoking cessation, or adopting new dietary habits, for which there is promising evidence.

Lifestyle Interventions for GERD

Lifestyle recommendations for GERD are primarily derived from epidemiological data and published case studies, though a few intervention trials have been performed. It is important to realize that while these data often lead to conflicting interpretation, individual differences in the relationship between lifestyle and GERD likely account for the heterogeneous outcomes of these studies.[12,35,36,43] In a post hoc analysis of the REQUEST (Re-assessment of quality of life on reflux esophagitis treatment) study performed in Japan, it was found that lifestyle modification (details not specified) plus lansoprazole (15 to 30 mg) was associated with significantly better health-related quality of life scores compared to those given lansoprazole and told to continue current lifestyle or those given no lifestyle instruction.[37] The following is a list of lifestyle-based recommendations that may be helpful to consider in patients suffering from GERD. The usefulness of each must be empirically determined.

Examples of Lifestyle Interventions
- Elevate the head of the bed six inches (using blocks under the bed posts rather than extra pillows as extra pillows may cause increased intra-abdominal pressure and exacerbate symptoms)
- Weight loss in obese and overweight persons
- Eat smaller meals or avoid consuming large quantities of fluids with meals
- Avoid large meals close to bedtime
- Avoid lying down immediately after eating a meal

- Avoid foods high in saturated fats and simple sugars
- Avoid caffeine
- Avoid beverages containing acid (red wine, carbonated beverages, orange juice, tomato juice, and other citrus fruits)
- Increase fiber intake
- Decrease alcohol intake
- Smoking cessation (In one recent study, smoking cessation [assisted with varenicline] was shown to improve GERD, reflux symptoms and health-related quality of life following one year of treatment)[38]
- Avoid strong mints that may relax the LES (enteric-coated peppermint capsule can be used)
- Avoid wearing tight clothing around abdomen

A cross-sectional study (n=1875) in Pakistan found a regular post-dinner walk was inversely related to GERD symptoms compared to lying down after dinner (OR: 0.66, 95% CI: 0.5-0.88), and a dinner-to-bedtime interval greater than three hours was associated with less GERD symptoms when compared to the GERD symptoms after a dinner-to-bedtime interval of an hour (for the third hour, OR: 0.55, 95% CI: 0.41-0.74; for the fourth hour, OR: 0.51, 95% CI: 0.37-0.71).[39]

Weight loss

A recent (2013) prospective longitudinal structured weight loss study has shown benefit for weight loss in overweight and obese subjects with GERD (BMI 25-39.9 kg/m²; average BMI at baseline: 34.7 ± 4.6 kg/m²).[40] Subjects were prospectively enrolled (n=332) and began a structured weight loss program for six months involving diet modification, physical activity incorporation, and behavioral change taught by a health educator in either a traditional face-to-face format or in a telephone conferencing format. Subjects met in person or over the phone weekly for one hour during the six months. During the weekly meetings, a patient behavior change lesson was taught for 30 minutes (including nutrition, physical activity and lifestyle modifications), weight measurements were made, physical activity was measured, and assessment of patient dietary compliance was completed. GERD status was measured by a validated reflux disease questionnaire at baseline and at follow up visits. At baseline, the prevalence of GERD was 37% (124/332). At the six month follow up period, there was no significant difference between the two groups (i.e., clinic face-to-face group vs. phone based weight loss program) in terms of weight loss or GERD symptom scores. The mean weight loss was 13.1 ± 7.7 kg, the mean decrease in waist circumference was 10.6 ± 9.1 cm, and the majority of subjects lost weight (97%). Further, weight loss, over a period of six months, resulted in a reduction of GERD symptoms for most of the subjects (81%) and complete resolution of symptoms in 65% of subjects. The overall change in GERD score from baseline (5.5 ± 4.3) to six months of follow up (1.8 ± 3.6) was significant (p<0.01).

There appeared to be a dose-response relationship between the degree of body weight lost and the resolution of GERD symptoms (r=0.17, p<0.05). A gender difference was found for the threshold weight loss for GERD symptom improvement; women experienced significant reduction in overall GERD score following a weight loss of 5 to 10% (p<0.05), whereas men had significant improvement of GERD symptoms after a weight loss of ≥ 10% of baseline body weight (p<0.01). Overall, this study shows promise for a structured lifestyle modification strategy (dietary modification, physical activity, and behavior change) for both weight loss and for improvement in GERD symptom severity.

Dietary Patterns

The Geneva Workshop Report consensus group agrees that most reflux is postprandial and avoidance of any foods/beverages that provoke reflux in an individual is, therefore, therapeutic.[41] Limited data are available comparing different dietary patterns with GERD-related outcomes; however, some evidence regarding the benefit of the Mediterranean diet and the low-carbohydrate diet for reducing GERD is emerging.

In a cross-sectional study performed in Albania (n=817, mean age: 50.2 ± 18.7 years), subjects were evaluated for GERD using the Montreal instrument for assessment of GERD, and subjects were interviewed about their dietary habits.[42] The dietary data were dichotomized into predominantly Mediterranean (frequent consumption of composite/traditional dishes, fresh fruit and vegetables, olive oil, and fish) or predominantly non-Mediterranean (frequent consumption of red meat, fried food, sweets, and junk/fast food). The investigators found the predominantly non-Mediterranean diet was

associated with greater risk of GERD (fully adjusted odds ratio = 2.3, 95% confidence interval = 1.2-4.5) when compared to the predominantly Mediterranean diet group while controlling for demographic and socioeconomic characteristics and lifestyle factors including eating habits (meal regularity, eating rate, and meal-to-sleep interval).

Early evidence from a Duke University report of five case studies showed promise for the adherence to a very low-carbohydrate diet (VLCD) in alleviating GERD symptoms.[43] This led to a number of intervention trials evaluating the role of various low-carbohydrate diets for the relief of GERD symptoms. Austin et al. completed a small-scale prospective study on eight obese (BMI > 30 kg/m^2) female subjects with GERD.[44] Subjects were allowed to consume unlimited amounts of meat and eggs, hard cheeses, and a specified amount of certain low-carbohydrate vegetables (a maximum of 20 g carbohydrates/day). Subjects were encouraged to drink six 8 oz. glasses of water daily and prohibited from drinking alcohol and caffeine. In these subjects, adherence to the VLCD significantly decreased the Johnson-DeMeester scores (mean score of 34.7 ± 10.1 before treatment versus 14.0 ± 3.7 after treatment, p=0.023), significantly decreased the percentage of time with a pH < 4.0 in the distal esophagus (5.1 ± 1.3% before the diet versus 2.5 ± 0.6% after the diet, p=0.022), and significantly improved subject GERD Symptom Assessment Scale – Distress Subscale (GSAS-ds) scores (p=0.0004). The authors noted the improvement of Johnson-DeMeester score following adherence to the VLCD in this small trial of obese women abstaining from alcohol and caffeine is similar to the magnitude reported with PPI treatment.[45] While the researchers limited the possibility of weight loss as a contributing factor (by assessing patients after an average of four days on the diet), the avoidance of alcohol and caffeine may have confounded the results as both alcohol and caffeine are known factors that exacerbate symptoms of GERD in some individuals.[2,46]

A more recent case-control study from a 16-week dietary intervention trial has evaluated the effects of carbohydrate and fat intake on GERD symptoms in 42 European-American and African-American obese women (BMI 30-39.9 kg/m^2).[47] Specifically, the researchers compared diets that contained 35% vs. 45% energy from carbohydrates, 48% versus 38% energy from fats (respectively), and a constant amount of protein (17% of energy). At baseline the prevalence of GERD was 20% for African-American women and 33.3% for European-American women. In this cohort, the GERD status of European-American women, but not African-American women, was significantly associated with total carbohydrate intake (r=0.34, p<0.001), added sugars intake (r=0.30, p=0.005), sucrose intake (r=0.33, p=0.001), glycemic load (r-0.34, p=0.001) and $HOMA_{IR}$ score (r=0.30, p=0.004). According to the authors' calculations, the odds of having GERD in these European-American women increased by 13% for every additional teaspoon (4.2 g) of sugar consumed. Resolution of GERD symptoms and discontinuation of GERD medication usage was statistically significant in the European-American group by the ninth week of diet adherence; the same results were obtained following the tenth week of the protocol for the African-American women. Adherence to the diet also led to weight loss (an average of 6.9 ± 3.3 kg in the European-American women, and an average of 6.5 ± 2.8 kg in the African American women), and reduced insulin resistance in women with GERD ($HOMA_{IR}$, p= 0.02).

Despite some epidemiological evidence that high-fat diets may be linked to GERD, many interventional dietary trials have not confirmed increasing dietary fat is problematic for GERD in healthy subjects.[48,49,50] One particular epidemiological study suggests a high-fat diet (high in saturated fat, cholesterol, or fat servings) is associated with GERD; however, it is unknown if this relationship is independent of obesity or not.[51] In this same study, dietary fiber was shown to reduce the risk of GERD symptoms.

Antacids

Antacids have been used for over 2,000 years for symptoms of heartburn, and include compounds such as bicarbonate salts (e.g., $NaHCO_3$, and Ca- or $MgCO_3$), alkali complexes of aluminum and/or magnesium (e.g., aluminum and magnesium hydroxides), aluminum and magnesium phosphates, and magnesium trisilicate.[62] Benefits of antacids include their rapid onset of action—the compounds act within minutes to elevate the gastric pH above 3.5, thereby offering symptomatic relief. Despite their rapid onset, use of antacids is limited by their short duration (about 20 minutes under fasting conditions and about 60 minutes following a meal),

which often requires repeated dosing.[64] While we do not advocate the long-term use of antacids to manage the symptoms of GERD, they may be a better option than PPIs or H2RAs for symptom relief while discovering successful lifestyle therapies, as they do not fundamentally alter the mechanism of acid production.

Melatonin

A bidirectional relationship has been proposed between GERD and sleep disturbance, whereby GERD may affect sleep quality (i.e., difficulty in falling asleep, sleep fragmentation, and early morning awakening). Disturbed sleep has been shown to intensify hyperalgesia of the esophagus when GERD subjects were challenged with an intraesophageal acid profusion stimulus.[52,53,54] In addition, night shift work has been associated with erosive esophagitis.[55] Remarkably, research has also shown subjects with GERD have significantly lower nocturnal serum melatonin levels compared to healthy controls (27.2 ± 8.5 pg/ml vs. 34.7 ± 4.8 pg/ml, respectively, p< 0.05); though subjects with NERD have significantly higher nocturnal melatonin serum levels than those with GERD (27.2 ± 8.5 pg/ml vs. 43.2 ± 10.8 pg/ml, respectively, p<0.01).[56] Consequently, melatonin has been researched for its potential therapeutic effect on GERD patients.

Melatonin is an important hormone for sleep and is secreted by the pineal gland. Most, however, do not know melatonin is also important for gut motility and is secreted by enterochromaffin cells (EC) in the gut, though the GI production of melatonin and its potential role as a protector of esophageal reflux is currently not well-understood.[57,58] Melatonin appears to modulate the LES by inhibitory action on gastric acid secretion. Melatonin also appears to stimulate the secretomotor neurons of the ENS, increasing bicarbonate secretion from enterocytes and thereby protecting the duodenumal epithelium against gastric acid.[59] In addition, melatonin may help avoid transient lower esophageal sphincter relaxation through its inhibition of nitric oxide biosynthesis.

Kandil et al. (2010) performed a clinical trial evaluating the protective role of melatonin against GERD.[60] Thirty-six subjects were placed into four groups: 1) healthy controls, 2) patients with GERD given 3 mg melatonin once daily at bedtime, 3) patients with GERD receiving omeprazole (20 mg bid), and 4) patients with GERD receiving both omeprazole and melatonin in the same doses as above. The patients were evaluated after four weeks and eight weeks of treatment. It should be noted that at baseline, the control group had higher levels of melatonin than all three GERD treatment groups. In both the eight-week melatonin group and the four-week melatonin plus omeprazole group, LES pressure, residual pressure, relaxation duration and relaxation percentage all improved significantly. Melatonin also increased esophageal pH (measured 5 cm above the LES), lowered basal acid output, and increased gastrin in the serum compared to baseline. The authors concluded melatonin could be used in the treatment of GERD either alone or in combination with omeprazole; the combination therapy may achieve clinical results quicker, as melatonin accelerates the healing effect of omeprazole and therefore shortens the duration of treatment and minimizes side effects. Currently, melatonin is the only compound shown in the literature to improve LES tone.

In a prospective, randomized, single-blind clinical trial, Pereira (2006) studied the effects of treatment with an amino acid and vitamin supplement containing melatonin (Group A) versus omeprazole monotherapy (Group B) on patient symptoms quantified using a five-point GERD symptom severity scale.[61] Group A consisted of 176 subject treated with melatonin (6 mg), tryptophan (200 mg), vitamin B12 (50 μg), methionine (100 mg), vitamin B6 (25 mg), betaine (100 mg) and folic acid (10 mg) given in one capsule once per day (recommended after evening meal). Group B (n=175) was treated with 20 mg omeprazole (recommended after evening meal). Following 40 days of treatment, all patients in Group A reported complete regression of symptoms, and 65.7% (115/175) of those in Group B reported similar symptom regression; there was a statistically significant difference between groups (p < 0.05).

Alginate
Alginates (alginic acids) are natural polysaccharide polymers of L-guluronic and D-mannuronic acid residues connected via 1:4 glycosidic linkages isolated from brown seaweed (Phacophycae) and available as OTC agents (combined with bicarbonates) for GERD symptom alleviation. Upon contact with gastric acid the alginate precipitates into a low density viscous gel.[62] Alginate compounds are commonly referred to as

"alginate raft-forming agents" because in the presence of gastric acid, a pH change triggers the sodium bicarbonate in the formulation to release carbon dioxide, which becomes trapped in the gel and floats atop the gastric contents, similar to a raft floating atop a pool of water. *In vitro* studies have shown calcium increases the alginate raft strength while aluminum (commonly used in antacid formulations) has been shown to reduce raft strength.[62]

Alginate compounds have been shown to be beneficial in improving GERD outcomes via interference with the acid pocket. The acid pocket is a mechanism implicated in postprandial GERD whereby a small "pocket" of gastric contents immediately distal to the cardia escapes the buffering effect of the meal and is vulnerable to reflux because of its proximity to the gastroesophageal junction.[63] Radiolabeled alginate-antacid studies in human GERD subjects (n=16) using scintigraphy and ^{111}In-labeled alginate-antacid have shown the alginate-antacid raft is able to localize to the postprandial acid pocket where it displaces the acid pocket below the diaphragm, and has been shown to significantly reduce acid reflux episodes and time to acid reflux compared to antacids alone (p=0.03 and p=0.01, respectively).[64] Similar to other antacids, alginate formulations are fast-acting, but alginate formulations offer a more prolonged treatment effect (up to four hours) compared to traditional antacids.[62] A recent meta-analysis evaluating fourteen studies (n= 2095) found alginate-based therapy for GERD increased the odds of symptom resolution when compared to placebo or antacids (OR: 4.42, 95% CI: 2.45-7.97).[65]

A double-blind parallel study randomized 195 NERD subjects to either four-week treatment with 20 ml sodium alginate suspension (3 times per day) or omeprazole 20 mg (once daily).[66] Upon intention-to-treat analysis, NERD symptomatic relief was similar in both the alginate treated group and the group treated with omeprazole (53.3% vs. 50.5%, respectively p=0.175), adverse events were similar as well (5.4% vs. 5.5% for sodium alginate vs. omeprazole). A study completed on Japanese subjects with NERD (n=76) randomized subjects to either four-week treatment with omeprazole (20 mg once daily) plus sodium alginate (30 mg qid) or omeprazole alone (20 mg once daily). After treatment, the group treated with the combination of PPI plus alginate formulation reported significantly more complete resolution of heartburn for at least seven consecutive days by the end of treatment (56.7%) compared to the omeprazole only group (25.7%).[67] One subject taking the combination of omeprazole and sodium alginate reported mild drug-related diarrhea that was not clinically significant.

Timing is important when taking an alginate formulation. The half-life of the alginate raft complex within the stomach has been shown to be maximized when administered 30 minutes following a meal compared to when fasting.[62] When administering an alginate formulation with a meal, it has been shown to mix with the meal contents and fail to form a raft. Therefore, it should be advised to administer alginate formulations 30 minutes following a meal for GERD outcomes. Alginate formulations have been used safely in children and pregnant women.[62] As with our recommendation with antacids generally, alginate formulas can be helpful to reduce GERD symptoms while discovering root causes and/or successful lifestyle interventions for the patient. They should not be viewed as a long-term therapy for GERD.

Herbal Remedies for GERD

Throughout the ages, numerous herbal remedies have been used in the attempt to reduce symptoms which are now defined as GERD. Western herbal approaches encourage the use of demulcent herbs for the rapid relief of heartburn symptoms. Demulcent herbs recommended for GERD include: Licorice root (*Glycyrrhiza glabra*), slippery elm bark (*Ulmus rubra*), and marshmallow root (*Althea officinalis*).[2,68,69] Bitter herbs given at low doses may be beneficial in increasing LES tone, improving saliva output, and accelerating gastric emptying; however, bitters may also increase acid production, which may be problematic in those with GERD. Gentle bitters such as globe artichoke leaf (*Cynara scolymus*) or yarrow (*Achillea millifolium*) may be more useful compared to stronger bitters such as gentian (*Gentiana lutia*) and wormwood (*Artemesia absinthium*). Bone and Mills offer a more comprehensive review of herbal approaches to GERD in their text, *Principles and Practice of Phytotherapy: Modern Herbal Medicine.*[68]

References

1. Vakil N, van Zanten SV, Kahrilas P, et al. The Montreal definition and classification of gastroesophageal reflux disease: a global evidence-based consensus. *Am J Gastroenterol.* 2006 Aug;101(8):1900-20; quiz 1943.
2. Hawrelak J. Gastro-oesophageal reflux disease. In: Wardle J, Sarris J. eds. *Clinical Naturopathy : An Evidence-based Guide to Practice.* 2 e. Sydney : Churchill Livingstone Australia, 2014.
3. Woodland P, Sifrim D. The refluxate: The impact of its magnitude, composition and distribution. *Best Pract Res Clin Gastroenterol.* 2010 Dec;24(6):861-71.
4. Harnik IG. In the Clinic. Gastroesophageal Reflux Disease. *Ann Intern Med.* 2015 Jul 7;163(1):ITC1.
5. de Bortoli N, Ottonello A, Zerbib F, et al. Between GERD and NERD: the relevance of weakly acidic reflux. *Ann N Y Acad Sci.* 2016 Jul 29.
6. Kee Song L, Topazian M. Gastrointestinal Endoscopy. In: Kasper D, Fauci A, Hauser S, Longo D, Jameson J, Loscalzo J. eds. *Harrison's Principles of Internal Medicine*, 19e. New York, NY: McGraw-Hill; 2015.
7. El-Serag HB, Sweet S, Winchester CC, Dent J. Update on the epidemiology of gastro-oesophageal reflux disease: a systematic review. *Gut.* 2014 Jun;63(6):871-80.
8. Icitovic N, Onyebeke LC, Wallenstein S, et al. The association between body mass index and gastroesophageal reflux disease in the World Trade Center Health Program General Responder Cohort. *Am J Ind Med.* 2016 Sep;59(9):761-6.
9. Chang P, Friedenberg F. Obesity and GERD. *Gastroenterol Clin North Am.* 2014 Mar;43(1):161-73.
10. Nilsson M, Johnsen R, Ye W, Hveem K, et al. Lifestyle related risk factors in the aetiology of gastro-oesophageal reflux. *Gut.* 2004 Dec;53(12):1730-5.
11. Hallan A, Bomme M, Hveem K, et al. Risk factors on the development of new-onset gastroesophageal reflux symptoms. A population-based prospective cohort study: the HUNT study. *Am J Gastroenterol.* 2015 Mar;110(3):393-400.
12. Festi D, Scaioli E, Baldi F, et al. Body weight, lifestyle, dietary habits and gastroesophageal reflux disease. *World J Gastroenterol.* 2009 Apr 14;15(14):1690-701.
13. Matsuki N, Fujita T, Watanabe N, et al. Lifestyle factors associated with gastroesophageal reflux disease in the Japanese population. *J Gastroenterol.* 2013 Mar;48(3):340-9.
14. Chua YC, Aziz Q. Perception of gastro-oesophageal reflux. *Best Pract Res Clin Gastroenterol.* 2010 Dec;24(6):883-91.
15. Lembo A, Zaman M, Jones M, Talley NJ. Influence of genetics on irritable bowel syndrome, gastro-oesophageal reflux and dyspepsia: a twin study. *Aliment Pharmacol Ther.* 2007 Jun 1;25(11):1343-50.
16. Bonfiglio F, Hysi PG, Ek W, Karhunen V, et al. A meta-analysis of reflux genome-wide association studies in 6750 Northern Europeans from the general population. *Neurogastroenterol Motil.* 2016 Aug 3. doi: 10.1111/nmo.12923.
17. Mohammed I, Cherkas LF, Riley SA, et al. Genetic influences in gastro-oesophageal reflux disease: a twin study. *Gut.* 2003 Aug;52(8):1085-9.
18. Malfertheiner M, Malfertheiner P, Costa SD, et al. Extraesophageal symptoms of gastroesophageal reflux disease during pregnancy. *Z Gastroenterol.* 2015 Sep;53(9):1080-3.
19. Bredenoord AJ, Pandolfino JE, Smout AJ. Gastro-oesophageal reflux disease. *Lancet.* 2013 Jun 1;381(9881):1933-42.
20. Boeckxstaens G, El-Serag HB, Smout AJ, et al. Symptomatic reflux disease: the present, the past and the future. *Gut.* 2014 Jul;63(7):1185-93.
21. Boeckxstaens GE. Review article: the pathophysiology of gastro-oesophageal reflux disease. *Aliment Pharmacol Ther.* 2007 Jul 15;26(2):149-60.
22. Mikami DJ, Murayama KM2. Physiology and pathogenesis of gastroesophageal reflux disease. *Surg Clin North Am.* 2015 Jun;95(3):515-25.
23. Vandenplas Y. Management of paediatric GERD. *Nat Rev Gastroenterol Hepatol.* 2014 Mar;11(3):147-57.
24. Farahmand F, Najafi M, Ataee P, et al. Cow's Milk Allergy among Children with Gastroesophageal Reflux Disease. *Gut Liver.* 2011 Sep;5(3):298-301.
25. Semeniuk J, Kaczmarski M. Gastroesophageal reflux (GER) in children and adolescents with regard to food intolerance. *Adv Med Sci.* 2006;51:321-6.
26. Ayazi S, Leers JM, Oezcelik A, et al. Measurement of gastric pH in ambulatory esophageal pH monitoring. *Surg Endosc.* 2009 Sep;23(9):1968-73.
27. Iwai W, Abe Y, Iijima K, et al. Gastric hypochlorhidria is associated with an exacerbation of dyspeptic symptoms in female patients. *J Gastroenterol.* 2013 Feb;48(2):214-21.
28. Martinucci I, de Bortoli N, Russo S, et al. Barrett's esophagus in 2016: From pathophysiology to treatment. *World J Gastrointest Pharmacol Ther.* 2016 May 6;7(2):190-206.

29.   Runge TM, Abrams JA, Shaheen NJ. Epidemiology of Barrett's Esophagus and Esophageal Adenocarcinoma. *Gastroenterol Clin North Am*. 2015 Jun;44(2):203-31.
30.   Spechler SJ, Souza RF. Barrett's esophagus. *N Engl J Med*. 2014 Aug 28;371(9):836-45.
31.   Kahrilas PJ, Hirano I. Diseases of the Esophagus. In: Kasper D, Fauci A, Hauser S, Longo D, Jameson J, Loscalzo J. eds. *Harrison's Principles of Internal Medicine*, 19e. New York, NY: McGraw-Hill; 2015.
32.   Kahrilas PJ, Boeckxstaens G. Failure of reflux inhibitors in clinical trials: bad drugs or wrong patients? *Gut*. 2012 Oct;61(10):1501-9. doi: 10.1136/gutjnl-2011-301898.
33.   Cicala M, Emerenziani S, Guarino MP, Ribolsi M. Proton pump inhibitor resistance, the real challenge in gastro-esophageal reflux disease. *World J Gastroenterol*. 2013 Oct 21;19(39):6529-35.
34.   Patrick L. Gastroesophageal reflux disease (GERD): a review of conventional and alternative treatments. *Altern Med Rev*. 2011 Jun;16(2):116-33.
35.   Ness-Jensen E, Hveem K, El-Serag H, et al. Lifestyle Intervention in Gastroesophageal Reflux Disease. *Clin Gastroenterol Hepatol*. 2016 Feb;14(2):175-82.e1-3.
36.   Kaltenbach T, Crockett S, Gerson LB. Are lifestyle measures effective in patients with gastroesophageal reflux disease? An evidence-based approach. *Arch Intern Med*. 2006 May 8;166(9):965-71.
37.   Kinoshita Y, Ashida K, Miwa H, Hongo M. The impact of lifestyle modification on the health-related quality of life of patients with reflux esophagitis receiving treatment with a proton pump inhibitor. *Am J Gastroenterol*. 2009 May;104(5):1106-11.
38.   Kohata Y, Fujiwara Y, Watanabe T, et al. Long-Term Benefits of Smoking Cessation on Gastroesophageal Reflux Disease and Health-Related Quality of Life. *PLoS One*. 2016 Feb 4;11(2):e0147860.
39.   Karim S, Jafri W, Faryal A, et al. Regular post dinner walk; can be a useful lifestyle modification for gastroesophageal reflux. *J Pak Med Assoc*. 2011 Jun;61(6):526-30.
40.   Singh M, Lee J, Gupta N, Gaddam S,et al. Weight loss can lead to resolution of gastroesophageal reflux disease symptoms: a prospective intervention trial. *Obesity (Silver Spring)*. 2013 Feb;21(2):284-90.
41.   [No authors listed]. An evidence-based appraisal of reflux disease management--the Genval Workshop Report. *Gut*. 1999 Apr;44 Suppl 2:S1-16.
42.   Mone I, Kraja B, Bregu A, et al. Adherence to a predominantly Mediterranean diet decreases the risk of gastroesophageal reflux disease: a cross-sectional study in a South Eastern European population. *Dis Esophagus*. 2015 Jul 14. doi: 10.1111/dote. 12384. [Epub ahead of print]
43.   Yancy WS Jr, Provenzale D, Westman EC. Improvement of gastroesophageal reflux disease after initiation of a low-carbohydrate diet: five brief case reports. *Altern Ther Health Med*. 2001 Nov-Dec;7(6):120, 116-9.
44.   Austin GL, Thiny MT, Westman EC, et al. A very low-carbohydrate diet improves gastroesophageal reflux and its symptoms. *Dig Dis Sci*. 2006 Aug;51(8):1307-12.
45.   Swiatkowski M, Budzyński J, Kłopocka M, et al. The effect of eight weeks of rabeprazole therapy on nitric oxide plasma level and esophageal pH and motility and motility nitric oxide plasma level in patients with erosive esophagitis. *Med Sci Monit*. 2004 Feb;10(2):CR46-51.
46.   Spantideas N, Drosou E, Bougea A, Assimakopoulos D. Gastroesophageal reflux disease symptoms in the Greek general population: prevalence and risk factors. *Clin Exp Gastroenterol*. 2016 Jun 21;9:143-9.
47.   Pointer SD, Rickstrew J, Slaughter JC, et al. Dietary carbohydrate intake, insulin resistance and gastro-oesophageal reflux disease: a pilot study in European- and African-American obese women. *Aliment Pharmacol Ther*. 2016 Sep 1. doi: 10.1111/apt.13784.
48.   Pehl C, Waizenhoefer A, Wendl B, et al. Effect of low and high fat meals on lower esophageal sphincter motility and gastroesophageal reflux in healthy subjects. *Am J Gastroenterol*. 1999 May;94(5):1192-6.
49.   Penagini R, Mangano M, Bianchi PA. Effect of increasing the fat content but not the energy load of a meal on gastro-oesophageal reflux and lower oesophageal sphincter motor function. *Gut*. 1998 Mar;42(3):330-3.
50.   Colombo P, Mangano M, Bianchi PA, Penagini R. Effect of calories and fat on postprandial gastro-oesophageal reflux. *Scand J Gastroenterol*. 2002 Jan;37(1):3-5.
51.   El-Serag HB, Satia JA, Rabeneck L. Dietary intake and the risk of gastro-oesophageal reflux disease: a cross sectional study in volunteers. *Gut*. 2005 Jan;54(1):11-7.
52.   Fujiwara Y, Arakawa T, Fass R. Gastroesophageal reflux disease and sleep disturbances. *J Gastroenterol*. 2012 Jul;47(7):760-9.
53.   Schey R, Dickman R, Parthasarathy S, et al. Sleep deprivation is hyperalgesic in patients with gastroesophageal reflux disease. *Gastroenterology*. 2007 Dec;133(6):1787-95.
54.   Lindam A, Ness-Jensen E, Jansson C, et al. Gastroesophageal Reflux and Sleep Disturbances: A Bidirectional Association in a Population-Based Cohort Study, The HUNT Study. *Sleep*. 2016 Jul 1;39(7):1421-7.
55.   Chung TH, Lee J, Kim MC. Impact of night-shift work on the prevalence of erosive esophagitis in shipyard male workers. *Int Arch Occup Environ Health*. 2016 Aug;89(6):961-6.
56.   Klupińska G, Wiśniewska-Jarosińska M, Harasiuk A, et al. Nocturnal secretion of melatonin in patients with upper digestive tract disorders. *J Physiol Pharmacol*. 2006 Nov;57 Suppl 5:41-50.
57.   Bertrand PP, Polglaze KE, Bertrand RL, et al. Detection of melatonin production from the intestinal epithelium using electrochemical methods. *Curr Pharm Des*. 2014;20(30):4802-6.
58.   de Oliveira Torres JD, de Souza Pereira R. Which is the best choice for gastroesophageal disorders: Melatonin or proton pump inhibitors? *World J Gastrointest Pharmacol Ther*. 2010 Oct 6;1(5):102-6.
59.   Sjöblom M, Flemström G. Melatonin in the duodenal lumen is a potent stimulant of mucosal bicarbonate secretion. *J Pineal Res*. 2003 May;34(4):288-93.
60.   Kandil TS, Mousa AA, El-Gendy AA, Abbas AM. The potential therapeutic effect of melatonin in Gastro-Esophageal Reflux Disease. *BMC Gastroenterol*. 2010 Jan 18;10:7.
61.   Pereira Rde S. Regression of gastroesophageal reflux disease symptoms using dietary supplementation with melatonin, vitamins and aminoacids: comparison with omeprazole. *J Pineal Res*. 2006 Oct;41(3):195-200.
62.   Mandel KG, Daggy BP, Brodie DA, et al. Review article: alginate-raft formulations in the treatment of heartburn and acid reflux. *Aliment Pharmacol Ther*. 2000 Jun;14(6):669-90.
63.   Mitchell DR, Derakhshan MH, Robertson EV, McColl KE. The Role of the Acid Pocket in Gastroesophageal Reflux Disease. *J Clin Gastroenterol*. 2016 Feb;50(2):111-9.
64.   Rohof WO, Bennink RJ, Smout AJ, et al. An alginate-antacid formulation localizes to the acid pocket to reduce acid reflux in patients with gastroesophageal reflux disease. *Clin Gastroenterol Hepatol*. 2013 Dec;11(12):1585-91; quiz e90.
65.   Leiman DA, Riff BP, Morgan S, et al. Alginate therapy is effective treatment for gastroesophageal reflux disease symptoms: a systematic review and meta-analysis. *Dis Esophagus*. 2016 Sep 26. doi: 10.1111/dote.12535.
66.   Chiu CT, Hsu CM, Wang CC, et al. Randomised clinical trial: sodium alginate oral suspension is non-inferior to omeprazole in the treatment of patients with non-erosive gastroesophageal disease. *Aliment Pharmacol Ther*. 2013 Nov;38(9):1054-64.
67.   Manabe N, Haruma K, Ito M, Takahashi N, et al. Efficacy of adding sodium alginate to omeprazole in patients with nonerosive reflux disease: a randomized clinical trial. *Dis Esophagus*. 2012 Jul;25(5):373-80.
68.   Bone K, Mills S. Herbal approaches to system dysfunctions. *Principles and practice of phytotherapy: Modern herbal medicine*, 2e. Edinburgh: Churchill Livingstone/Elsevier; 2013.
69.   Kiefer D. Gastroesophageal Reflux Disease. In: Rakel D ed. Integrative Medicine. Philadelphia, PA: Saunders; 2012.

Small Intestinal Bacterial Overgrowth

GI dysbiosis is described as any imbalance within the gut microbiota that leads to negative health consequences for the host (see also page 103). One particular form of dysbiosis is referred to as small intestinal bacterial overgrowth (SIBO), or alternatively, small bowel bacterial overgrowth (SBBO) or bacterial overgrowth of the small intestines (BOSI). This phenomenon has been described for decades and was classically associated with signs and symptoms of maldigestion/malabsorption (e.g., steatorrhea, B12 deficiency).[1] Today, SIBO is mostly defined by characteristic symptoms such as diarrhea, abdominal pain and bloating, symptoms that overlap significantly with the diagnostic criteria for IBS (see page 197 for discussion of IBS and SIBO). A similar, though much less studied phenomena called SIFO, or small intestinal fungal overgrowth (mostly linked to *Candida spp*), is likely co-incident with SIBO in many subjects and is especially linked with immunocompromised individuals.[2,3]

As the name implies, its most basic definition is fundamentally a quantitative overgrowth of bacteria within the small bowel. More specifically, it has been defined as 1×10^5 or more colony-forming units per milliliter (CFU/ml) of bacteria from small intestinal aspirate (duodenum/jejunum). This is roughly two-to-three orders of magnitude higher than the amount thought to be normal in these areas of the gut (see Figure 18, page 93). While this quantitative characterization is considered by some to be the "gold standard" definition of SIBO, there is still much debate about this.[4] Since this definition relies upon bacterial plate counts rather than metagenomics, it is highly skewed toward the minority of bacterial species that can be cultivated; and assumes the area of the aspirate collection is uniform in concentration with the entire small bowel. Others speculate that specific, unidentified species are the real culprit related to symptoms coincident with overgrowth, or that symptoms only exist when specific species of bacteria from the colon migrate into the small intestines. Furthermore, since this test is difficult, invasive and expensive to perform routinely in a clinical setting, simpler breath tests have become more popular in defining SIBO, creating a surrogate definition of SIBO (i.e., breath test positive).

Breath Tests for SIBO: Are They Diagnostic?

Since aspirating the small intestines for a bacterial plate count is not a routine procedure, a variety of breath tests using carbohydrate ingestion have been employed. The idea is based on the fact that when various carbohydrates (lactulose, glucose, xylose, etc.) are available to specific species of bacteria, hydrogen or methane gas will be produced during the fermentation of those carbohydrates (methane is actually produced by methanogenic bacteria using hydrogen formed by other bacteria). The measure (timing and quantity) of these gases in the patient's breath after consuming the test carbohydrate helps determine the location of the fermenting bacteria (small bowel or colon). Ghoshal et al., in their comparison of both breath tests with aspirate plating, describe the testing procedures as

follows[5] (different labs may have slight variations on these procedures):

Basal breath specimens were obtained after a 12 h fast; the patients avoided slowly absorbed carbohydrates (lentils, bread, potato, corn) and fiber the previous evening to avoid delayed excretion of hydrogen in the breath. Cigarette smoking and physical exercise were not permitted for 2 h before and during the test to prevent hyperventilation and consequent changes in breath hydrogen content. The patients then brushed their teeth, and rinsed their mouth with an antiseptic wash, followed by tap water, to eliminate an early hydrogen peak because of the action of oral bacteria on test sugars. An average of three values was considered as the basal breath hydrogen and methane levels. The patients were then asked to ingest 100 g glucose dissolved in 200 ml water or a 15 ml solution containing 10 g lactulose. Thereafter, breath hydrogen and methane were estimated every 15 min for 3 and 4 h during GHBT[glucose hydrogen breath test] and LHBT [laculose hydrogen breath test], respectively. An increase in hydrogen excretion, in ppm, following glucose or lactulose administration was calculated by subtracting the fasting value from the highest value of hydrogen obtained. A sustained increase in breath hydrogen (at least two consecutive readings) by 12 ppm above basal level following the administration of glucose was considered evidence of SIBO. A characteristic double peak or an early peak (increase in breath hydrogen 20 ppm above basal levels within 90 min) in breath hydrogen was considered SIBO. Fasting breath methane level of at least 10 ppm or increase by at least 10 ppm above basal after substrate ingestion was considered as a positive methane breath test.

Ghoshal et al. performed a comparison of each breath test and various interpretations (single peak, double peak; hydrogen and/or methane) with the "gold standard" microbial quantification of upper gut aspirates in 80 subjects with irritable bowel syndrome.[5] In this cohort of IBS subjects, 15 (19%) had SIBO as defined by an upper gut aspirate above 10^5 CFU/ml (18/80 had levels between 10^3 to10^5). Compared to this standard test (deemed to be 100% sensitive and 100% specific), each of the other breath tests were analyzed for their relative sensitivity (ability to correctly identify SIBO when present) and specificity (ability to accurately identify a SIBO-negative subject). They found that using the glucose hydrogen breath test (GBT), that only four of the 15 SIBO subjects had a positive breath test (27% sensitive), while none of the SIBO-negative subjects had a positive breath test (100% specific). The lactulose breath test (LBT) included two diagnostic categories; an early hydrogen peak detected one more SIBO patient than the GBT (5/15 or 33% sensitive), but incorrectly identified 23/65 non-SIBO subjects with a positive breath test (only 35% sensitive), while a double-peak was positive for only one (non-SIBO) subject (0% sensitivity, 98% specific). Using methane (alone) measures in the lactulose group also had limited sensitivity (13.3%) and specificity (41.3%).

These results clearly show what many have suggested: Breath tests are prone to misinterpretation or over-interpretation.[6,7,8] A Rome consensus conference, published some five years prior to the data described above, suggests the sensitivity and specificity of the lactulose and glucose breath tests are: for LBT, 52.4% and 85.7%, respectively; and for GBT, 62.5% and 81.8%, respectively.[9] The Rome Consensus statements related to SIBO are 1) *The jejunal aspirate culture is traditionally considered the gold standard diagnostic test for SIBO, despite some serious methodological limitations and lack of accessibility to clinical practice,* and 2) *Glucose Breath Test is the most accurate hydrogen breath test for non-invasive diagnosis of SIBO.* The addition of methane to hydrogen is helpful in capturing the overgrowth of methanogenic organisms common in about one in five subjects (i.e., improving sensitivity), though this may not increase the poor specificity of these tests.[10] Elevated methane-producing organisms increase the likelihood of constipation fivefold.[11]

The interpretation of these breath tests are dependent on the cut-offs used to define normal transit time and average fermentation in normal subjects. Since the average transit time is shorter in some populations, this is considered the main cause of frequent misinterpretation of an early hydrogen peak after lactulose ingestion, (see Figure 40).[12,13] In one study performed in India, comparing the LBT and the GBT in 175 IBS-D and 150 apparently healthy controls, the LBT was unable to differentiate between these two groups (34.3% and 30% positive breath test, respectively), while the GBT

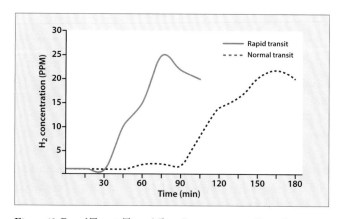

Figure 40: Bowel Transit Time Affects Interpretation of Lactulose Breath Test. The timing of lactulose fermentation is assumed to be early only if certain types of quantities of bacteria are in the small intestines (i.e., SIBO). However this assumes that the consumed lactulose would not reach the large intestines until at least 90 minutes after ingestion. A short bowel transit time will permit lactulose to reach the large intestines earlier, which many clinicians could inadvertently interpret as SIBO.

showed a statistical difference between these groups (6.2% and 0.66% positive breath test, respectively).[14] These differences also highlight the wide variability of the association between SIBO and IBS reported in the literature (see IBS and SIBO on page 197).

Breath Testing, Our Recommendation

Whether a positive breath test is diagnostic for SIBO or merely the evidence of elevated and early production of gas due to the fermentation of undigested carbohydrates may be an unimportant distinction, since both scenarios may contribute equally to the patient's signs and symptoms (gas, bloating, diarrhea, abdominal pain). And, with the exception of the use of antibiotics, which some clinicians may consider appropriate for a diagnosis of SIBO, the therapies for these are similar (see below). Clinicians should consider testing for SIBO when such a diagnosis is likely to alter their therapeutic strategy. Check with existing labs for their available test methods, substrates and cut-off points. One final note: Since breath testing is highly dependent on proper test methods, including pre-testing dietary restrictions, clinicians should be careful to ensure the patient understands these restrictions and is capable of performing the test as instructed.

PPI Use and SIBO

Low stomach acid (hypochlorhydria or achlorhydria) is thought to create an environment that allows for increase overgrowth of bacteria in the small intestines, especially when this condition is induced by drugs.[15,16] Therefore, the relationship between the use (or overuse) of proton-pump inhibitors (PPIs) as a contributing risk factor for SIBO is of concern to many. A recent systematic review and meta-analysis was conducted to evaluate the association between PPI use and SIBO, and found when SIBO was defined by duodenal or jujunal aspirate overgrowth, there was a strong association showing PPI users had a sevenfold higher incidence of SIBO.[17] However, while the risk for a positive breath test as a measure of SIBO in PPI users was nearly double (OR 1.93), this association did not reach statistical significance.

While some studies show no difference in the incidence of SIBO in those who use PPIs compared to subjects who do not, on balance, the majority of studies confirm this association, as does the physiology of an altered gastric and duodenal pH. In a study of 70 children (mean age 13.5 years) given 20 mg of omeprazole for four weeks who were glucose breath-test negative for SIBO at baseline, 21 of the 70 (30%) became breath-test positive after PPI use and an additional five more developed symptoms of SIBO while remaining breath-test negative.[18] The use of a probiotic (2 billion CFU/day of *L. rhamnosus* and *L. acidophilus*) in these children was not able to mitigate the PPI-induced SIBO. Therefore, unless their use is strongly indicated, there are many reasons to limit the use of PPIs in patients; the increased risk of small intestinal dysbiosis is merely one more. When possible, clinicians should help patients taper the use of PPIs and use therapies addressing the root cause of the condition for which the PPI was prescribed in the first place (see the negative consequences of PPI use and ways to taper patients off PPIs on page 219).

Prevention and Intervention Strategies for SIBO

Since the difference between a "normal" small intestinal microbiome and one defined as "SIBO" is difficult to define, it is not surprising that the majority of prevention and intervention strategies are also difficult to assess. The primary goal of most therapies is to eradicate the overgrowth (or at least the harmful and out-of-place organisms) while allowing the appropriate growth of the commensal organisms to thrive. This is typically attempted by limiting the environmental conditions for SIBO (avoiding PPIs and certain carbohydrates), directly altering the microbiota (antibiotics, probiotics) or by stimulating changes in bowel transit (laxatives, prokinetics, fiber supplementation).

Dietary Restriction

Since SIBO is characterized by altered fermentation of carbohydrates, many clinicians, nutritionists and dietitians recommend restriction of certain carbohydrates (fructose, lactose, FODMAPs, etc.). Surprisingly, we are not aware of any studies looking into the efficacy of these dietary approaches for non-IBS, SIBO-specific outcomes. One retrospective study suggests that in obese subjects, carbohydrate intake may influence their risk for SIBO.[19] Comparing 60 obese subjects with normal lean controls, 23.3% of the obese subjects had a positive glucose breath test, while only 6.6% of lean subjects had a positive breath test. Using diet recall, obese subjects with SIBO consumed statistically higher amounts of carbohydrates, refined sugars and less total and insoluble dietary fiber. These researchers did not further define these into FODMAP-related categories. Nonetheless, there is much promising data to recommend the FODMAP-restricted diet for subjects meeting the criteria for IBS, many of which may test positive for SIBO; so even without a base of evidence this dietary recommendation may be helpful in many patients with a positive SIBO breath test (see page 189 for discussion of IBS and page 236 for low FODMAP diet).

The use of prebiotics (e.g., inulin, FOS, etc.) in subjects with SIBO is controversial. By definition, these are complex carbohydrates that are substrates for bacterial fermentation, substances that many would recommend be restricted in SIBO subjects based on our recommendation above. We are aware of only one small uncontrolled pilot trial (n=20) that used 2.5 grams/day fructoligosaccharide (FOS) for seven days after a seven-day therapy of rifaximin in the treatment of breath-test positive subjects.[20] They reported a 66% improvement of symptoms from baseline after six months; however, since no rifaximin-only control group was used for comparison, the only conclusion we might make is that FOS did not appear to exacerbate the symptoms in this cohort. Whether these data are enough to temper the precaution to avoid even small amounts of prebiotics used as excipients with probiotics (i.e., synbiotics) is up to each clinician's own judgment.

Fiber supplements may be helpful in SIBO subjects with constipation, as they are in IBS-C, since many soluble and insoluble fiber supplements have more limited fermentation capacity and are likely to reach the colon before fermentation begins. Subjects (n=77) with a positive glucose breath test were randomized to either rifaximin (1,200 mg/day) or rifaximin and partially-hydrolyzed guar gum (5 g/day) for 10 days. Eradication (breath-test negative) was achieved in 61% of the rifaximin-only group and 87% in the rifaximin plus guar gum group (p=0.017). We suggest that fiber supplementation with guar or psyllium may be helpful in SIBO patients with constipation, though patients should be instructed to start with lower doses and gradually increase fiber intake while monitoring changes in GI symptoms.

Is Food Poisoning Involved in SIBO

See page 198 for discussion of how toxin exposure from food poisoning can alter gut motility and lead to IBS/SIBO symptoms

Dietary Supplementation of Nutrients

SIBO is characterized by nutrient deficiencies, especially fat malabsorption and some fat soluble vitamins (A, D, E), vitamin B12, iron, thiamin and nicotinamide.[21] Fat absorption is assumed to be compromised in some subjects with SIBO due to early bacterial deconjugation of bile acids which decreases the formation of micelles for fat absorption.[22] The supplementation of ox bile extracts and digestive enzymes containing pancrelipase or fungal-analog lipases are commonly recommended for SIBO patients (especially those with steatorrhea), though no research related to the efficacy of this recommendation has been performed (for discussion of enzyme or bile supplementation, see pages 37 and 42, respectively).

We also highly recommend that subjects with SIBO take a multivitamin/mineral supplement to ensure adequate intake/absorption of these other important nutrients known to be linked with SIBO. Since multivitamins often do not have adequate oral doses of vitamin B12 to overcome a chronic cobalamin deficiency, clinicians should consider additional supplementation with at least 1 mg of oral cobalamin. [For a complete discussion of B12 supplementation options, as well as our recommendations for the use of nutrients to supplement the diet, see our Standard Road map, *Supplementing Dietary Nutrients: A Guide for Healthcare Professionals* (Point Institute, 2014)].

Antimicrobials for SIBO

It is inevitable that any condition defined by an overgrowth of bacteria will be treated with an antimicrobial agent. Therefore, numerous clinical trials have been performed with a variety of different antibiotics, testing their efficacy in patients with SIBO. A recent meta-analysis of antibiotic therapy use for SIBO shows that, overall, normalization of breath test (i.e., positive at baseline, negative after therapy) using one of several antibiotics is about 50% (placebo average 10%).[23] The most commonly used antibiotic, by far, was rifaximin; which when used at 1,200 mg/day had an average of 60.8% rate of normalizing breath test (six studies at this dose, including 283 subjects).

There are many natural antimicrobial compounds that have been shown to be effective against many aerobic and anaerobic organisms from the human GI tract. However, few of these have been tested in the context of SIBO. One retrospective analysis of the use of several different commercially-available mixtures of herbal antimicrobial agents showed a rate of lactulose breath test normalization similar to rifaxamin.[24] While this was not a controlled trial (data extracted from patient charts) in which patients were given one of four different antimicrobial formulas with very different herbal mixtures, it does demonstrate that within the clinical setting, herbal antimicrobials may be equivalent to standard antibiotic treatment for SIBO.

Probiotic Therapy for SIBO

The supplementation of probiotics can be an important therapy for a number of gastrointestinal disorders involving dysbiosis (see extensive details on page 114). However, since SIBO is an overgrowth of bacteria in the small intestines and its symptoms are nominally related to excess fermentation, some clinicians are reluctant to recommend probiotics in subjects with a positive breath test indicating SIBO. Surprisingly, few studies have been designed to help answer this conundrum. Most published studies have been extremely small or uncontrolled (i.e., pilot studies).[25,26] Therefore, there is little available evidence to make specific recommendations for the use of probiotics for SIBO.

Anecdotal evidence suggests that subjects with SIBO should be given low doses of probiotics first (≤ 5 billion CFU/day) for a week or so to monitor any change of symptoms related to this therapy. This may require opening a capsule that contains a higher dose. Increasing the dose to 20 to 40 billion CFU/day should be done in a step-wise fashion as long as no increased symptoms accompany the stepped-up dosing. Our normal recommendation is a multi-strain probiotic (see page 127), a good place to start in all patients including those with SIBO. If mixed-strain products are associated with worsening symptoms, patients may want to consider using single-strain products to discover if one particular species or strain may be helpful. Once a patient is breath-test negative (or SIBO symptom-free), a mixed-strain probiotic given at 20 to 40 billion CFU/day should be recommended to help maintain normal microbiome.

References

1. Quigley EM. Small intestinal bacterial overgrowth: what it is and what it is not. *Curr Opin Gastroenterol*. 2014 Mar;30(2):141-6.
2. Erdogan A, Rao SS. Small intestinal fungal overgrowth. *Curr Gastroenterol Rep*. 2015 Apr;17(4):16.
3. Jacobs C, Coss Adame E, Attaluri A, et al. Dysmotility and proton pump inhibitor use are independent risk factors for small intestinal bacterial and/or fungal overgrowth. *Aliment Pharmacol Ther*. 2013 Jun;37(11):1103-11.
4. Grace E, Shaw C, Whelan K, Andreyev HJ. Review article: small intestinal bacterial overgrowth--prevalence, clinical features, current and developing diagnostic tests, and treatment. *Aliment Pharmacol Ther*. 2013 Oct;38(7):674-88.
5. Ghoshal UC, Srivastava D, Ghoshal U, Misra A. Breath tests in the diagnosis of small intestinal bacterial overgrowth in patients with irritable bowel syndrome in comparison with quantitative upper gut aspirate culture. *Eur J Gastroenterol Hepatol*. 2014 Jul;26(7):753-60.
6. Pimentel M. Breath Testing for Small Intestinal Bacterial Overgrowth: Should We Bother? *Am J Gastroenterol*. 2016 Mar;111(3):307-8.
7. Saad RJ, Chey WD. Breath testing for small intestinal bacterial overgrowth: maximizing test accuracy. *Clin Gastroenterol Hepatol*. 2014 Dec;12(12):1964-72.
8. Ghoshal UC. How to interpret hydrogen breath tests. *J Neurogastroenterol Motil*. 2011 Jul;17(3):312-7.
9. Gasbarrini A, Corazza GR, Gasbarrini G, et al. Methodology and indications of H2-breath testing in gastrointestinal diseases: the Rome Consensus Conference. *Aliment Pharmacol Ther*. 2009 Mar 30;29 Suppl 1:1-49.
10. Rana SV, Sharma S, Sinha SK, Kaur H, Sikander A, Singh K. Incidence of predominant methanogenic flora in irritable bowel syndrome patients and apparently healthy controls from North India. *Dig Dis Sci*. 2009 Jan;54(1):132-5.
11. Kunkel D, Basseri RJ, Makhani MD, et al. Methane on breath testing is associated with constipation: a systematic review and meta-analysis. *Dig Dis Sci*. 2011 Jun;56(6):1612-8.
12. Lu CL, Chen CY, Chang FY, Lee SD. Characteristics of small bowel motility in patients with irritable bowel syndrome and normal humans: an Oriental study. *Clin Sci (Lond)*. 1998 Aug;95(2):165-9.
13. Yu D, Cheeseman F, Vanner S. Combined oro-caecal scintigraphy and lactulose hydrogen breath testing demonstrate that breath testing detects oro-caecal transit, not small intestinal bacterial overgrowth in patients with IBS. *Gut*. 2011 Mar;60(3):334-40.
14. Rana SV, Sharma S, Kaur J, Sinha SK, Singh K. et al. Comparison of lactulose and glucose breath test for diagnosis of small intestinal bacterial overgrowth in patients with irritable bowel syndrome. *Digestion*. 2012;85(3):243-7.
15. Williams C. Occurrence and significance of gastric colonization during acid-inhibitory therapy. *Best Pract Res Clin Gastroenterol*. 2001 Jun;15(3):511-21.
16. Theisen J, Nehra D, Citron D, et al. Suppression of gastric acid secretion in patients with gastroesophageal reflux disease results in gastric bacterial overgrowth and deconjugation of bile acids. *J Gastrointest Surg*. 2000 Jan-Feb;4(1):50-4.
17. Lo WK, Chan WW. Proton pump inhibitor use and the risk of small intestinal bacterial overgrowth: a meta-analysis *Clin Gastroenterol Hepatol*. 2013 May;11(5):483-90.
18. Hegar B, Hutapea EI, Advani N, Vandenplas Y. A double-blind placebo-controlled randomized trial on probiotics in small bowel bacterial overgrowth in children treated with omeprazole. *J Pediatr (Rio J)*. 2013 Jul-Aug;89(4):381-7.
19. Ierardi E, Losurdo G, Sorrentino C, et al. Macronutrient intakes in obese subjects with or without small intestinal bacterial overgrowth: an alimentary survey. *Scand J Gastroenterol*. 2016 Mar;51(3):277-80.
20. Rosania R, Giorgio F, Principi M, et al. Effect of probiotic or prebiotic supplementation on antibiotic therapy in the small intestinal bacterial overgrowth: a comparative evaluation. *Curr Clin Pharmacol*. 2013 May;8(2):169-72.
21. DiBaise, J. K. Nutritional consequences of small intestinal bacterial overgrowth. *Practical Gastroenterology*. 2008; 32(12): 15-28.
22. Kim YS, Spritz N, Blum M, et al. The role of altered bile acid metabolism in the steatorrhea of experimental blind loop. *J Clin Invest*. 1966 Jun;45(6):956-62.
23. Shah SC, Day LW, Somsouk M, Sewell JL. Meta-analysis: antibiotic therapy for small intestinal bacterial overgrowth. *Aliment Pharmacol Ther*. 2013 Oct;38(8):925-34.
24. Chedid V, Dhalla S, Clarke JO, et al. Herbal therapy is equivalent to rifaximin for the treatment of small intestinal bacterial overgrowth. *Glob Adv Health Med*. 2014 May;3(3):16-24.
25. Khalighi AR, Khalighi MR, Behdani R, et al. Evaluating the efficacy of probiotic on treatment in patients with small intestinal bacterial overgrowth (SIBO)--a pilot study. *Indian J Med Res*. 2014 Nov;140(5):604-8.
26. Chen WC, Quigley EM. Probiotics, prebiotics & synbiotics in small intestinal bacterial overgrowth: opening up a new therapeutic horizon! *Indian J Med Res*. 2014 Nov;140(5):582-4.

Low FODMAP Diet

The acronym, FODMAP, stands for **F**ermentable **O**ligosaccharides (e.g., fructans), **D**isaccharides (e.g., lactose), **M**onosaccharides (i.e., fructose) **a**nd **P**olyols (e.g., sorbitol, xylitol, mannitol, etc.). These represent a heterogeneous group of short-chain carbohydrate molecules that are poorly absorbed along the GI tract in certain individuals.[1] Consumption of FODMAPs has been associated with increased luminal distention, leading to symptoms of abdominal bloating, pain and altered bowel habits in certain individuals. These symptoms may lead to the diagnostic signature of IBS or other functional gastrointestinal disorders.[2,3,4]

There are several proposed mechanisms by which FODMAPs induce these symptoms. First, the absorption of some FODMAP components may be delayed or extremely poor. For instance, disaccharides (e.g., lactose) may be inadequately hydrolyzed in the small intestine by brush border enzymes, or monosaccharides (e.g., fructose in excess of glucose) may have a low absorptive capacity, leaving excess FODMAP solutes in the lumen of the small intestine. These solutes create an osmotic potential, forcing water to enter the lumen to maintain osmotic homeostasis, which contributes to abdominal bloating, distention, and pain in those with visceral hypersensitivity. Secondly, because of the slow absorption or malabsorption of FODMAPs, bacteria present within the colonic microbiome readily ferment the substrates into short-chain fatty acids (e.g., butyrate, propionate, acetate) and gases (e.g., hydrogen, carbon dioxide, and methane in some individuals). Thirdly, FODMAPs have been shown to change motility; fructose-sorbitol ingestion has been shown to reduce orocecal transit time in healthy subjects.[5]

What is the Low FODMAP Diet?

According to Mansueto et al., beginning in the 1980s, researchers observed that consumption of poorly absorbed, short-chain carbohydrates was associated with induction of GI symptoms.[4] Eventually, in 2005, a research team at Monash University in Australia used the term FODMAP to categorize and characterize these symptom-provoking food components. The group suggested a diet low in FODMAP foods may be of benefit for GI symptom relief in those with functional and organic GI disorders such as IBS and IBD.[6] Since 2005, research exploring the low FODMAP diet for GI symptom relief has been very active.

Although some studies have been cited as having low methodological quality, partly due to the complexity of dietary intervention studies, most published research has shown benefit for the low FODMAP diet in IBS.[7,8,9,14] A recent systematic review and meta-analysis by Marsh et al. (2016) showed benefit for the low FODMAP diet for functional gastrointestinal symptoms including: abdominal pain, bloating, distension, constipation, diarrhea and flatulence.[10] The British Dietetic Association recently (2016) updated their evidence-based guidelines for the dietary management of IBS in adults and included a recommendation for the low FODMAP diet in these patients; additionally, national guidelines from Japan and the United Kingdom recommend the low FODMAP diet in IBS management.[11,12,13] (see this and other therapies for IBS on page 189).

Implementation of the Low FODMAP Diet

Partly owing to risk for nutritional inadequacy following the low FODMAP diet, the complexity of the diet, and the paucity of evidence surrounding self-directed patient administration of the diet, it is widely cited that implementation of the low FODMAP diet should be done under the supervision of a dietitian, nutritionist, or other healthcare provider educated in this diet.[14] In most studies, implementation of the low FODMAP diet by a healthcare provider has been in a one-on-one setting where the educator provides individualized dietary advice while ensuring nutritional adequacy within the overall diet (often by providing reference materials to the patient). However, evidence is now emerging for greater cost benefits and clinical effectiveness of the use of group-based low FODMAP dietary education and implementation.[15]

Essentially, the low FODMAP diet is an "elimination and re-challenge" diet, where patients identify foods in their current diet that are high in FODMAPs and replace them with alternatives low in FODMAPs (see Table 9 for list).[16] The elimination portion of the diet begins with the "induction phase" where the patient adheres to a stringent and restricted diet, eliminating all high FODMAP foods for four to six weeks.[17] It should be noted that the length of the "induction phase" is not defined by the evidence from clinical trials. In fact, many clinical studies report subjects experience symptom reduction after about seven days; however, De Giorgio et al. explain that an extended induction period (i.e., four to six weeks) is proposed to allow the patient time to learn the diet and ensure symptomatic persistence of the effect.[1]

The status of symptoms at the end of the "induction phase" determines whether or not a re-challenge phase is necessary. If an adherent patient's GI symptoms are not improved following the "induction phase," the patient should discontinue the low FODMAP diet and seek other dietary or appropriate therapies. However, if the patient experiences symptom improvement after eliminating foods high in FODMAPs, then the patient is advised to follow an individualized, "step-down" food reintroduction plan to determine tolerance of certain FODMAP-containing foods. Different groups of FODMAPs (i.e., monosaccharides, polyols, oligosaccharides) may have different osmotic and fermentative potential based largely on their molecular weight and degree/rate of absorption, resulting in heterogeneity among different FODMAP components. At the same time, there may be heterogeneity in individual response to different FODMAP components or FODMAP-containing foods across individuals. The goal of the reintroduction, or re-challenge, phase is to diversify and minimize unnecessary dietary restriction for an individual as much as possible, and restrict only to the level needed for symptomatic control.

TYPES OF SUGARS	HIGH FODMAP FOODS	LOW FODMAP ALTERNATIVES
Oligosaccharides	**Fruits:** Watermelon, white peaches, persimmon, prunes, nectarines and most dried fruit	**Fruits:** Banana, most berries (except boysenberries and blackberries), grapes, lemon juice, lime juice, mandarin, orange, kiwifruit, pineapple, passion fruit, and rhubarb
	Vegetables: Onion, garlic, artichokes, leeks, beetroot, savoy cabbage and peas (except sugar-snap peas)	**Vegetables:** Capsicum, bok choy, green beans, parsnip, silverbeet, cucumber, carrots, celery, eggplant, lettuce, potatoes, yams, tomatoes, and zucchini
	Legumes: Red kidney beans (boiled), baked beans, and soya beans (boiled)	
	Grains: Wheat-, rye-, and barley-based products	**Grains:** Wheat-free grains/flour, gluten-free bread or cereal products, and quinoa
	Fibers: FOS and GOS	
Disaccharides	**Lactose:** Dairy products: cows/goat milk, and yogurt	**Lactose-free:** Almond or rice-based milk, yogurt and ice cream, hard cheese, feta and cottage cheese
Monosaccharides	**Fruits:** Apples, pears, watermelon, mango, cherries, boysenberries and fruit juice from high-fructose foods	**Fruits:** Banana, grapes, honeydew melon, kiwifruit, lemon juice, lime juice, mandarin, orange, passion fruit, paw paw, and most berries (except boysenberries and blackberries)
	Vegetables: Asparagus and sugar-snap peas	**Vegetables:** Green beans, broccoli, Brussels sprouts, carrots, eggplant
	Sweeteners: Honey, high-fructose corn syrup , fructose (in excess of glucose)	**Sweeteners:** Maple syrup
Polyols	**Fruits:** Apples, pears, avocado, apricots, blackberries, nectarines, peaches, plums, prunes, and watermelon	**Fruits:** Banana, grapes, honeydew melon, kiwifruit, lemon juice, lime juice, mandarin, orange, passion fruit, and paw paw
	Vegetables: Sweet potato, mushrooms, cauliflower, and snow peas	**Vegetables:** Green beans, broccoli, Brussels sprouts, carrots, eggplant
	Sweeteners: Mannitol and Sorbitol	**Sweeteners:** Maple syrup, and sugar (sucrose)

Table 9: **Basic list of Foods high or low in FODMAPs.** Modified from Nanayakkara WS, Skidmore PM, O'Brien L, et al. Efficacy of the low FODMAP diet for treating irritable bowel syndrome: the evidence to date. *Clin Exp Gastroenterol.* 2016 Jun 17;9:131-42, (licensed under a Creative Commons Attribution 3.0 License) and Monash University. Low FODMAP Diet Application. iPhone version accessed September 23, 2016.

Additional information regarding the low FODMAP diet is available on the Monash University website; the group also has created a database of FODMAP foods available as a mobile application called the "Monash University Low FODMAP Diet App." The app is frequently updated and contains a convenient list of foods high and low in FODMAPs (as of July 2016, the app costs $7.99 USD).[18] According to Nanayakkara et al., research is underway to compile a comprehensive nutrient composition database for FODMAPs.[16]

Limitations of the Low FODMAP Diet:

One of the most commonly cited limitations of the low FODMAP diet is the unknown effects that long-term adherence to the diet may pose on the microbiome, as many "prebiotic fibers" would be limited when following a low FODMAPs. Staudacher et al. showed the low FODMAP diet was able to better manage IBS symptoms after four weeks of fermentable carbohydrate restriction; however, the low FODMAP diet was also associated with a decreased abundance of *Bifidobacteria*.[19] The group also found calcium intake was lower in the low FODMAP diet group (p=0.012), which may have been due to reduction in food selection (e.g., dairy intake). Another more recent trial found a low FODMAP diet (3.05 g/day FODMAPs content) was associated with a significant reduction in total bacterial abundance (p<0.001) but significantly increased bacterial diversity (p<0.001) compared to a typical Australian diet (23.7 g/day FODMAPs content).[20] Other limitations include the perceived difficulty of adhering to the diet, and the nutritional adequacy of the diet (e.g., calcium intake). Based on these limitations, especially the unknown effects that low FODMAP diets may pose on an individual's microbiome, this diet is not recommended to the general population without GI symptoms. For symptomatic individuals, it is recommended to restrict the diet only to the level of symptom control, reintroducing as many components as symptomatically feasible. The diet should not be used as a long-term dietary strategy.

References

1. De Giorgio R, Volta U, Gibson PR. Sensitivity to wheat, gluten and FODMAPs in IBS: facts or fiction? *Gut.* 2016 Jan;65(1):169-78.
2. Fedewa A, Rao SS. Dietary fructose intolerance, fructan intolerance and FODMAPs. *Curr Gastroenterol Rep.* 2014 Jan;16(1):370.
3. El-Salhy M, Gundersen D.Diet in irritable bowel syndrome. *Nutr J.* 2015 Apr 14;14:36.
4. Mansueto P, Seidita A, D'Alcamo A, Carroccio A. Role of FODMAPs in Patients With Irritable Bowel Syndrome. *Nutr Clin Pract.* 2015 Oct;30(5):665-82.
5. Madsen JL, Linnet J, Rumessen JJ. Effect of nonabsorbed amounts of a fructose-sorbitol mixture on small intestinal transit in healthy volunteers. *Dig Dis Sci.* 2006 Jan;51(1):147-53.
6. Gibson PR, Shepherd SJ. Personal view: food for thought--western lifestyle and susceptibility to Crohn's disease. The FODMAP hypothesis. *Aliment Pharmacol Ther.* 2005 Jun 15;21(12):1399-409.
7. Shepherd SJ, Halmos E, Glance S. The role of FODMAPs in irritable bowel syndrome. *Curr Opin Clin Nutr Metab Care.* 2014 Nov;17(6):605-9.
8. Khan MA, Nusrat S, Khan MI, Nawras A, Bielefeldt K. Low-FODMAP Diet for Irritable Bowel Syndrome: Is It Ready for Prime Time? *Dig Dis Sci.* 2015 May;60(5):1169-77.
9. Tuck CJ, Muir JG, Barrett JS, Gibson PR. Fermentable oligosaccharides, disaccharides, monosaccharides and polyols: role in irritable bowel syndrome. *Expert Rev Gastroenterol Hepatol.* 2014 Sep;8(7):819-34.
10. Marsh A, Eslick EM, Eslick GD. Does a diet low in FODMAPs reduce symptoms associated with functional gastrointestinal disorders? A comprehensive systematic review and meta-analysis. *Eur J Nutr.* 2016 Apr;55(3):897-906.
11. McKenzie YA, Bowyer RK, Leach H, et al. British Dietetic Association systematic review and evidence-based practice guidelines for the dietary management of irritable bowel syndrome in adults (2016 update). *J Hum Nutr Diet.* 2016 Jun 8. doi: 10.1111/jhn.12385. [Epub ahead of print]
12. National Institute for Health and Clinical Excellence (2015) Irritable bowel syndrome in adults. Diagnosis and management of irritable bowel syndrome in primary care. Clinical Guideline 61 Update 2015. Available at: http://www.nice.org.uk/Guidance/CG61
13. Fukudo S, Kaneko H, Akiho H, et al. Evidence-based clinical practice guidelines for irritable bowel syndrome. *J Gastroenterol.* 2015 Jan;50(1):11-30.
14. Staudacher HM, Irving PM, Lomer MC, Whelan K. Mechanisms and efficacy of dietary FODMAP restriction in IBS. *Nat Rev Gastroenterol Hepatol.* 2014 Apr;11(4):256-66.
15. Whigham L, Joyce T, Harper G, et al. Clinical effectiveness and economic costs of group versus one-to-one education for short-chain fermentable carbohydrate restriction (low FODMAP diet) in the management of irritable bowel syndrome. *J Hum Nutr Diet.* 2015 Dec;28(6):687-96.
16. Nanayakkara WS, Skidmore PM, O'Brien L, et al. Efficacy of the low FODMAP diet for treating irritable bowel syndrome: the evidence to date. *Clin Exp Gastroenterol.* 2016 Jun 17;9:131-42.
17. Gibson PR, Varney J, Malakar S, Muir JG. Food components and irritable bowel syndrome. *Gastroenterology.* 2015 May;148(6):1158-74.e4.
18. http://www.med.monash.edu/cecs/gastro/fodmap/
19. Staudacher HM, Lomer MC, Anderson JL, et al. Fermentable carbohydrate restriction reduces luminal bifidobacteria and gastrointestinal symptoms in patients with irritable bowel syndrome. *J Nutr.* 2012 Aug;142(8):1510-8.
20. Halmos EP, Christophersen CT, Bird AR, et al. Diets that differ in their FODMAP content alter the colonic luminal microenvironment. *Gut.* 2015 Jan;64(1):93-100.

Candida Overgrowth in the GI Tract and Beyond

Candidiasis is the term used to describe overgrowth of the yeast *Candida albicans* and similar species (*C. glabrata, C. tropicalis, C. parapsilosis*, and *C. krusei*) in the GI tract or other mucosal tissues.[1,2] *Candida* is a normal inhabitant of the GI tract in humans, as well as the mucus membranes of other orifices, such as the mouth, nose and vagina, where it is often deemed a commensal organism.[3] In fact, *Candida* species are the dominant genera within the human mycobiome.[4] When *Candida* grows as a single-celled "yeast" organism, it is generally not considered to be a pathogen. However, when *Candida* undergoes a phenotypic switch to its sessile, biofilm-forming hyphae form, it is considered a pathogen and difficult to remove.[5,6] Though these features are not necessary for invasive behavior, and *Candida* biofilm have not yet been demonstrated in the GI tract, agents that inhibit this phenotypic switch are considered important for inhibiting *Candida* overgrowth outside the GI tract (e.g., mouth, vagina) and especially on implanted devices.[7,8]

During times of immune suppression/compromise, critical illness or GI microbiota disruption (i.e., antibiotic use) *Candida* can become an opportunistic pathogen as the yeast alters its invasive characteristics and migrates from the GI tract to colonize other tissues.[9,10] The oldest description of a *Candida* infection is oral thrush, which is common in immune-compromised individuals.[11] Recurrent vulvovaginal candidiasis is experienced by millions of women worldwide, and along with thrush, is the most common form of extra-gastrointestinal candidiasis seen by the clinician.[12] Candidemia, the invasion of live *Candida* in the blood or other tissue, is rare, severe and should result in immediate hospitalization (although the patient is likely to already be hospitalized as this is frequently a nosocomial infection).[13] Finally, *Candida* is often found on dental devices (e.g., dentures, implants) or other implants within the gastrointestinal, genitourinary tract or elsewhere, often resulting in continued re-infections in individuals treated for *Candida* overgrowth (some of these can be serious candidemia when involving cardiovascular implants).[14,15]

**Candida* overgrowth is commonly related to the following:*

- Antibiotic use, either long-term use (acne, otitis media, sinusitis, etc.) or short-term, high-dose use (surgery, UTI, etc.).[16,17,18,19]
- High consumption of sugars, white flour, pastries, etc., are assumed to increase the growth of *Candida* in the GI tract and mouth. These assumptions are based on *Candida*'s use of simple sugars as an energy source, though studies examining the effect of *Candida* growth following increased sugar intake have had equivocal results.[20,21]
- Compromised immune system (HIV/AIDS, organ transplant, chemotherapy).[22]
- Chronic HPA axis activation/stress (which suppresses the immune system)[23,24]
- *Clostridium difficile* infection[25]
- Inflammatory bowel disease[26,27,28]

Diagnosing GI Overgrowth of *Candida*

While oral or vaginal *Candida* overgrowth is common and easily diagnosed, overgrowth within the GI tract often goes unrecognized or is attributed to other causes. Such causes may be concomitant with *Candida* overgrowth, including dyspepsia (gas, bloating), bacterial dysbiosis, SIBO or IBD symptoms. Other non-GI symptoms often related to *Candida* overgrowth may include mental fog, muscle/joint weakness or pain, general fatigue, and skin irritations. These symptoms are a result of yeast growth (and their metabolites), as well as the death of yeast organisms. These processes put additional burden on the detoxification capacity of the liver, which is responsible for transforming yeast metabolites into harmless substances for elimination.

Once an individual has *Candida* overgrowth, reoccurrence is quite common. Patients will often need to maintain a consistent and vigilant lifestyle management program to prevent repeated incidence of candidiasis. Likewise, strategies to increase immune system and GI barrier function should be considered as an ongoing strategy after implementing a strategy to reduce *Candida* overgrowth (unlike with *H. pylori*, eradication is not the goal of therapy).

The relative abundance of *Candida spp.* can be determined using analysis of the fecal mycobiome (often part of a comprehensive stool analysis or CDSA™). When these measures show an increased abundance of *Candida* in the stool, it suggests (along with history and symptom questionnaires) that *Candida* overgrowth may be contributing to the patient's poor health. There are times when additional sample testing for *Candida* can

be performed; usually to determine more specific species or susceptibility to antifungal agents. These might also be utilized if the stool culture within the CDSA™ shows only modest *Candida* growth but symptoms and history (past or concomitant yeast infections) suggest *Candida* involvement.

These tests typically analyze serum or saliva for antibodies (IgA, IgG, or IgM) to *Candida* peptides or cell-wall components that cross-react to prepared anti-*Candida* antibodies.[29,30,31] Positive reactivity to these tests suggests that the gut-associated immune system has had frequent encounters with invasive *Candida* organisms within the GI mucosa, though it does not indicate live *Candida* within the blood. Ask your lab for additional *Candida* test information if you suspect *Candida* that is not confirmed by stool culture analysis.

Treating Chronic *Candida* Overgrowth: A Lifestyle and Nutrient Approach[†]

The diagnosis and treatment of *Candida* overgrowth has been a concern of integrative medicine clinicians for many years, even when there was little confirmation in the literature as to its importance. In fact, several texts related to treating *Candida* were very popular within the integrative community for decades.[32,33]

Treating *Candida* overgrowth requires a team effort on behalf of both clinician and patient. It is not possible to completely eliminate *Candida*, as it is a ubiquitous and commensal organism. The goals are to eliminate its invasive activity, maintain appropriately low growth of *Candida*, increase beneficial commensal microbiota, and improve immune system and intestinal barrier function to restore vital GI function and health.

Anti-*Candida* diet: As with much of the microbiota living in the GI tract, dietary habits are probably the single greatest contributor to the growth of *Candida* and other fungi. Since *Candida* is a simple yeast organism that thrives on simple sugars, the primary focus of anti-*Candida* diets has been the limitation of simple sugars from the diet. Patients with *Candida* overgrowth are therefore advised to limit the intake of all simple sugars. This includes soft drinks, juices, most

breads, pastries, candy and fruits with mostly simple sugars. Hidden sugar in foods such as condiments and salad dressings, and the like should also be limited.

For the most part, there is strong agreement for the limitation of sugar as the basis of the dietary approach to limit *Candida* overgrowth as older reports have suggested connections between dietary intake of sugars and increased prevalence of *Candida* overgrowth.[34,35,36] Unfortunately, there is limited published clinical research confirming the use of dietary restriction of simple sugars as a therapeutic intervention for *Candida* overgrowth. Studies in neutropenic mice inoculated with *Candida albicans* and given either glucose, xylitol or no additional carbohydrates in their water have been tested for both *Candida* growth and invasive behavior.[37] Mice given glucose had significantly higher levels of *Candida* growth in their GI tracts ($p \leq 0.05$) and significantly more invasive *Candida* in the GI mucosa ($p = 0.00006$). And while other *in vitro* tests have implicated simple sugars in helping *Candida* bind to human tissues, a study attempting to elicit *Candida* overgrowth in healthy subjects using increased intakes of dietary sugars failed to show a statistical increase in *Candida* overgrowth.[20,38]

[†] This chapter describes the treatment of chronic *Candida* overgrowth in the gut caused by poor lifestyle habits and weakened immune system function. These therapies are not adequate, and should not be relied upon, to treat invasive candidiasis or candidemia, which require serious systemic antifungal agents. Also, since the purpose of this chapter is to evaluate the lifestyle and nutrient approaches for reducing chronic Candida overgrowth, the role of antifungal pharmaceuticals is not discussed in this chapter. The clinician should evaluate this information and apply it as they deem appropriate in relation to their knowledge and experience related to antifungal pharmaceuticals.

We should note that this study was performed in healthy subjects with no overt immune or gastrointestinal symptoms and no baseline overgrowth of Candida in the gut.[21] However, subgroup analysis did show a significant, although moderate, increase in fecal measures of C. albicans during the high-sugar-diet period in those subjects with elevated mouth wash measures of Candida at baseline; suggesting that those subjects with a propensity for increased Candida overgrowth may be more susceptible to increased gastrointestinal overgrowth with added simple sugars in their diet. Therefore, unless otherwise contraindicated, dietary restriction of simple sugars is likely to help reduce Candida overgrowth in vulnerable patients.

The restriction or inclusion of other dietary components is also widely debated amongst clinicians and patients (especially through internet discussion groups). Commonly restricted foods include yeast-fermented foods and beverages, coffee and other caffeinated beverages, dairy products, corn, alcohol, and potatoes.[39]

Several medium chain fatty acids have been shown to have anti-fungal activity and may help limit Candida overgrowth. In particular, the saturated fatty acids caprylic acid (8:0, octanoic acid), capric acid (10:0, decanoic acid), undecylenic acid (11:0) and lauric acid (12:0) are known to inhibit the growth or virulence of Candida albicans.[40,41,42,43] These fatty acids are found in various food sources, though they are particularly high in coconut oil, which has demonstrated in vitro anti-Candida activity.[44,45] So far, there are no published reports of coconut oil being tested in clinical trials of human subjects with oral, vaginal or GI overgrowth of Candida. Therefore, it is difficult to make specific recommendations concerning the amount of coconut oil to add to the diet for an anti-Candida benefit. There is, however, a recent animal study that effectively lowered GI colonization of Candida albicans when mice were switched from a diet containing fats from soy or beef tallow to the same diet containing coconut oil.[46] The use of coconut oil or concentrated salts of these fatty acids (e.g., caprylic acid, capric acid, undecylenic acid) may help reduce the growth and invasive characteristics of Candida in vulnerable subjects.

Natural Antifungal Agents

Numerous antifungal agents (pharmaceutical and natural) have been described as limiting the growth and/or conversion to the hyphae form of Candida, though the majority of data is based on cell culture/in vitro studies. Check with your laboratory or guideline recommendations for appropriate doses and regimens of pharmaceutical antifungals.[47,48,49] Many natural compounds (primarily plant or fungal-derived chemicals) have been demonstrated to inhibit the growth of Candida albicans and other Candida species. Though few have been tested in controlled clinical trials, many of these have been used for decades within the integrative medicine community to help reduce the burden of GI Candida and related overgrowth in mucosal tissues (e.g., thrush, vulvovaginitis). As we briefly outline some of the more commonly used agents here, we should note these should not be considered reliable agents when attempting to treat life-threatening or complex invasive situations involving Candida or other fungi.

Plant Essential Oils

Some of the most studied and potent natural antifungal agents are found in the essential oil of several common botanicals, including oregano, thyme, cloves, cinnamon, and melaleuca, though hundreds of botanicals and their compounds have been evaluated.[50,51] Extracts and concentrates containing compounds such as carvacrol, thymol, eugenol, cinnamaldehydes and others have been specifically tested and shown to inhibit the growth of Candida spp in vitro.[52,53]

Carvacrol is a phenolic compound found in the essential oil of **oregano** (Origanum vulgare), **thyme** (Thymus vulgaris) and other plants in the mint family. It is a potent antimicrobial agent and, along with thymol, has been shown to induce membrane destabilization and alter the immune-evading properties of Candida albicans and related fungal species.[54,55,56] Though extracts of oregano are known to have antifungal activity, studies have shown this activity correlates strongly with carvacrol content.[57] In an animal model of oral and vaginal Candida overgrowth, carvacrol and eugenol (via mouthwash or intravaginal injections) prevented the growth and/or invasive hyphae forms better than nystatin.[58,59] Carvacrol and eugenol have also been shown to increase the susceptibility of Candida to fluconazole by destabilizing its biofilm.[60]

Eugenol is a phenylpropene compound found primarily in the essential oil of **clove** (*Syzygium aromaticum*), though it is also found in other spices.[61] Clove extracts have been shown to have strong growth inhibitory activity against a number of *Candida* isolates; in many cases this activity is superior to nystatin.[62] As mentioned above, eugenol has been confirmed to be one of the most potent anti-*Candida* components of clove.[63] Clove oil and eugenol have been shown to have antifungal activities against several different fungi, including fluconazole-resistant *Candida* strains.[64] Eugenol has also been shown to inhibit *Candida* biofilm formation.[65]

Thyme (*Thymus vulgaris*) is closely related to oregano and has also been shown to contain potent antifungal activity, mostly associated with its volatile oil component **thymol** (an isomer of carvacrol). Thymol has been studied, often with carvacrol and eugenol, and shown to have potent anti-*Candida* properties, frequently having similar or superior activity compared to pharmaceutical antifungal agents.[66,67,68] Thymol has been shown to inhibit the formation of the hyphae form, an action that may be enhanced by adding eugenol.[69] Thymol is also a potent inhibitor of *Candida* biofilm formation.[70] A commercially available vaginal douche product containing carvacrol, thymol and eugenol has been shown to be effective for vaginal candidiasis, though the product only appears to be available in Italy.[71]

Cinnamon (*Cinnamomum cassia* and related species) and its essential oils, extracts, and compounds have also been evaluated for anti-*Candida* activity, in particular the compound **cinnamaldehyde**.[72,73,74] These studies have confirmed potent anti-*Candida* properties related to essential oil preparations of cinnamon, and fungicidal, fungistatic, hyphae-inhibiting and biofilm-inhibiting activities of cinnamaldehyde.[75,76,77,78]

Finally, essential oil preparations of **tea tree** (*Melaleuca alternifolia*) are well-known for their antifungal properties, and have been shown to possess potent anti-*Candida* activities.[79] Mechanistic studies suggest tea tree oil and its major constituent **terpinen-4-ol** work to destabilize the fungal membrane, similar to the other essential oils mentioned.[80,81] Small clinical trials have shown that dilute solutions of tea tree oil are able to reduce *Candida* growth in immunocompromised patients or subjects with denture stomatitis.[82,83,84]

On the one hand, these and other essential oils represent some of the most potent natural antifungal agents tested, though almost no studies have been published on their ingestion for reducing gastrointestinal overgrowth of *Candida*. Furthermore, depending on how concentrated the essential oil preparation may be, these products can be strong irritants to mucosal membranes. We suggest using dilute preparations (drops added to water) to swallow or rinse (for oral *Candida*), or the use of soft gel encapsulated products delivering essential oils directly to the gut. These soft gels may need to be prepared with additional hardening agents, as essential oils may weaken or dissolve standard soft gel capsules. Common side effects include temporary warm sensation in the gut and smell of essential oil on the breath.

Other Botanical and Phytochemicals

Due to the growing resistance to pharmaceutical antifungal agents, a large number of plants and their phytochemicals have been tested for fungicidal and fungistatic activities against *Candida spp*. While this list of plants and plant compounds is rather long, we will discuss a few that are likely to be commonly available in foods or dietary supplements, several of which are commonly used by integrative clinicians.

Plant roots containing **berberine alkaloids** (berberine, hydrastine, etc.) have been used as antimicrobial and antifungal agents in most of the regions they have been discovered. These include **goldenseal** (*Hydrastis canadensis*), **barberry** (*Berberis vulgaris*), **Oregon grape** (*Mahonia aquifolium*), **Indian Barberry** *(Berberis aristata)*, and **Chinese goldenthread** (*Coptis chinensis*, the primary commercial source of berberine with Indian Barberry). Berberine has been extensively tested and shown to contain numerous mechanisms for inhibiting the growth and pathogenicity of *Candida* and other yeast species.[85,86] Berberine has also been shown to increase the antifungal potency of fluconazole and other similar agents.[87,88,89]

Garlic (*Allium sativum*) preparations and phytonutrients have also been renowned for their antimicrobial and antifungal properties, including notable anti-*Candida* effects.[90,91,92] Although human clinical trials using garlic preparations (extracts in tablets), have shown limited benefit, we recommend the increased use of garlic (and other spices with antifungal effects) in the diet as often as possible in subjects prone to *Candida* overgrowth.[93,94]

Preparations of both **olive leaf and oil** (*Olea europaea*) and their phenolic compound **hydroxytyrosol** have been investigated for their anti-*Candida* activity with promising results.[95,96,97,98] Also, plants with high levels of **tannins (tannic acid)** have been noted for their antifungal effects, some of which have been shown to have anti-*Candida* activities. However, most of the plants tested are not represented in the diet or commonly available as dietary supplement ingredients. In addition, many **plant flavonoids** have been shown to inhibit the growth, biofilm formation, or invasive characteristics of *Candida*.[99,100] These should be consumed as part of a diverse, phytonutrient-rich diet. Finally, the polyphenol-rich plant resin collected as bee **propolis** has also been shown to have potent anti-*Candida* effects.[101,102] Various preparations of propolis are available as dietary supplement ingredients and may be a helpful addition for reducing *Candida* overgrowth.

There are many other plants and phytochemicals with anti-*Candida* properties. However, unlike many of those listed here, they have little historical use amongst Western medicinal practitioners treating patients with *Candida* overgrowth. Ironically, the majority of the research on all the plants and phytochemicals described above is currently being performed in Asia or South America; very little has been published from Western nations. In addition, while *in vitro* tests of these botanicals are often performed in comparison to pharmaceutical antifungal agents, there are very few clinical trials upon which to formulate specific dosing recommendations (see summary below for basic recommendations).

Probiotics and *Candida* Overgrowth

Candida overgrowth in the gut and elsewhere represents a specific form of dysbiosis for which added friendly bacteria in the form of probiotic therapy may prove beneficial. The added connection between antibiotic use and *Candida* overgrowth further strengthens this premise. Several clinical trials have been performed in subjects with oral or vaginal candidiasis using common probiotic strains or combinations of strains with some beneficial success, though measures of fecal *Candida* are not always reported. Several studies have shown that probiotics delivered directly to oral tissue can reduce the overgrowth of oral *Candida*. One study

used tablets/lozenges held in the mouth delivering a mixture of *B. longum*, *L. bulgaricus*, *S. thermophilus* three times per day,[103] one study provided two different strains of *L. reuteri* in a lozenge given twice daily,[104] and a third study provided probiotics added to cheese that was chewed and swallowed.[105]

The use of probiotics consumed orally or inserted into the vagina has been shown to alter the vaginal microbiota, reducing measures of vulvovaginal candidiasis.[106,107] Clinical trials using direct applications of probiotics have been effective using *L. fermentum* and *L. acidophilus*, and also a multi-strain combination of *L. acidophilus*, *L. rhamnosus*, *S. thermophilus*, and *L. bulgaricus*. In addition, oral consumption of probiotics have been shown to reduce vaginal candidiasis, including studies using *L. rhamnosus* and *L.reuteri*,[108] or *L. rhamnosus* alone.[109]

Finally, the use of oral probiotic therapy in preterm neonates or children in pediatric intensive care units to prevent *Candida* overgrowth has also been tested and found to prevent the gastrointestinal overgrowth of *Candida*. A variety of strains have been used, though the most common are *L.reuteri*, *L. rhamnosus*, *S. boulardii*, *L. acidophilus*, *B. bifidum*, *B. longum*, and *S. thermophilus*.[110,111,112,113]

This wide range of positive clinical data, along with a host of *in vitro* anti-candicidal activity associated with specific probiotic species, strengthens the general recommendation for the use of oral probiotics as an adjunct therapy for candidiasis. Though specific strain and dose recommendations are difficult, we suggest including a mixed strain probiotic that contains multiple species of *Lactobacilli* and the yeast probiotic *S. boulardii*. Therapeutic and prophylactic doses of 20 to 40 billion CFU/day are likely to be a good starting point, though no dose-response studies in humans have yet been published.

Limiting the Die-off (Herxheimer) Reaction

The overgrowth of *Candida* creates a host of symptoms that may be different in each individual. However, an overly aggressive anti-*Candida* protocol can initiate a "die-off" reaction, often called the Jarisch-Herxheimer response (often simply "Herxheimer reaction") in some patients. This response was classically noted as an immunological reaction to the treatment of syphilis, with symptoms ranging from nausea, GI upset, diarrhea, skin reactions, headaches, fatigue and "flu-like" symptoms.[114] It is presumed that the reaction is due to the elevated burden upon the liver and immune system in dealing with dead *Candida* particles and metabolites, though this has rarely been described in clinical studies specifically as a "Herxheimer" reaction.

Clinicians should be aware that some patients may experience significant symptoms when initially implementing regimens designed to reduce *Candida* overgrowth. For this reason, clinicians should consider reducing the doses of various antifungal agents (natural or pharmaceutical) and slowly increasing the dose of these agents over a five- to 10-week period. Furthermore, in keeping with other suggestions made throughout this Road map, clinicians should consider comprehensive support for the immune and detoxification systems prior to or during an anti-*Candida* protocol. Finally, clinicians should ensure that once the burden of *Candida* overgrowth is reduced, that a gut repair protocol is implemented to help heal the gut barrier that may have been compromised during the *Candida* overgrowth or treatment process (see page 153 for suggestions).

Formulary and Protocol Suggestion for *Candida* Overgrowth

- Encapsulated product with mixed anti-*Candida* ingredients: caprylic/undecylenic acid, berberine, powdered plant extracts, etc. To prevent die-off reaction, start first week or two at low dose, increasing dose as necessary in stepwise fashion over the course of the protocol (five to eight weeks).

- Soft gel product containing potent antifungal essential oils: clove (eugenol), thyme (thymol), oregano (carvacrol). This type of product can be added to an encapsulated product protocol. These are potent volatile oils; soft gel capsules should be swallowed, never chewed. Encapsulated/soft gel products can also be used during maintenance/prophylactic protocol.

- Probiotic product: Comprehensive strain product (5+ strains) delivering 20 to 40 billion CFUs in several capsules (or sachets) throughout the day. High-dose products (>100 billion CFUs) may be considered for short-term use, especially if pharmaceutical antifungal or antibiotics have been used in the patient.

References

1. Hani U, Shivakumar HG, Vaghela R, et al. Candidiasis: a fungal infection--current challenges and progress in prevention and treatment. *Infect Disord Drug Targets*. 2015;15(1):42-52.
2. Turner SA, Butler G. The Candida pathogenic species complex. *Cold Spring Harb Perspect Med*. 2014 Sep 2;4(9):a019778.
3. Neville BA, d'Enfert C, Bougnoux ME. Candida albicans commensalism in the gastrointestinal tract. *FEMS Yeast Res*. 2015 Nov;15(7). pii: fov081.
4. Mukherjee PK, Sendid B, Hoarau G, et al. Mycobiota in gastrointestinal diseases. *Nat Rev Gastroenterol Hepatol*. 2015 Feb;12(2):77-87.
5. Palková Z, Váchová L. Yeast cell differentiation: Lessons from pathogenic and non-pathogenic yeasts. *Semin Cell Dev Biol*. 2016 Sep;57:110-9.
6. Sudbery PE. Growth of Candida albicans hyphae. *Nat Rev Microbiol*. 2011 Aug 16;9(10):737-48.
7. Harriott MM, Noverr MC. Importance of Candida-bacterial polymicrobial biofilms in disease. *Trends Microbiol*. 2011 Nov;19(11):557-63.
8. Sardi JC, Scorzoni L, Bernardi T, et al. Candida species: current epidemiology, pathogenicity, biofilm formation, natural antifungal products and new therapeutic options. *J Med Microbiol*. 2013 Jan;62(Pt 1):10-24.
9. Lagunes L, Rello J. Invasive candidiasis: from mycobiome to infection, therapy, and prevention. *Eur J Clin Microbiol Infect Dis*. 2016 Aug;35(8):1221-6.
10. Eggimann P, Garbino J, Pittet D. Epidemiology of Candida species infections in critically ill non-immunosuppressed patients. *Lancet Infect. Dis*. 2003;3:685–702.
11. Millsop JW, Fazel N. Oral candidiasis. *Clin Dermatol*. 2016 Jul-Aug;34(4):487-94.
12. Sobel JD. Recurrent vulvovaginal candidiasis. *Am J Obstet Gynecol*. 2016 Jan;214(1):15-21.
13. Antinori S, Milazzo L, Sollima S, Galli M, Corbellino M. Candidemia and invasive candidiasis in adults: A narrative review. *Eur J Intern Med*. 2016 Jul 6. pii: S0953-6205(16)30198-4.
14. Cuéllar-Cruz M, Vega-González A, Mendoza-Novelo B, et al. The effect of biomaterials and antifungals on biofilm formation by Candida species: a review. *Eur J Clin Microbiol Infect Dis*. 2012 Oct;31(10):2513-27.
15. Cauda R. Candidaemia in patients with an inserted medical device. *Drugs*. 2009;69 Suppl 1:33-8.
16. Shankar J, Solis NV, Mounaud S, et al. Using Bayesian modelling to investigate factors governing antibiotic-induced Candida albicans colonization of the GI tract. *Sci Rep*. 2015 Feb 3;5:8131.
17. Jensen JU, Hein L, Lundgren B, et al. Invasive Candida infections and the harm from antibacterial drugs in critically ill patients: data from a randomized, controlled trial to determine the role of ciprofloxacin, piperacillin-tazobactam, meropenem, and cefuroxime. *Crit Care Med*. 2015 Mar;43(3):594-602.
18. Mason KL, Erb Downward JR, Mason KD, et al. Candida albicans and bacterial microbiota interactions in the cecum during recolonization following broad-spectrum antibiotic therapy. *Infect Immun*. 2012 Oct;80(10):3371-80.
19. Gillies M, Ranakusuma A, Hoffmann T1, et al. Common harms from amoxicillin: a systematic review and meta-analysis of randomized placebo-controlled trials for any indication. *CMAJ*. 2015 Jan 6;187(1):E21-31.
20. Pizzo G, Giuliana G, Milici ME, Giangreco R. Effect of dietary carbohydrates on the in vitro epithelial adhesion of Candida albicans, Candida tropicalis, and Candida krusei. *New Microbiol*. 2000 Jan;23(1):63-71.
21. Weig M, Werner E, Frosch M, Kasper H. Limited effect of refined carbohydrate dietary supplementation on colonization of the gastrointestinal tract of healthy subjects by Candida albicans. *Am J Clin Nutr*. 1999 Jun;69(6):1170-3.
22. Saunus JM, Kazoullis A, Farah CS. Cellular and molecular mechanisms of resistance to oral Candida albicans infections. *Front Biosci*. 2008 May 1;13:5345-58.
23. Ehrström SM, Kornfeld D, Thuresson J, Rylander E. Signs of chronic stress in women with recurrent candida vulvovaginitis. *Am J Obstet Gynecol*. 2005 Oct;193(4):1376-81.

24. Ehrström S, Kornfeld D, Rylander E. Perceived stress in women with recurrent vulvovaginal candidiasis. *J Psychosom Obstet Gynaecol.* 2007 Sep;28(3):169-76.
25. Russo A, Falcone M, Fantoni M, et al. Risk factors and clinical outcomes of candidaemia in patients treated for Clostridium difficile infection. *Clin Microbiol Infect.* 2015 May;21(5):493.e1-4.
26. Sokol H, Leducq V, Aschard H, et al. Fungal microbiota dysbiosis in IBD. *Gut.* 2016 Feb 3. pii: gutjnl-2015-310746.
27. Chehoud C, Albenberg LG, Judge C, et al. Fungal Signature in the Gut Microbiota of Pediatric Patients With Inflammatory Bowel Disease. *Inflamm Bowel Dis.* 2015 Aug;21(8):1948-56.
28. Kumamoto CA. Inflammation and gastrointestinal Candida colonization. *Curr Opin Microbiol.* 2011 Aug;14(4):386-91.
29. Kondori N, Edebo L, Mattsby-Baltzer I. Circulating beta (1-3) glucan and immunoglobulin G subclass antibodies to Candida albicans cell wall antigens in patients with systemic candidiasis. *Clin Diagn Lab Immunol.* 2004 Mar;11(2):344-50.
30. Jaijakul S, Vazquez JA, Swanson RN, et al. (1,3)-β-D-glucan as a prognostic marker of treatment response in invasive candidiasis. *Clin Infect Dis.* 2012 Aug;55(4):521-6.
31. Pitarch A, Nombela C, Gil C. Prediction of the clinical outcome in invasive candidiasis patients based on molecular fingerprints of five anti-Candida antibodies in serum. *Mol Cell Proteomics.* 2011 Jan;10(1):M110.004010.
32. Crook, William G. *The Yeast Connection: A Medical Breakthrough.* New York: Vintage, 1986. Print.
33. Trowbridge J and Walker M. *The Yeast Syndrome: How to help your doctor identify & treat the real cause of your yeast-related illness.* New York: Bantam Books. 1986.
34. Cormane RH, Goslings WR. Factors influencing the growth of Candida albicans (in vivo and in vitro studies). *Sabouraudia.* 1963 Oct;3(1):52-63.
35. Olsen I, Birkeland JM. Initiation and aggravation of denture stomatitis by sucrose rinses. *Scand J Dent Res* 1976;84:94–7.
36. Reed BD, Slattery ML, French TK. The association between dietary intake and reported history of Candida vulvovaginitis. *J Fam Pract* 1989;29:509–15.
37. Vargas SL, Patrick CC, Ayers GD, Hughes WT. Modulating effect of dietary carbohydrate supplementation on Candida albicans colonization and invasion in a neutropenic mouse model. *Infect Immun.* 1993 Feb;61(2):619-26.
38. Samaranayake LP, MacFarlane TW. The effect of dietary carbohydrates on the in-vitro adhesion of Candida albicans to epithelial cells. *J Med Microbiol.* 1982 Nov;15(4):511-7.
39. Martins N, Ferreira IC, Barros L, Silva S, Henriques M. Candidiasis: predisposing factors, prevention, diagnosis and alternative treatment. *Mycopathologia.* 2014 Jun;177(5-6):223-40.
40. Hayama K, Takahashi M, Yui S, Abe S. Inhibitory effects of several saturated fatty acids and their related fatty alcohols on the growth of Candida albicans. *Drug Discov Ther.* 2015 Dec;9(6):386-90.
41. Bergsson G, Arnfinnsson J, Steingrímsson O, Thormar H. In vitro killing of Candida albicans by fatty acids and monoglycerides. *Antimicrob Agents Chemother.* 2001 Nov;45(11):3209-12.
42. Shi D, Zhao Y, Yan H, et al. Antifungal effects of undecylenic acid on the biofilm formation of Candida albicans. *Int J Clin Pharmacol Ther.* 2016 May;54(5):343-53.
43. McLain N, Ascanio R, Baker C, et al. Undecylenic acid inhibits morphogenesis of Candida albicans. *Antimicrob Agents Chemother.* 2000 Oct;44(10):2873-5.
44. Ogbolu DO, Oni AA, Daini OA, Oloko AP. In vitro antimicrobial properties of coconut oil on Candida species in Ibadan, Nigeria. *J Med Food.* 2007 Jun;10(2):384-7.
45. Shino B, Peedikayil FC, et al. Comparison of Antimicrobial Activity of Chlorhexidine, Coconut Oil, Probiotics, and Ketoconazole on Candida albicans Isolated in Children with Early Childhood Caries: An In Vitro Study. *Scientifica (Cairo).* 2016;2016:7061587.
46. Gunsalus KT, Tornberg-Belanger SN, Matthan NR, et al. Manipulation of Host Diet To Reduce Gastrointestinal Colonization by the Opportunistic Pathogen Candida albicans. *mSphere.* 2015 Nov 18;1(1). pii: e00020-15.
47. De Cremer K, Staes I, Delattin N, et al. Combinatorial drug approaches to tackle Candida albicans biofilms. *Expert Rev Anti Infect Ther.* 2015 Aug;13(8):973-84.
48. Cui J, Ren B, Tong Y, Dai H, Zhang L. Synergistic combinations of antifungals and anti-virulence agents to fight against Candida albicans. *Virulence.* 2015;6(4):362-71.
49. Tagliaferri E, Menichetti F. Treatment of invasive candidiasis: between guidelines and daily clinical practice. *Expert Rev Anti Infect Ther.* 2015 Jun;13(6):685-9.
50. Pauli A. Anticandidal low molecular compounds from higher plants with special reference to compounds from essential oils. *Med Res Rev.* 2006 Mar;26(2):223-68.
51. Bona E, Cantamessa S, Pavan M, et al. Sensitivity of Candida albicans to essential oils: are they an alternative to antifungal agents? *J Appl Microbiol.* 2016 Aug 29. doi: 10.1111/jam.13282.
52. Rajkowska K, Kunicka-Styczyńska A, Maroszyńska M. Selected Essential Oils as Antifungal Agents Against Antibiotic-Resistant Candida spp.: In Vitro Study on Clinical and Food-Borne Isolates. *Microb Drug Resist.* 2016 Apr 19. [Epub ahead of print]
53. Soares IH, Loreto ÉS, Rossato L, et al. In vitro activity of essential oils extracted from condiments against fluconazole-resistant and -sensitive Candida glabrata. *J Mycol Med.* 2015 Sep;25(3):213-7.
54. Khan A, Ahmad A, Ahmad Khan L, et al. Effect of two monoterpene phenols on antioxidant defense system in Candida albicans. *Microb Pathog.* 2015 Mar;80:50-6.
55. Gallucci MN, Carezzano ME, Oliva MM, et al. In vitro activity of natural phenolic compounds against fluconazole-resistant Candida species: a quantitative structure-activity relationship analysis. *J Appl Microbiol.* 2014 Apr;116(4):795-804.
56. Ahmad A, Khan A, Akhtar F, et al. Fungicidal activity of thymol and carvacrol by disrupting ergosterol biosynthesis and membrane integrity against Candida. *Eur J Clin Microbiol Infect Dis.* 2011 Jan;30(1):41-50.
57. Vale-Silva L, Silva MJ, Oliveira D, et al. Correlation of the chemical composition of essential oils from Origanum vulgare subsp. virens with their in vitro activity against pathogenic yeasts and filamentous fungi. *J Med Microbiol.* 2012 Feb;61(Pt 2):252-60.
58. Chami F, Chami N, Bennis S, Evaluation of carvacrol and eugenol as prophylaxis and treatment of vaginal candidiasis in an immunosuppressed rat model. *J Antimicrob Chemother.* 2004 Nov;54(5):909-14.
59. Chami N, Chami F, Bennis S, Trouillas J, Remmal A. Antifungal treatment with carvacrol and eugenol of oral candidiasis in immunosuppressed rats. *Braz J Infect Dis.* 2004 Jun;8(3):217-26.
60. Doke SK, Raut JS, Dhawale S, Karuppayil SM. Sensitization of Candida albicans biofilms to fluconazole by terpenoids of plant origin. *J Gen Appl Microbiol.* 2014;60(5):163-8.
61. Pramod K, Ansari SH, Ali J. Eugenol: a natural compound with versatile pharmacological actions. *Nat Prod Commun.* 2010 Dec;5(12):1999-2006.
62. Mansourian A, Boojarpour N, et al. The comparative study of antifungal activity of Syzygium aromaticum, Punica granatum and nystatin on Candida albicans; an in vitro study. *J Mycol Med.* 2014 Dec;24(4):e163-8.
63. Chami N, Bennis S, Chami F, et al. Study of anticandidal activity of carvacrol and eugenol in vitro and in vivo. *Oral Microbiol Immunol.* 2005 Apr;20(2):106-11.
64. Pinto E, Vale-Silva L, Cavaleiro C, Salgueiro L, et al. Antifungal activity of the clove essential oil from Syzygium aromaticum on Candida, Aspergillus and dermatophyte species. *J Med Microbiol.* 2009 Nov;58(Pt 11):1454-62.
65. He M, Du M, Fan M, Bian Z. In vitro activity of eugenol against Candida albicans biofilms. *Mycopathologia.* 2007 Mar;163(3):137-43.
66. de Castro RD, de Souza TM, et al. Antifungal activity and mode of action of thymol and its synergism with nystatin against Candida species involved with infections in the oral cavity: an in vitro study. *BMC Complement Altern Med.* 2015 Nov 24;15:417.
67. de Vasconcelos LC, Sampaio FC, et al. Cell viability of Candida albicans against the antifungal activity of thymol. *Braz Dent J.* 2014;25(4):277-81.
68. Guo N, Liu J, Wu X, et al. Antifungal activity of thymol against clinical isolates of fluconazole-sensitive and -resistant Candida albicans. *J Med Microbiol.* 2009 Aug;58(Pt 8):1074-9.
69. Braga PC, Sasso MD, Culici M, Alfieri M. Eugenol and thymol, alone or in combination, induce morphological alterations in the envelope of Candida albicans. *Fitoterapia.* 2007 Sep;78(6):396-400.
70. Braga PC, Culici M, Alfieri M, Dal Sasso M. Thymol inhibits Candida albicans biofilm formation and mature biofilm. *Int J Antimicrob Agents.* 2008 May;31(5):472-7.
71. Sosto F, Benvenuti C; CANVA Study Group. Controlled study on thymol + eugenol vaginal douche versus econazole in vaginal candidiasis and metronidazole in bacterial vaginosis. *Arzneimittelforschung.* 2011;61(2):126-31.
72. Pires RH, Montanari LB, Martins CH, et al. Anticandidal efficacy of cinnamon oil against planktonic and biofilm cultures of Candida parapsilosis and Candida orthopsilosis. *Mycopathologia.* 2011 Dec;172(6):453-64.
73. Ooi LS, Li Y, Kam SL, Wang H, Wong EY, Ooi VE. Antimicrobial activities of cinnamon oil and cinnamaldehyde from the Chinese medicinal herb Cinnamomum cassia Blume. *Am J Chin Med.* 2006;34(3):511-22.

74. Quale JM, Landman D, Zaman MM, et al. In vitro activity of Cinnamomum zeylanicum against azole resistant and sensitive Candida species and a pilot study of cinnamon for oral candidiasis. *Am J Chin Med*. 1996;24(2):103-9.

75. Taguchi Y, Hasumi Y, Abe S, Nishiyama Y. The effect of cinnamaldehyde on the growth and the morphology of Candida albicans. *Med Mol Morphol*. 2013 Mar;46(1):8-13.

76. Taguchi Y, Hasumi Y, Hayama K, et al. Effect of cinnamaldehyde on hyphal growth of C. albicans under various treatment conditions. *Med Mycol J*. 2012;53(3):199-204.

77. Shreaz S, Bhatia R, Khan N, et al. Spice oil cinnamaldehyde exhibits potent anticandidal activity against fluconazole resistant clinical isolates. *Fitoterapia*. 2011 Oct;82(7):1012-20.

78. Pires RH, Montanari LB, Martins CH, et al. Anticandidal efficacy of cinnamon oil against planktonic and biofilm cultures of Candida parapsilosis and Candida orthopsilosis. *Mycopathologia*. 2011 Dec;172(6):453-64.

79. Ninomiya K, Maruyama N, Inoue S, et al. The essential oil of Melaleuca alternifolia (tea tree oil) and its main component, terpinen-4-ol protect mice from experimental oral candidiasis. *Biol Pharm Bull*. 2012;35(6):861-5.

80. Li WR, Li HL, Shi QS, Sun TL, et al. The dynamics and mechanism of the antimicrobial activity of tea tree oil against bacteria and fungi. *Appl Microbiol Biotechnol*. 2016 Oct;100(20):8865-75.

81. Hammer KA, Carson CF, Riley TV. Antifungal effects of Melaleuca alternifolia (tea tree) oil and its components on Candida albicans, Candida glabrata and Saccharomyces cerevisiae. *J Antimicrob Chemother*. 2004 Jun;53(6):1081-5.

82. Vazquez JA, Zawawi AA. Efficacy of alcohol-based and alcohol-free melaleuca oral solution for the treatment of fluconazole-refractory oropharyngeal candidiasis in patients with AIDS. *HIV Clin Trials*. 2002 Sep-Oct;3(5):379-85.

83. Jandourek A, Vaishampayan JK, Vazquez JA. Efficacy of melaleuca oral solution for the treatment of fluconazole refractory oral candidiasis in AIDS patients. *AIDS*. 1998 Jun 18;12(9):1033-7.

84. Catalán A, Pacheco JG, Martínez A, Mondaca MA. In vitro and in vivo activity of Melaleuca alternifolia mixed with tissue conditioner on Candida albicans. *Oral Surg Oral Med Oral Pathol Oral Radiol Endod*. 2008 Mar;105(3):327-32.

85. da Silva AR, de Andrade Neto JB1, da Silva CR, et al. Berberine Antifungal Activity in Fluconazole-Resistant Pathogenic Yeasts: Action Mechanism Evaluated by Flow Cytometry and Biofilm Growth Inhibition in Candida spp. *Antimicrob Agents Chemother*. 2016 May 23;60(6):3551-7.

86. Dhamgaye S, Devaux F, Vandeputte P, et al. Molecular mechanisms of action of herbal antifungal alkaloid berberine, in Candida albicans. *PLoS One*. 2014 Aug 8;9(8):e104554.

87. Wei GX, Xu X, Wu CD. In vitro synergism between berberine and miconazole against planktonic and biofilm Candida cultures. *Arch Oral Biol*. 2011 Jun;56(6):565-72.

88. Li DD, Xu Y, Zhang DZ, Quan H, et al. Fluconazole assists berberine to kill fluconazole-resistant Candida albicans. *Antimicrob Agents Chemother*. 2013 Dec;57(12):6016-27.

89. Iwazaki RS, Endo EH, Ueda-Nakamura T, et al. In vitro antifungal activity of the berberine and its synergism with fluconazole. *Antonie Van Leeuwenhoek*. 2010 Feb;97(2):201-5.

90. Iciek M, Kwiecień I, Włodek L. Biological properties of garlic and garlic-derived organosulfur compounds. *Environ Mol Mutagen*. 2009 Apr;50(3):247-65.

91. Li WR, Shi QS, Dai HQ, et al. Antifungal activity, kinetics and molecular mechanism of action of garlic oil against Candida albicans. *Sci Rep*. 2016 Mar 7;6:22805.

92. Khodavandi A, Harmal NS, Alizadeh F, et al. Comparison between allicin and fluconazole in Candida albicans biofilm inhibition and in suppression of HWP1 gene expression. *Phytomedicine*. 2011 Dec 15;19(1):56-63.

93. Ebrahimy F, Dolatian M, Moatar F, Majd HA. Comparison of the therapeutic effects of Garcin(®) and fluconazole on Candida vaginitis. *Singapore Med J*. 2015 Oct;56(10):567-72.

94. Watson CJ, Grando D, Fairley CK, et al. The effects of oral garlic on vaginal candida colony counts: a randomised placebo controlled double-blind trial. *BJOG*. 2014 Mar;121(4):498-506.

95. Pereira AP, Ferreira IC, Marcelino F, et al. Phenolic compounds and antimicrobial activity of olive (Olea europaea L. Cv. Cobrançosa) leaves. *Molecules*. 2007 May 26;12(5):1153-62.

96. Zorić N, Kopjar N, Kraljić K, et al. Olive leaf extract activity against Candida albicans and C. dubliniensis - the in vitro viability study. *Acta Pharm*. 2016 Sep 1;66(3):411-21.

97. Zoric N, Horvat I, Kopjar N, et al. Hydroxytyrosol expresses antifungal activity in vitro. *Curr Drug Targets*. 2013 Aug;14(9):992-8.

98. Goel N, Rohilla H, Singh G, Punia P. Antifungal Activity of Cinnamon Oil and Olive Oil against Candida Spp. Isolated from Blood Stream Infections. *J Clin Diagn Res*. 2016 Aug;10(8):DC09-11.

99. Seleem D, Pardi V, Murata RM. Review of flavonoids: A diverse group of natural compounds with anti-Candida albicans activity in vitro. *Arch Oral Biol*. 2016 Aug 27. pii: S0003-9969(16)30227-8.

100. Shahzad M, Sherry L, Rajendran R, et al. Utilising polyphenols for the clinical management of Candida albicans biofilms. *Int J Antimicrob Agents*. 2014 Sep;44(3):269-73.

101. Tobaldini-Valerio FK, Bonfim-Mendonça PS, et al. Propolis: a potential natural product to fight Candida species infections. *Future Microbiol*. 2016 Aug;11:1035-46.

102. das Neves MV, da Silva TM, et al. Isoflavone formononetin from red propolis acts as a fungicide against Candida sp. *Braz J Microbiol*. 2016 Jan-Mar;47(1):159-66.

103. Li D, Li Q, Liu C, Lin M, et al. Efficacy and safety of probiotics in the treatment of Candida-associated stomatitis. *Mycoses*. 2014 Mar;57(3):141-6.

104. Kraft-Bodi E, Jørgensen MR, Keller MK, et al. Effect of Probiotic Bacteria on Oral Candida in Frail Elderly. *J Dent Res*. 2015 Sep;94(9 Suppl):181S-6S.

105. Hatakka K, Ahola AJ, Yli-Knuuttila H, et al. Probiotics reduce the prevalence of oral candida in the elderly--a randomized controlled trial. *J Dent Res*. 2007 Feb;86(2):125-30.

106. Reid G, Burton J, Hammond JA, Bruce AW. Nucleic acid-based diagnosis of bacterial vaginosis and improved management using probiotic lactobacilli. *J Med Food*. 2004 Summer;7(2):223-8.

107. Reid G, Charbonneau D, Erb J, et al. Oral use of Lactobacillus rhamnosus GR-1 and L. fermentum RC-14 significantly alters vaginal flora: randomized, placebo-controlled trial in 64 healthy women. *FEMS Immunol Med Microbiol*. 2003 Mar 20;35(2):131-4.

108. Martinez RC, Franceschini SA, et al. Improved treatment of vulvovaginal candidiasis with fluconazole plus probiotic Lactobacillus rhamnosus GR-1 and Lactobacillus reuteri RC-14. *Lett Appl Microbiol*. 2009 Mar;48(3):269-74.

109. Bohbot JM, Cardot JM. Vaginal impact of the oral administration of total freeze-dried culture of LCR 35 in healthy women. *Infect Dis Obstet Gynecol*. 2012;2012:503648.

110. Demirel G, Celik IH, Erdeve O, et al. Prophylactic Saccharomyces boulardii versus nystatin for the prevention of fungal colonization and invasive fungal infection in premature infants. *Eur J Pediatr*. 2013 Oct;172(10):1321-6.

111. Kumar S, Bansal A, Chakrabarti A, Singhi S. Evaluation of efficacy of probiotics in prevention of candida colonization in a PICU-a randomized controlled trial. *Crit Care Med*. 2013 Feb;41(2):565-72.

112. Romeo MG, Romeo DM, Trovato L, et al. Role of probiotics in the prevention of the enteric colonization by Candida in preterm newborns: incidence of late-onset sepsis and neurological outcome. *J Perinatol*. 2011 Jan;31(1):63-9.

113. Manzoni P, Mostert M, Leonessa ML, et al. Oral supplementation with Lactobacillus casei subspecies rhamnosus prevents enteric colonization by Candida species in preterm neonates: a randomized study. *Clin Infect Dis*. 2006 Jun 15;42(12):1735-42.

114. Belum GR, Belum VR, Chaitanya Arudra SK, Reddy BS. The Jarisch-Herxheimer reaction: revisited. *Travel Med Infect Dis*. 2013 Jul-Aug;11(4):231-7.

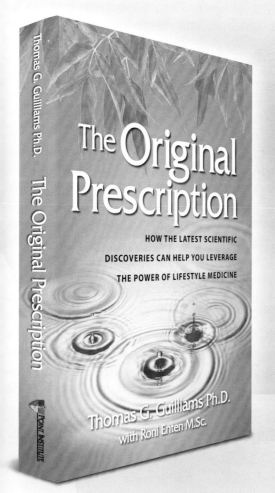
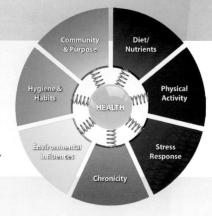

Supplementing Dietary Nutrients
A Guide for Healthcare Professionals

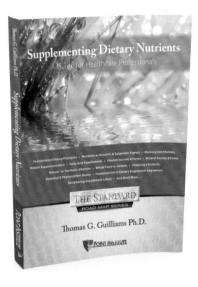

Written from an industry insider's perspective, this up-to-date reference guide answers challenging questions related to nutrition and dietary supplement use in clinical practice:

- How can nutrients serve as genomic and epigenetic signals?

- What are proven dietary patterns?

- Natural verses synthetic vitamins?

- Whole food verses isolates?

- What is the regulatory climate of dietary supplements?

- How are USRDAs determined and are they adequate?

"With more than 20 years of research that validates the need for nutritional therapy for the management of chronic disease like diabetes, cancer, and heart disease, it is time for healthcare professionals to get trained and patients to become informed. This easy-to-use resource is a must-have to make the process simple and attainable."

Shilpa P. Saxena, M.D.
Chief of Medicine | n1health

"This book provides accurate and beautifully condensed information on supplements that will enhance the knowledge of all practitioners. I highly recommend it as part of your library."

Mark Houston MD MS MSc FACP FAHA FASH FACN
Associate Clinical Professor of Medicine | Vanderbilt Medical School | Director, Hypertension Institute of Nashville

"Dr. Guilliams' work is essential for all who want to better understand nutrients and supplementation in a practical and meaningful way. I recommend it for clinicians and clients alike to go beyond the surface and begin this important dialogue."

Robert Bonakdar MD FAAFP ABIHM
Director of Pain Management | Scripps Center for Integrative Medicine
Founder and Co-Director | Scripps Natural Supplements: An Evidence Based Update Conference

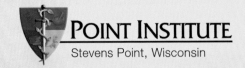

POINT INSTITUTE
Stevens Point, Wisconsin

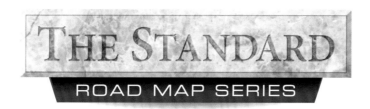

THE STANDARD
ROAD MAP SERIES

Principles and Protocols for Healthcare Professionals

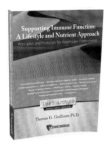

Supporting Immune Function:
A Lifestyle and Nutrient Approach
Principles and Protocols for Healthcare Professionals

This guide summarizes the latest knowledge concerning clinically-relevant immune system function (including autoimmune dysfunctions). Evidence for lifestyle and nutrient interventions affecting immune functions will be discussed in detail; along with suggested protocols for improving immune function related to both acute and chronic immune challenges.

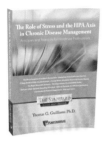

The Role of Stress and the HPA Axis
in Chronic Disease Management
Principles and Protocols for Healthcare Professionals

This guide outlines the evidence connecting HPA axis and neurotransmitter dysfunction with a wide-range of chronic diseases. Different testing and protocol strategies will be reviewed, allowing the clinician to design a diagnostic and treatment strategy that suits their practice and patients. Intervention strategies will emphasize lifestyle, nutritional and nutraceutical therapies.

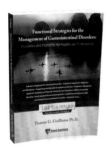

Functional Strategies for the Management
of Gastrointestinal Disorders
Principles and Protocols for Healthcare Professionals

This guide outlines the basic functions and dysfunctions of the GI-system, as viewed through the lens of functional medicine. Protocols are based upon rebuilding each of the functions of the GI tract; focusing on evidence-based therapies using lifestyle and nutraceutical interventions.

Coming Soon!

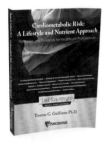

Cardiometabolic Risk:
A Lifestyle and Nutrient Approach
Principles and Protocols for Healthcare Professionals

This guide discusses the relationship between lifestyle inputs and the mechanisms that drive both type 2 diabetes and cardiovascular events. Strategies to help assess patient's insulin resistance, inflammatory status and lipid metabolism will be coupled with evidence-based implementation strategies that include diet, exercise, stress-control and nutraceutical interventions.

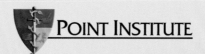

POINT INSTITUTE